Encyclopedia of Myeloid Leukemia

Volume II

Encyclopedia of Myeloid Leukemia

Volume II

Edited by **Matthew Griffin**

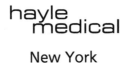

New York

Published by Hayle Medical,
30 West, 37th Street, Suite 612,
New York, NY 10018, USA
www.haylemedical.com

Encyclopedia of Myeloid Leukemia
Volume II
Edited by Matthew Griffin

International Standard Book Number: 978-1-63241-172-3 (Hardback)

Contents

Preface

This book is a contribution by various experts from around the world, including America, Europe, Africa and Asia who have worked in the fields of myeloid cell biology and myeloid leukemia pathogenesis. The book aims to provide reviews about new developments in the fields of basic science of acute myeloid leukemia (AML) and chronic myeloid leukemia (CML). This book includes the particulars of leukemia biology and pathogenesis and presents a comprehensive summary of the research activities in the same field.

This book unites the global concepts and researches in an organized manner for a comprehensive understanding of the subject. It is a ripe text for all researchers, students, scientists or anyone else who is interested in acquiring a better knowledge of this dynamic field.

I extend my sincere thanks to the contributors for such eloquent research chapters. Finally, I thank my family for being a source of support and help.

Editor

Vav1: A Key Player in Agonist-Induced Differentiation of Promyelocytes from Acute Myeloid Leukemia (APL)

Valeria Bertagnolo, Federica Brugnoli and Silvano Capitani
University of Ferrara, Section of Human Anatomy,
Department of Morphology and Embryology,
Italy

1. Introduction

Acute promyelocytic leukemia (APL) is the M3 subtype of acute myeloid leukemia (AML), characterized by aberrant hyperproliferation of progenitors originally committed to terminal differentiation into granulocytes but blocked at the promyelocytic stage. Although clinical studies have introduced treatments employing arsenic trioxide, anthracyclines and anti-CD33 monoclonal antibodies, all-*trans* retinoic acid (ATRA)-based therapy represents, until today, the standard cure of APL patients (Lo-Coco & Ammatuna, 2006; Tallman, 2007). ATRA treatment of APL constitutes, at present, the only example of successful differentiation therapy of a human cancer, in which tumor cells are induced to complete their maturation to neutrophils. Studies on both APL blasts and APL-derived cell lines have elucidated that ATRA acts throughout a complex network that includes the degradation of the PML/RARα fusion protein and the activation of RARα-mediated gene transcription (Breitman et al., 1980; Lanotte et al., 1991; Yang et al., 2003). In addition, it has been reported that ATRA- and phorbol 12-myristate 13-acetate (PMA)-mediated differentiation of human myeloid leukemia cell lines results in changes of their sensitivity to chemotherapeutic drugs, suggesting that advantages in the cure of APL and other malignancies could be obtained by combining differentiating agents and conventional anticancer drugs (Jasek et al., 2008; Kogan, 2009; Nasr et al., 2008).

Even if the mechanism by which ATRA interacts with its receptor located on specific DNA sequences is well known, the events mediated by the ATRA target genes, able to elicit the integrated signaling networks that promote maturation of tumoral promyelocytes, have not been fully clarified and are currently under study to also identify specific molecular targets for new therapies of APL.

One of the proteins up-regulated by ATRA in APL-derived cells and that resulted chiefly involved in the maturation program of tumoral promyelocytes is Vav1, the sole member of the Vav family of proteins physiologically expressed only in haematopoietic cells, where it works as an important signal transducer in immune response (Katzav, 2009; Tybulewicz, 2005). Relevant insights into the function of Vav1 in hematopoietic cells have been provided by studies with knockout mice, demonstrating that the targeted down-modulation of Vav1 compromises maturation of both lymphoid and myeloid cells (Zhang et al., 1994). In particular, a severe impairment of IL-2 production and calcium mobilization in response to external stimuli has been found in T and B cells (Fujikawa et al., 2003; Haubert & Weckbecker, 2010) and the defective motility observed in the Vav1-/- neutrophils, concomitant with the decrease in migration, has been demonstrated to reduce the capacity for an innate immune response (Phillipson et al., 2009). Vav1 has a critical role also in regulating the acquisition by macrophages of maturation-related competence, as demonstrated by the smaller adhesive area, the reduced motility and the lower migration speed of macrophages from Vav1-deficient mice (Hall et al., 2006; Wells et al., 2005). More recently, Vav1 activity has been demonstrated to be required specifically for SDF1α-dependent perivascular homing and subsequent engraftment of hematopoietic stem cells (Sanchez-Aguilera et al., 2011). In both lymphoid and myeloid cells, Vav1 is involved in the dynamic regulation of the filamentous actin cytoskeleton, critical to numerous physical cellular processes, including adhesion, migration and phagocytosis (Cougoule et al., 2006; Stricker et al., 2010).

Vav1 contains an array of structural motifs that enable it to play a role in several distinct cell functions, like cytoskeletal reorganization and regulation of gene expression during proliferation, maturation, and apoptosis of hematopoietic cells (Clevenger et al., 1995; Fischer et al., 1998; Kong et al., 1998). The Vav1 domains include a DH region which exhibits a GDP/GTP exchange activity for the RhoA, Rac1 and CDC42 small GTPases, a PH domain interacting with phosphoinositides, two SH3 domains and one SH2 domain mediating protein-protein interactions, a CH domain that functions as an actin-binding motif and an AC region that contains 3 regulatory tyrosines. Vav1 also possesses 2 putative nuclear localization signals, indicative for a role of the protein also inside the nuclear compartment (Bustelo, 2001).

In both myeloid and lymphoid cells, the best known function of Vav proteins is the guanosine exchange factor (GEF) for small G proteins which is modulated, at variance with the other exchange factors for Rho/Rac in humans, by phosphorylation on tyrosine residues (Bustelo, 2002). However, some functions of Vav1 in hematopoietic cells are independent of its GEF activity and are attributed to its ability to interact with a number of signalling molecules, in both cytoplasm and nucleus. In particular, inside the nuclear compartment Vav1 seems to play its most intriguing role as part of transcriptionally active complexes (Houlard et al., 2002) and by interacting with components of the DNA-dependent protein kinase complex as well as with hnRNP proteins (Romero et al., 1996, 1998).

In addition to the role played in the acquisition of a mature phenotype by normal hematopoietic cells, Vav1 has been found to promote the agonist-induced completion of the differentiation program of tumoral myeloid precursors. In cell lines derived from APL patiens treated with differentiating agents Vav1 plays indeed multiple roles aimed to regulate different aspects of maturation along the neutrophilic and the monocytic/macrophagic lineages. Since Vav1 may be recruited by various differentiating agents and plays a central role in the completion of the differentiation program of leukemic promyelocytes along diverse hematopoietic lineages, it might be considered a common target for developing new therapeutic strategies for the different subtypes of myeloid leukemias.

2. Vav1 and netrophil-like phenotypical maturation

Promyelocytes derived from APL, which are blocked at different steps of their neutrophil differentiation, contain levels of Vav1 variably lower than those found in mature neutrophils. Treatments with differentiating doses of ATRA induce a significant increase of Vav1 expression in primary blasts obtained from the bone marrow of APL patients as well as in the APL-derived cell lines HL-60 and NB4. A similar increase of Vav1 is observed when normal CD34+ hematopoietic progenitors are treated with a cytokine cocktail promoting granulocytic differentiation, clearly indicating that an adequate expression of Vav1 has to be achieved along with neutrophil maturation of both normal precursors and poorly differentiated neoplastic cells (Bertagnolo et al., 2005). These evidence, obtained in a variety of normal and neoplastic cells under different experimental conditions, ascribe to Vav1 the potential role of a ubiquitous key player in the path leading myeloid precursors to acquire the mature phenotype of differentiated neutrophils.

The issue of whether the increase of Vav1 observed in differentiation of tumoral promyelocytes is merely designed to the function of the protein in mature cells or, more intriguingly, it is functionally relevant to the maturation mechanism, has been addressed by studies in which the expression of Vav1 was forcedly modulated. The experiments have been performed in ATRA treated HL-60 and NB4 cells, which are blocked at different levels of granulocytic differentiation, and thus constitute models well suited to better understand the role of Vav1 in the maturation process. As a consequence of Vav1 over-expression during ATRA treatment of both cell lines, the expression of the myeloid surface marker CD11b increases, indicating that Vav1 supports the role of ATRA in regulating the maturation process. On the other hand, the sole over-expression of Vav1 is capable to significantly induce the expression of CD11b only in HL-60 cells, that, compared to NB4 cells, are blocked to a less differentiated stage (Bertagnolo et al., 2005). This suggests the existence of a direct and ATRA-independent role of Vav1 in regulating the expression of CD11b, at least in cells that are blocked at early stages of the neutrophilic maturation.

Neutrophils radically change in shape during development and functional life (Sanchez & Wangh, 1999). Accordingly, profound rearrangements of the cell morphology take place throughout differentiation of myeloid precursors along the granulocytic lineage, and the nucleus is the cell compartment that undergoes the biggest architectural changes by a mechanism still largely unknown. Modifications of the nuclear shape constitute one of the markers of neutrophil maturation of tumoral promyelocytes and are particularly evident after treatment with ATRA of HL-60 cells, according to the notion that this cell type is blocked at an early stage of maturation. On the other hand, the sole over-expression of Vav1 is unable to induce nuclear modifications in both HL-60 and NB4 cells, indicating that other ATRA-induced events are required to regulate the maturation-related rearrangements of cell morphology (Bertagnolo et al, 2005).

The use of siRNAs specific for Vav1 unequivocally demonstrates that Vav1 is not dispensable for the progression of tumoral promyelocytes along the granulocytic lineage. In fact, the down-modulation of Vav1 expression during ATRA treatment of both HL-60 and NB4 cells counteracts the agonist-induced increase of CD11b expression and prevents the maturation-related modifications of cell/nucleus morphology, definitely assigning to Vav1 a crucial role in regulating phenotypical maturation of APL-derived cells (Bertagnolo et al, 2005, 2008).

2.1 Tyrosine phosphorylation of Vav1

In parallel with the increase of Vav1 expression, ATRA treatment of HL-60 and NB4 cells also induces Vav1 tyrosine phosphorylation. Since, in the whole cell, the rise of the phosphosphorylation level is almost proportional to the increase in total Vav1 amount, ATRA seems to ensure to differentiating cells the achievement of an adequate amount of tyrosine phosphorylated Vav1, according with the functions of Vav1 in mature neutrophils. On the other hand, the accumulation of tyrosine-phosphorylated Vav1 inside the nuclear compartment seems to be a distinctive feature of the differentiation process induced by ATRA in APL-derived cells (Bertagnolo et al., 2005). In fact, a progressive increase of tyrosine phosphorylated Vav1 inside the nucleus accompanies the agonist-induced maturation (Bertagnolo et al., 1998), indicative of a specific role of tyrosine phosphorylated Vav1 inside the nuclear compartment. The tyrosine phosphorylation level of nuclear Vav1 reaches a maximum in ATRA-treated NB4 cells, which constitute the cell model with the most advanced level of neutrophil maturation among APL-derived precursors (Bertagnolo et al., 2005), clearly correlating tyrosine phosphorylated Vav1 with the maturation-related events that occur inside the nuclear compartment and opening the question of which kinase/s is/are involved in this process.

In both myeloid and lymphoid cells, Vav1 is phosphorylated in tyrosine/s by receptors with intrinsic tyrosine kinase activity or by membrane and/or cytoplasmic tyrosine kinases of the Syk/Zap70, Src and Jak families (Bustelo, 2002). More recently, also the c-Abl kinase has been reported to be specifically involved in regulating the activity of Vav1 in integrin-mediated neutrophil adhesion (Cui et al., 2009). Recruitment and phosphorylation of Vav1 depend on its ability to interact with a number of signalling proteins by means of its various domains. In particular, the interaction between the SH2 domain of Vav1 and phosphorylated proteins is thought to serve for recruitment of activated kinases, which in turn can phosphorylate Vav1 (Bustelo, 2002). The Syk/ZAP-70 family of tyrosine kinases constitutes an example of proteins that contain two SH2 domains, a tandem sequence that might confer high specificity in tyrosine kinase- mediated signalling. In addition, both ZAP-70 and Syk contain a consensus binding sequence for the Vav1 SH2 domain that seems to be critical for antigen receptor-mediated signal transduction (Ottinger et al., 1998).

Experiments performed with HL-60 cells have demonstrated the association of tyrosine phosphorylated Syk with the Vav1-SH2 domain, in both whole cell and nuclear compartment, as a consequence of ATRA treatment (Bertagnolo et al., 2001). These data are in agreement with the notion that activation of Syk occurs in differentiating HL-60 cells (Qin & Yamamura, 1997) and mature neutrophils, in which it regulates migration (Schymeinsky et al., 2006) and the formation of lamellipodia during phagocytosis (Shi et al., 2006). While in whole HL-60 cells the Vav1/Syk association takes place regardless of their phosphorylation level and of ATRA treatment, the formation of Vav1/Syk complexes inside the nuclear compartment strongly increases during the differentiation process, suggesting a specific role for this tyrosine kinase in the nucleus. The role of Syk in phosphorylating Vav1 has been demonstrated by means of *in vitro* assays (Bertagnolo et al., 2001) and confirmed by the use of a pharmacological model of Syk inhibition, in which both HL-60 and NB4 cells were treated with Piceatannol (Bertagnolo et al., 2001, 2008), a tyrosine kinase inhibitor with a reported selectivity for Syk (Law et al, 1999; Seow et al., 2002).

The Syk-dependent tyrosine phosphorylation of Vav1 during the ATRA-induced phenotypical differentiation is not relevant for the expression of the surface marker CD11b, as indicated by the use of Piceatannol in both HL-60 and NB4 cells, but seems to play a crucial role in regulating the reorganization of cell architecture. In fact, when Piceatannol is administered in combination with ATRA, the modifications of nuclear morphology typical of granulocytic differentiation are almost completely abrogated, similarly to what observed when the expression of Vav1 is down-modulated during the differentiation treatment (Bertagnolo et al., 2008). However, since Piceatannol fails to abrogate completely the ATRA-induced tyrosine phosphorylation of Vav1 in both HL-60 and NB4 cells (Bertagnolo et al., 2008), other kinase/s, in addition to Syk, are probably recruited by ATRA in these cell models.

The results from these inhibition studies support the hypothesized action model that requires tyrosine phosphorylated Vav1 in maturation of tumoral myeloid precursors. Nevertheless, the issue needs further investigations, in order to identify the kinase/s involved. In fact, by extending the analysis to other tyrosine kinase inhibitors, it has been found that PP1 and AG490, inhibitors of Src and Jak tyrosine kinase families, respectively, did not affect to any significant extent the tyrosine phosphorylation of Vav1 (Bertagnolo et al., 2004), leaving open the question of which other tyrosine kinases, in addition to Syk, phosphorylate Vav1 during maturation of tumoral promyelocytes.

2.1.1 Participation to protein complexes with signaling molecules

In addition to the obvious interaction with tyrosine kinases, the optimal phosphorylation of Vav1 seems to require the association with adaptor molecules that facilitate the spatial proximity between Vav1 and the upstream kinases. These associations also depend on the tyrosine phosphorylation of the involved proteins and often require the engagement of either the SH3 or the SH2 domains of Vav1 as interacting motifs (Bustelo, 2002). In this context, SLP-76, an adaptor protein predominantly expressed in T cells and myeloid cells and which is a substrate for ZAP-70 and Syk tyrosine kinases, has been reported to associate, via tyrosine-phosphorylated residues in its NH2-terminal domain, with the SH2 domain of Vav1 after ligation of the T-cell antigen receptor (Tuosto et al., 1996; Pauker & Barda-Saad,, 2011). SLP-76 was also described as an important adaptor molecule that is regulated by Syk in C-reactive protein-stimulated platelets (Gross et. al, 1999) and that plays a critical role in FcRI-mediated activation of mast cells *in vivo* and *in vitro* (Pivniouk et al., 1999).

Some of the Vav1-interacting molecules play a role in down modulation of Vav1 signals. A potential negative regulator of Vav1 is Cbl, which down-modulates Syk/ZAP-70 and other protein tyrosine kinases (Lupher et al., 1999). Cbl associates with Vav1 upon T-cell receptor stimulation of primary murine lymphocytes and Jurkat T cells. This interaction appears to require the whole SH3-SH2-SH3 COOH-terminal domain of Vav1 and a proline-rich sequence of Cbl and seems to inhibit the Vav1-dependent signal transduction (Bustelo et al., 1997). Very recently, Chiang & Hodes (2011) have demonstrated a role of Cbl in repressing signaling events that can mediate thymic differentiation in the absence of Vav1, since Cbl inactivation rescued defective T cell development in Vav1-/- mice.

The molecules involved in the recruitment and phosphorylation of Vav1 during the ATRA-dependent granulocytic differentiation of tumoral promyelocytes were investigated in HL-60 cells by using GST-fusion NH2-terminal and COOH-terminal Vav1-SH3 and GST-fusion Vav1-SH3-SH2-SH3 proteins. One of the proteins interacting with Vav1 in HL-60 cells is the adaptor molecule Cbl, present only in the cytoplasm and strongly phosphorylated in response to ATRA treatment. The Vav1/Cbl interaction in HL-60 cells occurs also in control conditions and requires the entire SH3-SH2-SH3 domain of Vav1 (Bertagnolo et al., 2001).

The adaptor protein SLP-76 has been also identified as a phosphorylated protein interacting with the SH3-SH2-SH3 fragment of Vav1 in both cells and nuclei of HL-60 after ATRA treatment. Similarly to Cbl, SLP-76 associates with Vav1 also in control conditions, without quantitative changes due to the differentiation process. Vav1-associated SLP-76 was more abundant in nuclei than in whole cell lysates, indicating a preferential association into the nucleus of these two molecules, in contrast with an exclusive cytoplasmic distribution of Vav1/Cbl complexes (Bertagnolo et al., 2001).

The interaction of Vav1 with Cbl and SLP-76 in HL-60 cells may be correlated to the transmembrane signaling mediated by CD38, an early biomarker of ATRA-induced differentiation in the HL-60 cell line, in which it may play a causal role in myeloid differentiation (Lamkin et al., 2006). A correlation between Vav1 and CD38-activated signaling has been recently demonstrated by experiments in which the expression of a cytosolic deletion mutant of CD38 caused failure to up-regulate ATRA-induced proteins such as CD11b, Vav1 and Fgr, this latter able to phosphorylate Vav1 after ATRA treatment of HL-60 cells (Congleton et al., 2011).

Exclusive of the ATRA treatment of HL-60 seems to be the compartmentalized association between Vav1 and interacting proteins during ATRA treatment, since Cbl/Vav1 complexes are located in the cytoplasm while SLP-76/Vav1 complexes reside in the inner nuclear compartment. This suggests that Vav1 is recruited by one or more signal transduction cascades, starting from cell membrane and directed to the nucleus and involving the two adaptor proteins Cbl and SLP-76, which may then discretely regulate the amount of Vav1 in the cytoplasmic and nuclear compartments (Fig. 1).

The Vav1-associated protein complexes identified in HL-60 cells also contain the tyrosine kinase Syk. In particular, Vav1/Cbl/Syk complexes have been found in cytoplasm whereas Vav1/SLP-76/Syk complexes have been demonstrated inside the nuclear compartment. These associations are present in control conditions and result strongly increased after ATRA treatment (Bertagnolo et al., 2001). This suggests that, during the maturation of APL-derived myeloid precursors, a sequence of signals originated from membrane receptors and directed to the nuclear compartment is ended to regulate the amount of tyrosine phosphorylated Vav1 inside the nucleus (Fig. 1) and that this pathway may involve the negative regulation of Cbl on Vav1 activity.

In both cells and nuclei of HL-60 cells, other signalling molecules associate with Vav1 as a consequence of ATRA treatment. They include the γ1 isoform of PI-PLC and the p85 regulatory subunit of PI3K. In particular, ATRA treatment increases the binding of tyrosine-phosphorylated Vav1 to both N-terminal and C-terminal SH2 domains of p85 (Bertagnolo et al., 1998). Since Vav1 is the only member of the Vav1/PLC-γ1/PI3K complex to possess a nuclear localization sequence (Bustelo, 2001), it is conceivable that Vav1 is directly involved in regulating the amount of PLC-γ1 and PI3K inside the nuclear compartment.

2.1.2 Phosphorylation of Vav1 on Tyr745

Vav1 contains 31 tyrosine residues whose phosphorylation was originally investigated almost exclusively in relation to the function of Vav1 as a GEF. A crucial role in this context seems to be played by Tyr174 in both lymphoid and myeloid cells, even if other mechanisms have emerged in the last few years as regulators of Vav1 GEF activity, and recent data suggest that Tyr174 is coversely involved in roles of Vav1 not mediated by GEF activity (Katzav, 2009). In addition to Tyr174, other conserved residues, Tyr142 and Tyr160, have been described to be phosphorylated in activated Vav1. It has also been suggested that phosphorylation of the tyrosines located inside the acidic region of Vav1 may allow Tyr142, Tyr160, and Tyr174 to become docking sites for kinases, which can then phosphorylate additional tyrosine residues in Vav proteins (Miletic et al., 2006; Yu et al., 2010). Recently, several of the tyrosine residues at the carboxyl terminus of Vav1 have been shown to be phosphorylated in cancer cells, raising the possibility that also these tyrosine residues play an important role in Vav1 function (Lazer et al., 2010).

The residue Tyr174, phosphorylated by members of Syk/Zap70 and Src tyrosine kinase families, plays a central role in regulating GEF activity of Vav1 in mature neutrophils, including β2 integrin-mediated neutrophil migration *in vitro* and neutrophil recruitment during the inflammatory response *in vivo* (Schymeinsky et al., 2006). In APL-derived cells, ATRA induces the phosphorylation of Tyr174 in NB4 but not in HL-60 cells and independently of the activity of Syk (Bertagnolo et al., 2011). Both cytofluorimetrical analysis of CD11b expression and migration assays on NB4 cells over-expressing the Tyr174Phe-mutated Vav1 have ruled out any relevant role for this tyrosine residue in supporting the activity of ATRA in this cell line (Bertagnolo et al., 2010). Since phosphorylation of Tyr174 in neutrophils has been mainly associated to the GEF activity of Vav1 in mature cells, these findings suggest that the ATRA-induced phosphorylation of Tyr174 occurs in parallel with differentiation and may constitute a marker of the acquisition of a mature phenotype. This hypothesis is confirmed by the failure of ATRA in inducing the phosphorylation of Tyr174 in HL-60 cells, that reach indeed only a partially differentiatiated phenotype (Bertagnolo et al., 2011).

Since the phosphorylation of Vav1 on the Tyr174 residue seems unrelated to the path by which tyrosine phosphorylated Vav1 affects the ATRA-induced maturation of APL-derived cells, proteomic studies have been undertaken to identify other tyrosine residues phosphorylated after ATRA treament in both HL-60 and NB4 cells. Mass spectra analysis performed on Vav1 immunoprecipitated from NB4 whole cells identified Tyr745 as an ATRA-induced phosphorylated residue, within a highly conserved Vav1 sequence. The analysis of maturation-related features in differentiating NB4 cells over-expressing the Tyr745Phe-mutated form of Vav1 have clearly shown that phosphorylation of this tyrosine residue is crucial in regulating CD11b expression as well as in promoting the acquisition of migratory capabilities (Bertagnolo et al., 2010). Even if Tyr745 has never been correlated with the known roles of Vav1, multiple sequence alignment analysis of proteins from different species indicates that this is a highly conserved aminoacid, likely involved in physiological roles of Vav1.

Inhibition studies have ruled out the role of Syk in phosphorylating Tyr745 as a consequence of ATRA treatment and, at present, no data are available about the involved tyrosine kinase. This is in part due to the fact that analysis performed with softwares designed to predict cell signaling interactions using short sequence motifs failed to recognize the Tyr745 of Vav1 as a putative phosphorylation site by the known tyrosine kinases. However, some tyrosine residues of Vav1 are not surface exposed and/or may be involved in intramolecular interactions, thereby precluding their tyrosine phosphorylation and impairing their recognition by the data base analysis. Since Tyr745 is located inside a short helix on the SH2 domain of Vav1, its phosphorylation could be an event secondary to phosphorylation of other tyrosine residues, which may induce conformational changes of Vav1 allowing Tyr745 to become accessible to a specific tyrosine kinase.

2.1.3 GEF activity

The best known function of tyrosine phosphorylated Vav1 is a catalytic role as a GEF towards the Rho family of GTPases, in which Tyr174 is crucial. Tyr174 lies within an α-helix and binds directly with the GTPase interaction pocket of the DH domain, blocking access to substrate and inhibiting Vav1 GEF activity. Phosphorylation releases Tyr174 from the binding pocket, relieving the auto-inhibition (Bustelo et al., 2001). The activity of the DH domain is also regulated by the CH domain, as deletion of this domain results in constitutively active GEF activity. It has been suggested that the Vav1 CH domain can bind to the C1 region, occluding the DH domain and blocking access to GTPases. CH–C1 interaction apparently stabilizes the inhibitory Tyr174–DH interaction. In addition, the PH domain regulates Vav1 catalytic activity by interaction with two inositol lipids: phosphatidylinositol 4, 5- bisphosphate (PIP$_2$) and phosphatidylinositol 3, 4, 5-trisphosphate (PIP$_3$). Whereas the binding of PIP$_3$ moderately enhances the in vitro GEF activity of Vav1, binding to PIP$_2$ has an inhibitory effect. Consistent with this model, Vav1 carrying a single mutation in its PH domain is constitutively active and induces cytoskeleton rearrangements as a consequence of Rac activation. Deletions of C1 domain or mutations that disrupt its structural integrity inhibit Vav1 GEF activity. High resolution X-ray structure of DH–PH–C1 domains suggests that PH and C1 domains contribute to GEF activity by stabilizing the DH domain structure and not through direct contacts with GTPases (Bustelo, 2002).

GEF activity of Vav1 has long been regarded as the key for transferring the signal from activated receptors to the cytoskeleton. Among the molecules constituting the cytoskeleton architecture, actin seems to be a preferred target of the Vav1-dependent GEF activity. Several partners are involved in the pathway by which Vav1 affects actin cytoskeleton. It has been reported that Vav1 is a preferential exchange factor for Rac1, which in turn may activate phosphatidylinositol-4-phosphate (PIP) 5-kinase which phosphorylates PIP to PIP$_2$. PIP$_2$ may function as an activator of actin-binding proteins, like talin and vinculin, that attach the cytoskeleton to the cell membrane. Another potential target for the GEF activity of Vav1, Cdc42, may activate the WASP protein, a key mediator of actin polymerization (Hornstein et al., 2004). Finally, Vav1-activated small G proteins play an essential role in regulating actin cytoskeleton dynamics by also interacting with the p21-activated serine-threonine kinase (PAK) family of actin-regulatory enzymes (Daniels & Bokoch, 1999).

In both lymphoid and myeloid cells, like other proteins with a GEF activity, Vav1 mediates a number of cytoskeletal-associated cellular processes, being an essential part of the molecular link connecting activated receptors to the actin cytoskeleton. A consistent number of studies (reviewed in Hornstein et al., 2004) have reported the role of Vav1 in the formation of immunological synapse and in phagocytosis of T cells. In non adherent neutrophils, stimulation of chemoattractant receptors induces a complex sequence of events: actin reorganization, shape changes, development of polarity and reversible adhesion, all culminating in chemotaxis. The complex signaling mechanisms that regulate neutrophil migration are well studied, and Vav1 appears to be a major point of the inhibitory crosstalk between adhesion receptors and cytokine receptors (Gakidis et al., 2004). In particular, the activity of Vav1 as GEF for Rac2 is inhibited in adherent cells, as a possible consequence of the activation by adhesion of one or more tyrosine phosphatases responsible of dephosphorylating Vav1. On the other hand, experiments performed with Vav1-/- mice have demonstrated that motility and mobilization into peripheral blood induced in neutrophils by FMLP are significantly reduced, as well as the generation of filamentous actin (Kim et al., 2003). Studies performed in a rat model have demonstrated that the M-CSF-induced chemotaxis of bone marrow macrophages is initiated by the 3-phosphoinositide-dependent GEF activity of Vav1 on Rac (Vedham et al., 2005).

In APL-derived HL-60 cells, ATRA treatment induces an increase of total GEF activity, not attributable to Vav1, as deduced by *in vitro* assays on Ras/Rac small G proteins performed on Vav1 immunoprecipitated from both whole cells and isolated nuclei (Bertagnolo et al., 2001). This implies that, in this cell model, the Syk-dependent tyrosine phosphorylation of Vav1 is not ended to regulate its GEF activity and that alternative pathways have to be considered to explain the mechanism by which Vav1 affects the organization of cytoskeleton and nucleoskeleton during maturation of tumoral promyelocytes.

2.2 GEF-independent activity of phosphorylated Vav1
2.2.1 Regulation of actin cytoskeleton
In addition to act as a GEF, Vav1 may mediate actin reorganization through other, GEF-independent mechanisms. The presence in its structure of a number of tyrosines and domains potentially involved in protein-protein interactions suggests for Vav1 a role in actin polymerization as an adapter protein that links signaling and cytoskeletal molecules. In T cells, Vav1 binds constitutively Talin and Vinculin, anchoring the actin cytoskeleton to the plasma membrane, and the cytoskeletal protein Zyxin (Hornstein et al., 2004). In the same cell model, a direct link between Vav1 and dynamin 2 (Dyn2), a component of the cytoskeletal regulators, has also been demonstrated (Gomez et al., 2005).

A mechanism by means of which tyrosine-phosphorylated Vav1 regulates cytoskeleton of ATRA-treated tumoral promyelocytes, identified in HL-60 cells, implies the interaction of Vav1 with the p85 regulatory subunit of PI3K. Studies aimed to establish the functional meaning of this interaction have demonstrated that, in maturing myeloid precursors, PI3K activity closely depends on its association with tyrosine phosphorylated Vav1 and that when Vav1/PI3K interaction and/or PI3K activity are abrogated, the phenotypic differentiation of ATRA-treated HL-60 is compromised (Bertagnolo et al., 1999, 2004). These evidence assign to Vav1/PI3K interaction a prominent function in the regulation of cytoskeleton alternative to the described role of 3-phosphoinositides on GEF activity of Vav1 (Han et al., 1998).

Also actin participates in the ATRA-induced protein complexes containing Vav1 and PI3K in HL-60 cells. Remarkably, when the association between Vav1 and PI3K is inhibited, the formation of PI3K/actin complexes is reduced, suggesting that the interaction of PI3K with Vav1 is essential for its association with actin (Bertagnolo et al., 2004). Since the recovery of 3-phosphoinositides is strongly reduced when the Vav1-dependent PI3K/actin interaction is abrogated, it can be concluded that Vav1 regulates the physical contact of PI3K with their cytoskeleton-associated substrates. These observations suggest that in addition to playing a regulatory role in Vav1 activation, PI3K activity may itself be regulated by Vav1.

PI3K is likely to play essential roles in granulocytic differentiation of tumoral myeloid precursors, considering that both down-modulation of its expression and pharmacological inhibition of its activity during ATRA treatment significantly reduce the tendency of HL-60 cells to acquire the differentiated phenotype (Bertagnolo et al., 1999). The response to ATRA and the downstream effects of PI3K observed during the induced differentiation support the notion that PI3K is recruited in the path controling cytoskeleton in mature granulocytes. In fact, PI3K is activated in response to chemotactic factors in murine and human neutrophils (Cicchetti et al., 2002; Niggli & Keller, 1997; Stephens et al., 2002) in which newly produced PIP_3 is involved in determining the localization and possibly the crosslinking/stabilization of actin filaments (Chen et al., 2003; Hannigan et al., 2002; Wang et al., 2002). In vitro experiments have demonstrated that PI3K may affect actin-related modifications of cytoskeleton also by directly affecting PAK kinase activity (Menard & Mattingly, 2004). PI3K has a more general influence on cytoskeleton by determining the amount of the inositol-containing lipids, that have emerged as major players in regulating actin assembly at several levels and with different mechanisms, including the direct interaction with cytoskeletal proteins, such as vinculin and gelsolin (Janmey et al., 1999, Takenawa & Itoh, 2001).

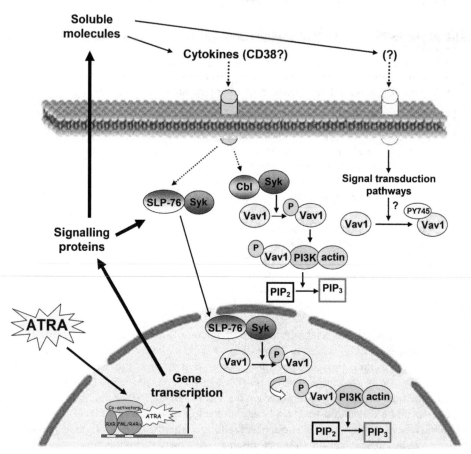

Fig. 1. Schematic representation of the recruitment and phosphorylation of Vav1 in ATRA-treated promyelocytes.

Since, in ATRA-treated promyelocytes, both PI3K activity and the modifications of the nucleus architecture depend on the formation of Vav1/PI3K complexes, Vav1 may be important for targeting PI3K to its nuclear substrates. The association of Vav1 with other lipid modifying enzymes, including specific PI-PLC isoforms (Bertagnolo et al., 1998;), suggests a more general role of Vav1 in determining the composition of the actin-associated phosphoinositide pool and, ultimately, in regulating actin polymerization in differentiating HL-60 cells.

2.2.2 Regulation of gene expression

Microarray analysis performed on APL-derived cell lines has identified several genes whose expression is modified by ATRA treatment, including genes for a number of cytokines, in turn involved in the differentiative program of tumoral promyelocytes (Hsu et al., 1999; Visani et al., 1996). As a consequence of ATRA administration, tyrosine-phosphorylated Vav1 accumulates inside the nuclear compartment of APL-derived cells and becomes involved in the changes of nuclear morphology. Since local reorganization of nuclear architecture is required for both transcription and post-transcriptional events, it is conceivable that Vav1 plays a role in regulating ATRA-related gene expression.

An array analysis performed on HL-60 cells focussed on genes coding for cytokines and cytokine receptors indicates that the inhibition of the Syk-dependent tyrosine-phosphorylation of Vav1 during ATRA treatment prevents the ATRA-induced expression of 8 genes (Bertagnolo et al., 2005). Among them, the thymosin beta-10 (TMSB10) gene has been found, encoding for a small G-actin binding protein that induces depolymerization of intracellular F-actin pools and thus deeply affects actin architecture (Liu et al., 2004; Rho et al., 2004). Tyrosine-phosphorylated Vav1 is also involved in regulating the ATRA-induced expression of the gene for Notch homolog, that codifies for a molecule playing a role in mediating cell fate decisions during hematopoiesis (Ohishi et al., 2003) and whose signaling might be necessary for the proliferation and survival of AML cells, possibly through the maintenance of the expression of c-Myc and Bcl2, as well as the phosphorylation of the Rb protein (Li et al., 2010). The involvement of Vav1 in regulating ATRA-dependent expression of cytokines and/or growth factors has been ascertained by silencing Vav1 during ATRA admistration, further confirming that the increase of Vav1 expression is not an epiphenomenon but constitutes a key event able to actually promote the granulocytic maturation of tumoral myeloid precursors.

The evidence that Vav1 has a role in regulating ATRA-dependent gene expression in APL-derived cells suggests the participation of Vav1 to transcriptional complexes activated by ATRA, also considering that, in both myeloid and lymphoid cells, Vav1 seems to be involved in regulating DNA transcription, by direct interaction with, or as a facilitator of, transcription factors (Katzav, 2004). In particular, Vav1 regulates Nuclear Factor of Activated T-cells (NFAT), Activator Protein-1 (AP-1) and Nuclear Factor κB (NF-κB) in T-cells in response to TCR stimulation, and exerts a specific role in regulating the CREB-dependent gene transcription (Haubert & Weckbecker, 2010; Schneider & Rudd, 2008). Direct evidence for the presence of Vav1 as a component of an active transcriptional complex has been reported by Houlard et al. (2002) demonstrating the participation of Vav1 in complexes with NFAT and NF-kB-like, as facilitator of their transcriptional activity.

In APL-derived cells, nuclear Vav1 associates with PU.1 (Brugnoli et al., 2010), a transcription factor induced by ATRA and able to play a crucial role in the completion of granulocytic differentiation of APL-derived myeloid precursors (Mueller et al., 2006). In particular, the down-modulation of PU.1 by means of specific siRNAs has allowed to establish that, like in other tumoral myeloid precursors (Denkinger et al., 2002), PU.1 regulates the expression of Vav1 induced by ATRA in NB4 cells (Brugnoli et al., 2010).

In AML-derived myeloid precursors, PU.1 represents a major determinant of the myeloid expression of CD11b (Kastner & Chan, 2008; Pahl et al., 1993), an integrin receptor whose surface expression increases concurrently with CD11b mRNA levels during myeloid differentiation of APL-derived cell lines (Barber et al., 2008). Chromatin immunoprecipitation (ChIP) experiments performed on NB4 cells treated with ATRA have demonstrated that PU.1 is recruited to its consensus sequence within the *CD11b* promoter (Brugnoli et al., 2010). Since the over-expression of PU.1 might influence phenotype and restore differentiation of primary myeloid leukemic blasts (Durual et al., 2007), and its silencing counteracts the ATRA ability to induce the expression of the granulocytic marker CD11b (Mueller et al., 2006), PU.1 may be used by ATRA to promote CD11b expression during the late stages of the maturation of APL-derived cells. This is confirmed by *in vitro* experiments demonstrating the formation of PU.1-containing complexes on the *CD11b* promoter (Brugnoli et al., 2010).

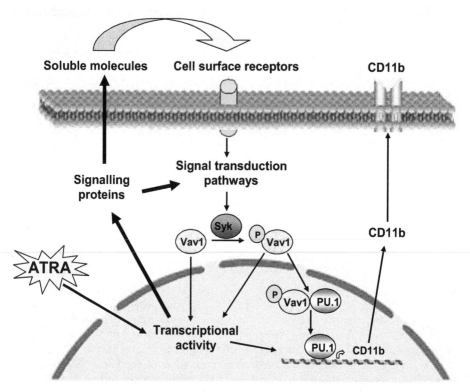

Fig. 2. Schematic representation of the involvement of Vav1 in regulating gene expression in differentiating promyelocytes.

Also Vav1 is recruited to the PU.1 consensus sequence on the *CD11b* promoter in untreated NB4 cells. ATRA treatment, by inducing an increase in Syk-dependent tyrosine phosphorylation of Vav1, displaces this protein from existing molecular complexes on the *CD11b* promoter. Accordingly, the specific inhibition of Syk activity is accompanied by the appearance of a Vav1-containing complex (Brugnoli et al., 2010). The participation of Vav1 to molecular complexes including PU.1 has been ruled out by EMSA experiments. On the other hand, both expression and tyrosine phosphorylation levels of Vav1 seem to play a role in regulating the formation of PU.1-containing complexes. In fact, when the amount of Vav1 is forcedly reduced or its tyrosine phosphorylation is inhibited during the differentiation treatment, the formation of a PU.1-containing complex is negatively affected (Brugnoli et al.,

2010). It is then conceivable that Vav1, and in particular tyrosine-phosphorylated Vav1, regulates the recruitment of PU.1 to its consensus sequence on the *CD11b* promoter region and, possibly, the expression of this surface antigen.

3. Vav1 and protein expression

Proteome analysis currently provides the opportunity to identify global changes in gene expression by directly measuring protein amount. A number of recent studies have used this approach to evaluate protein expression during differentiation/apoptosis induced by different agonists in APL-derived cells. In particular, it has been reported that ATRA modulates the expression level of structural and signal transduction proteins as well as of molecules involved in the different phases of protein synthesis (Dong et al, 2006; Harris et al., 2004; Wan et al., 2001; Wang et al., 2004;).

On the basis of the evidence that inside the nucleus of a number of different cell lines, including APL-derived cells, Vav1 participates to molecular complexes with DNA-related proteins (Brugnoli et al., 2010; Houlard et al., 2002; Romero et al., 1998) a more general role of Vav1 in regulating events ended to control protein expression can be hypothesized. 2D electrophoresis followed by mass spectrometry have established that, in both HL-60 and NB4 cells, the down-modulation of Vav1 abrogates the capacity of ATRA of modulating the expression of proteins associated to cytoskeleton and involved in proliferation and of apoptosis-related proteins, as well as of molecules implicated in metabolism, synthesis, folding and degradation of proteins (Bertagnolo et al., 2008). The majority of the identified proteins are affected by Vav1 down-modulation only in one of the two analyzed cell lines, according to the notion that HL-60 and NB4 cells, even if both derived from patients with APL, show peculiar genotypic and phenotypic profiles (Barber et al., 2008). Interestingly, in NB4 cells, the lack of Vav1 affects the ATRA-dependent expression of the Splicing factor, arg/ser rich 3 (Sfrs3), a member of SR proteins, known as non-snRNP splicing factors, that may affect both constitutive and alternative splicing of mRNA (Sanford et al., 2005). This evidence further supports the role of Vav1 in regulating the ATRA-dependent gene expression.

Some of the identified proteins are differentially expressed, as a consequence of Vav1-down-modulation during ATRA treatment, in both cell lines, suggesting that they may constitute a common part of the signalling activated by ATRA in APL-derived promyelocytes. Notably, this group of proteins includes the ε isoform of the 14-3-3 family of proteins, specifically involved in the caspase networks (Liou et al., 2007). The increased expression of 14-3-3ε in both HL-60 and NB4 cells when Vav1 is down-modulated during ATRA treatment suggests that the amount of Vav1 may be critical in determining the mechanism of caspase activation in APL.

Vav1 also affects the ATRA-dependent expression of α-enolase, a multifunction protein involved in glycolysis and up-regulated in the sera of a number of cancer patients, in which it seems to have a role in tumorigenesis (Zou et al., 2005). α-enolase is expressed at high levels in most AML subtypes in which it might contribute to the adverse evolution of the disease (Lopez-Pedrera et al., 2006). Since down-modulation of Vav1 during ATRA treatment of APL-derived cells reduces the expression of α-enolase (Bertagnolo et al., 2008), it has been suggested that Vav1 promotes the differentiation of tumoral promyelocytes by also targeting metabolic pathways.

The proteasome component "splice isoform 2 subunit $\alpha3$" is down-modulated as well in HL-60 and NB4 cells under the same experimental conditions (Bertagnolo et al., 2008). Since proteasome is the major cellular proteolytic machinery responsible for degradation of normal and damaged proteins (Von Mikecz, 2006), Vav1 may also be involved in regulating protein degradation during ATRA dependent maturation of tumoral promyelocytes.

Also the component of microtubules α-tubulin is affected by down-modulation of Vav1 during ATRA treatment (Bertagnolo et al., 2008), indicating that Vav1, in addition to regulate cytoskeleton reorganization, takes part to the profound architectural changes of differentiating promyelocytes by regulating the expression of cytoskeleton components.

4. Vav1 and monocytic/macrophagic differentiation

The human promyelocytic leukemia cell lines HL-60 and NB4 can be differentiated either toward neutrophils by ATRA or to monocytes/macrophages by PMA (Murao et al., 1983; Song & Norman, 1998). PMA is a stable analogue of 2, 3-diacylglycerol that induces, even if with dynamics not identical in HL-60 and NB4 cells, morphological and functional changes related to monocyte maturation, accompanied by a loss of proliferative capacity (Jasek et al., 2008). Immunochemical and immunocytochemical analysis demonstrate that the expression of Vav1 increases also during the PMA-induced acquisition of a monocyte-like phenotype of HL-60 and NB4 cells (Bertagnolo et al., 2011). This is consistent with the notion that also mature monocytes express Vav1 and that proper amounts of the protein are necessary for their inflammation related functions (Bhavsar et al., 2009; Hall et al., 2006). In the same cell types, PMA also induces a relevant increase of tyrosine phosphorylation of Vav1. On the other hand, and in contrast to what observed in the ATRA-treatment of the same cell line, no role for Syk was demonstrated in this event (Bertagnolo et al., 2011), consistent with the notion that, at least in HL-60 cells, Syk might exert a narrower role, restricted to directing cells toward granulocyte differentiation (Qin & Yamamura, 1997). In both HL-60 and NB4 cells, PMA induces a relevant increase of tyrosine phosphorylation of Vav1 on the Tyr174 residue (Bertagnolo et al., 2011), according to the GEF role played by Vav1 in myeloid cells. These results are also in agreement with other data indicating that, in macrophage-like differentiated HL-60 cells, the activity of Syk is ended to regulate the roles played by mature cells in immune response, including their complement-mediated phagocytosis, in which the kinase regulates both actin dynamics and the Vav1-RhoA activation pathway (Shi et al., 2006).

Also in differentiation of APL-derived cells to monocytes/macrophages, a crucial role for Vav1 in determining the acquisition of maturation-related features has been demonstrated by silencing the expression of Vav1 induced by PMA (Bertagnolo et al., 2011). Under these conditions, the expression of CD11b, which is induced by PMA and constitutes a marker also for monocyte differentiation, is significantly reduced, similarly to what demonstrated during the treatment with ATRA of HL-60 and NB4 cells (Bertagnolo et al. 2011). This suggests that, in differentiating APL-derived cells, Vav1 plays a role in regulating the expression of the CD11b surface antigen regardless the agonist employed and the maturation lineage. Since in NB4 cells treated with ATRA Vav1 is recuited to protein/DNA complexes on the CD11b promoter (Brugnoli et al., 2010), it can be speculated that Vav1 plays a specific role in driving the expression of CD11b as part of the transcriptional machinery also during the differentiation of NB4 cells along the monocytic/macrophagic lineage.

Also cell adhesion is affected by down-modulation of Vav1 during PMA treatment of HL-60 and NB4 cells, in terms of both number of adherent cells and of adhesion area of cells that remain attached to the flask bottom. These results are in agreement with the data obtained with macrophages from Vav1-/- mice, showing a smaller adhesive area or a decreased adhesion efficiency (Wells et al., 2005).

4.1 Regulation of actin

As above reported, the main known functional role of tyrosine phosphorylated Vav1 is to regulate cytoskeleton reorganization, a phenomenon at the basis of both adhesion and migration of monocytes/macrophages. Vav1 regulates cell architecture not only by means of its GEF activity but also by interacting with proteins in turn involved in cytoskeleton reorganization. In addition, in both HL-60 and NB4 cells, Vav1 affects the ATRA-induced expression of the microtubule component α-tubulin.

Contrarily to what observed during granulocytic differentiation, Vav1 down-modulation does not have any effect on expression and architectural organization of α-tubulin during PMA-induced monocytic/macrophagic maturation of NB4 cells (Bertagnolo et al., 2011). This indicates that, during the maturation process of APL-derived cells, Vav1 exerts an agonist- and lineage-specific role in regulating α-tubulin. From a more general point of view, concerning microtubule organization, it can be speculated that the role of Vav1 is restricted to the control of the motility of mature cells, as also suggested by the evidence that changes in microtubule dynamics contribute to the reduced migration speed of Vav1-/- macrophages in response to CSF-1 (Wells et al., 2005).

In living cells, the F-actin cytoskeleton encompasses a variety of different structures that are essential for many different aspects of cell physiology. In particular, dynamic modulation of the filamentous actin cytoskeleton is critical to numerous physical cellular processes, including adhesion, migration and phagocytosis, all requiring precise regulation of cell shape (Stricker et al., 2010). Recent data demonstrate that Vav proteins, including Vav1, are required for actin cytoskeleton reorganization during migration of macrophages, by coupling RhoA and Rac1 activity to adhesion receptors (Bhavsar et al., 2009). Also in ATRA-induced maturation of cells derived from APL Vav1 seems to regulate actin organization.

In HL-60 and NB4 cells treated with PMA, an unprecedented involvement of Vav1 in regulating the increase of actin expression has been shown very recently (Bertagnolo et al., 2011), that constitutes a further confirmation that Vav1, besides being involved in the formation of filaments, takes part to cytoskeleton reorganization as a modulator of protein expression.

The modifications of cell shape in the different cell processes seem to be regulated by the existence of the F-actin cortex, a thin, membrane-bound F-actin network (Stricker et al., 2010). Defective actin-cap formation has been found in lymphocytes from a Vav-deficient mice, clearly correlating Vav1 activity with the regulation of cell shape (Holsinger et al., 1998). Furthermore, a recent work in which adhesive micropatterned surfaces have been used to control the overall shape of fibroblasts, has demonstrated that the shape of the nucleus is tightly regulated through a perinuclear actin cap, which is located above and around the interphase nucleus (Khatau et al., 2009). A wide variety of contractile F-actin networks with different architectures and polarity have also been found near cell adhesion surfaces, correlated with the migratory capability of adherent cells (Stricker et al., 2010). By means of confocal analysis of PMA-treated adherent NB4 cells, it has been demonstrated the existence of an agonist-induced F-actin network, in which F-actin colocalyzes with Vav1, that sharply defines the cytoplasmatic cell border, accumulates inside thin and long cell processes and surrounds the nuclear compartment (Bertagnolo et al., 2011). Since the existence of cytoplasmatic processes in PMA-treated adherent cells are indicative of migratory activity (Stricker et al., 2010), Vav1/F-actin co-localization in cytoplasm protrusions is suggestive of a synergy of the two molecules in controling cell motility. This is in agreement with the role described for Vav proteins in the maintenance of normal morphology and migratory behaviour in macrophages (Bhavsar et al., 2009). The strong Vav1/F-actin co-localization observed at the nuclear periphery and, in particular, in the region above the nucleus, suggests that the two proteins may cooperate in regulating the shape of the nucleus through an actin filament structure similar to the perinuclear actin cap described by Khatau et al. (2009). On the other hand, the role of Vav1 in modulating cell adhesion of PMA-treated cells seems to be related to its ability to regulate expression of integrins, like CD11b, rather than to a direct effect on actin-based cytoskeleton.

5. Conclusion

The present review focuses on the role of the multidomain protein Vav1 in promoting and sustaining the completion of the differentiation program of tumoral promyelocytes. Vav1 is a key protein in the ATRA- and PMA-induced maturation of APL-derived cells, since either its down-modulation or over-expression respectively prevents or potentiates the ability of these agonists to induce the acquisition of a mature phenotype. Alternatively to the best known function of Vav1 as a GEF for small G proteins, ended to regulate cell shape by affecting actin assembly, other mechanisms by which Vav1 affects myeloid differentiation have been described, reflecting the great interactive and regulatory potential of Vav1, which make the full understanding of its functions a very difficult, yet fascinating story.

An example of the complex role played by Vav1 during myeloid differentiation of APL-derived cells is the interaction of Vav1 with various lipid-modifying enzymes ended to regulate the pool of phosphoinositides associated to cytoskeleton. The resulting modifications of actin cytoskeleton contribute to the changes of cellular and nuclear shape occurring in differentiating tumoral promyelocytes (Fig. 3).

The participation of Vav1 to molecular complexes with other adaptor proteins differently distributed in the cytoplasm and in the nucleus suggests the existence of a signal sequence originated from membrane receptors and directed to the nuclear compartment. Inside the nucleus of APL-derived cells, Vav1 seems to play its most intriguing role by regulating the expression of CD11b, a surface marker of both granulocyte and monocyte differentiation, and of a number of ATRA-modulated proteins (Fig. 3). The nuclear issue assumes thus great relevance, confering to Vav1 compartimentalized strategic roles in regulating the maturation process of tumoral promyelocytes.

The bulk of the studies reviewed here are mostly concerned with two cell lines, HL-60 and NB4, derived from APL patients, driven to achieve differentiation by treatment with drugs of the retinoids or phorbol esters families. Even though a better understanding of the functional engagement of Vav1 will be required before converting scientific achievements into clinical advances, Vav1 might be considered a common target for developing new therapeutic strategies for the different subtypes of myeloid leukemias.

In addition, it can be speculated that the identified pathways involving Vav1 are of more general interest and may be potentially extended also outside the haemopoietic/immunological systems.

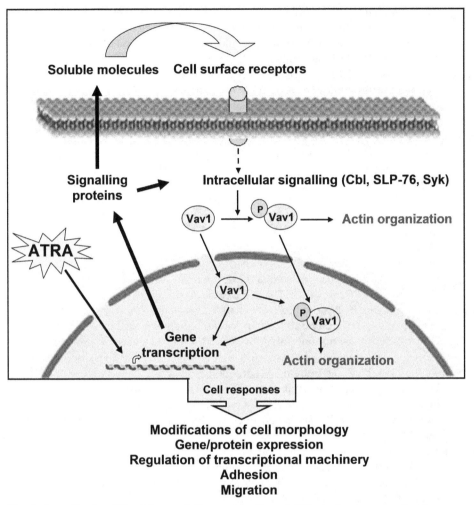

Fig. 3. Overall role of Vav1 in regulating maturation of APL-derived promyelocytes.

6. Acknowledgments

The authors are supported by MIUR (Cofin 2008 and FIRB Accordi di Programma 2010), MAE (Italy-Croatia bilateral project 2009-2011) and by University of Ferrara (Italy).

7. References

Barber, N., Belov, & L., Christopherson, R.I. (2008). All-trans retinoic acid induces different immunophenotypic changes on human HL60 and NB4 myeloid leukaemias. *Leukemia Research*, Vol.32, No.2, (February 2008), pp. 315-322.

Bertagnolo, V., Marchisio, M., Volinia, S., Caramelli, E. & Capitani, S. (1998). Nuclear association of tyrosine-phosphorylated Vav to phospholipase C-gamma1 and phosphoinositide 3-kinase during granulocytic differentiation of HL-60 cells. *FEBS Letters*, Vol.441, No.3, (December 1998), pp. 480-484.

Bertagnolo, V., Neri, L.M., Marchisio, M., Mischiati, C. & Capitani, S. (1999). Phosphoinositide 3-kinase activity is essential for all-trans-retinoic acid-induced granulocytic differentiation of HL-60 cells. *Cancer Research*, Vol. 59, No.3, (February 1999), pp. 542-546.

Bertagnolo, V., Marchisio, M., Brugnoli, F., Bavelloni, A., Boccafogli, L., Colamussi, M.L., & Capitani, S. (2001). Requirement of tyrosine-phosphorylated Vav for morphological differentiation of all-trans-retinoic acid-treated HL-60 cells. *Cell Growth & Differentiation*, Vol.12,No.4, (April 2001), pp. 193-200.

Bertagnolo, V., Brugnoli, F., Marchisio, M., Celeghini, C., Carini, C., & Capitani, S. (2004). Association of PI 3-K with tyrosine phosphorylated Vav is essential for its activity in neutrophil-like maturation of myeloid cells. *Cellullar Signaling*, Vol.16, No.4, (April 2004), pp. 423-433.

Bertagnolo, V., Brugnoli, F., Mischiati, C., Sereni, A., Bavelloni, A., Carini, C., & Capitani, S. (2005). Vav promotes differentiation of human tumoral myeloid precursors. *Experimental Cell Research*, Vol.306, No.1, (May 2005), pp. 56-63.

Bertagnolo, V., Grassilli, S., Bavelloni, A., Brugnoli, F., Piazzi, M., Candiano, G., Petretto, A., Benedusi, M., & Capitani, S. (2008). Vav1 modulates protein expression during ATRA-induced maturation of APL-derived promyelocytes: a proteomic-based analysis. *Journal of Proteome Research*, Vol. 7, No.9, (September 2008), pp. 3729-3736.

Bertagnolo, V., Grassilli, S., D'Aguanno, S., Brugnoli, F., Bavelloni, A., Faenza, I., Nika, E., Urbani, A., Cocco, L., & Capitani, S. (2010). Mass spectrometry-based identification of Y745 of Vav1 as a tyrosine residue crucial in maturation of acute promyelocytic leukemia-derived cells. *Journal of Proteome Research*, Vol.9, No.2, (February 2010), pp. 752-760.

Bertagnolo, V., Nika, E., Brugnoli, F., Bonora, M., Grassilli, S., Pinton, P., & Capitani, S. (2011). Vav1 is a crucial molecule in monocytic/macrophagic differentiation of myeloid leukemia-derived cells. *Cell and Tissue Research*, [Epub ahead of print], (June 2011), DOI: 10.1007/s00441-011-1195-5.

Bhavsar, P.J., Vigorito, E., Turner, M., & Ridley, A.J. (2009). Vav GEFs regulate macrophage morphology and adhesion-induced Rac and Rho activation. *Experimental Cell Research*, Vol.315, No.19, (November 2009), pp. 3345-3358.

Breitman, T.R., Selonick, S.E., & Collins, S.J. (1980). Induction of differentiation of the human promyelocytic leukemia cell line (HL-60) by retinoic acid. *Proceedings of the National Academy of Sciences of the United States of America*, Vol.77, No.5, (May 1980), pp. 2936-2940.

Brugnoli, F., Lambertini, E., Varin-Blank, N., Piva, R., Marchisio, M., Grassilli, S., Miscia, S., Capitani, S., & Bertagnolo, V. (2010). Vav1 and PU.1 are recruited to the CD11b promoter in APL-derived promyelocytes: role of Vav1 in modulating PU.1-containing complexes during ATRA-induced differentiation. *Experimental Cell Research*, Vol.316, No.1, (January 2010), pp. 38-47.

Bustelo, X. R., Crespo, P., Lopez-Barahona, M., Gutkind, J. S., & Barbacid, M. (1997). Cbl-b, a member of the Sli-1/c-Cbl protein family, inhibits Vav-mediated c-Jun N-terminal kinase activation. *Oncogene*, Vol.15, No.21, (November 1997), pp. 2511–2520, 1997.

Bustelo, X.R. (2001). Vav proteins, adaptors and cell signaling. *Oncogene*, Vol.20, No.44, (October 2001), pp. 6372-6381.

Bustelo, X.R. (2002). Regulation of Vav proteins by intramolecular events. *Frontiers in Biosciences*, Vol.7, (January 2002), pp. 24-30.

Chen, L., Janetopoulos, C., Huang, Y.E., Iijima, M., Borleis, J., & Devreotes, P.N. (2003). Two phases of actin polymerization display different dependencies on PI(3,4,5)P3 accumulation and have unique roles during chemotaxis. *Molecular Biology of the Cell*, Vol.14, No.12, (December 2003), pp. 5028-5037.

Chiang, J., & Hodes, R.J. (2011). Cbl Enforces Vav1 Dependence and a Restricted Pathway of T Cell Development. *PLoS ONE*, Vol.6, No.4, (April 2011), e18542.

Cicchetti, G., Allen, P.G., & Glogauer, M. (2002). Chemotactic signaling pathways in neutrophils: From receptor to actin assembly. *Critical Reviews in Oral Biology & Medicine*, Vol.13, No.3, (May 2002), pp. 220–228.

Clevenger, C.V., Ngo, W., Sokol, D.L., Luger, S.M. & Gewirtz, A.M. (1995). Vav is necessary for prolactin-stimulated proliferation and is translocated into the nucleus of T-cell line. *The Journal of Biological Chemistry*, Vol.270, No.22, (June 1995), pp. 13246-13253.

Congleton, J., Jiang, H., Malavasi, F., Lin, H., & Yen, A. (2011). ATRA-induced HL-60 myeloid leukemia cell differentiation depends on the CD38 cytosolic tail needed for membrane localization, but CD38 enzymatic activity is unnecessary. *Experimental Cell Research*, Vol.317, No.7, (April 2011), pp. 910-919.

Cougoule, C., Hoshino, S., Dart, A., Lim, J., & Caron, E. (2006). Dissociation of recruitment and activation of the small G-protein Rac during Fcgamma receptor-mediated phagocytosis. *The Journal of Biological Chemistry*, Vol.281, No.13, (March 2006), pp. 8756-8764.

Cui, L., Chen, C., Xu, T., Zhang, J., Shang, X., Luo, J., Chen, L., Ba, X., & Zeng, X. (2009). c-Abl kinase is required for beta 2 integrin-mediated neutrophil adhesion. *Journal of Immunology*, Vol.182, No.5, (March 2009), pp. 3233–3242.

Daniels, R.H., & Bokoch, G.M. (1999). p21-activated protein kinase: a crucial component of morphological signaling? *Trends in Biochemical Sciences*, Vol.24, No.9, (September 1999), pp. 350-355.

Denkinger, D.J., Lambrecht, T.Q., Cushman-Vokoun, & A.M., Kawahara, R.S. (2002). PU.1 regulates the expression of the vav proto-oncogene. *Journal of Cellular Biochemistry*, Vol.84, No.4, (January 2002), pp. 772-783.

Dong, H., Ying, T., Li, T., Cao, T., Wang, J., Yuan, J., Feng, E., Han, B., Hua, F., Yang, Y., Yuan, J., Wang, H., & Xu, C. (2006). Comparative proteomic analysis of apoptosis induced by sodium selenite in human acute promyelocytic leukemia NB4 cells. *Journal of Cellular Biochemistry*, Vol.98, No.9, (August 2006), pp. 1495-1506.

Durual, S., Rideau, A., Ruault-Jungblut, S., Cossali, D., Beris, P., Piguet, V., & Matthes T. (2007). Lentiviral PU.1 overexpression restores differentiation in myeloid leukemic blasts. *Leukemia*, Vol.21, No.5, (May 2007), pp. 1050-1059.

Fischer, K.D., Kong, Y.Y., Nishina, H., Tedford, K., Marengère, L.E., Kozieradzki, I., Sasaki, T., Starr, M., Chan, G., Gardener, S., Nghiem, M.P., Bouchard, D., Barbacid, M., Bernstein, A., & Penninger, J.M. (1998). Vav is a regulator of cytoskeletal reorganization mediated by the T-cell receptor. *Current Biology*, Vol.8, No.10, (May 1998), pp. 554-562.

Fujikawa, K., Miletic, A.V., Alt, F.W., Faccio, R., Brown, T., Hoog, J., Fredericks, J., Nishi, S., Mildiner, S., Moores, S.L., Brugge, J., Rosen, F.S., & Swat, W. (2003) Vav1/2/3-null mice define an essential role for Vav family proteins in lymphocyte development and activation but a differential requirement in MAPK signaling in T and B cells. *The Journal of Experimental Medicine*, Vol.198, No.10, (November 2003), pp. 1595-1608.

Gakidis, M.A., Cullere, X., Olson, T., Wilsbacher, J.L., Zhang, B., Moores, S.L., Ley, K., Swat, W., Mayadas, T., & Brugge, J.S. (2004). Vav GEFs are required for beta2 integrin-dependent functions of neutrophils. *The Journal of Cell Biology*, Vol.166, No.2, (July 2004), pp. 273-282.

Gomez, T. S., Hamann, M. J., McCarney, S., Savoy, D. N., Lubking, C. M., Heldebrant, M. P., Labno, C. M., McKean, D. J., McNiven, M. A., Burkhardt, J. K. & Billadeau, D. D. (2005). Dynamin 2 regulates T cell activation by controlling actin polymerization at the immunological synapse. *Nature Immunology*, Vol.6, No.3, (March 2005), pp. 261-270.

Gross, B. S., Ran Lee, J., Clements, J. L., Turner, M., Tybulewicz,V. L. J., Findell, P. R., Koretzky, G. A., & Watson, S. P. (1999). Tyrosine phosphorylation of SLP-76 is downstream of Syk following stimulation of the collagen receptor in platelets. *The Journal of Biological Chemistry*, Vol.274, No.9, (February 1999), pp. 5963-5971.

Hall, A.B., Gakidis, M.A., Glogauer, M., Wilsbacher, J.L., Gao, S., Swat, W., & Brugge, J.S. (2006). Requirements for Vav guanine nucleotide exchange factors and Rho GTPases in FcgammaR- and complement-mediated phagocytosis. *Immunity*, Vol.24, No.3, (March 2006), pp. 305-316.

Han, J., Luby-Phelps, K., Das, B., Shu, X., Xia, Y., Mosteller, R.D., Krishna, U.M., Falck, J.R., White, M.A., & Broek, D. (1998). Role of substrates and products of PI 3-kinase in regulating activation of Rac-related guanosine triphosphatases by Vav. *Science*, Vol.279, No.5350, (January 1998), pp. 558-560.

Hannigan, M., Zhan, L., Li, Z., Ai, Y., Wu, D., Huang, C.K. (2002). Neutrophils lacking phosphoinositide 3-kinase gamma show loss of directionality during N-formyl-Met-Leu-Phe-induced chemotaxis. *Proceedings of the National Academy of Sciences of the United States of America*, Vol.99, No.6, (March 2002), pp. 3603-3608.

Harris, M.N., Ozpolat, B., Abdi, F., Gu, S., Legler, A., Mawuenyega, K.G., Tirado-Gomez, M., Lopez-Berestein, G., & Chen, X.(2004). Comparative proteomic analysis of all-trans-retinoic acid treatment reveals systematic posttranscriptional control mechanisms in acute promyelocytic leukemia. *Blood*, Vol.104, No.5, (September 2004), pp. 1314-1323.

Haubert, D., & Weckbecker, G. (2010). Vav1 couples the T cell receptor to cAMP response element activation via a PKC-dependent pathway. *Cellular Signaling*, Vol.22, No.6, (June 2010), pp. 944-954.

Holsinger, L.J., Graef, I.A., Swat, W., Chi, T., Bautista, D.M., Davidson, L., Lewis, R.S., Alt, F.W., & Crabtree, G.R. (1998). Defects in actin-cap formation in Vav-deficient mice implicate an actin requirement for lymphocyte signal transduction. *Current Bioloogy*, Vol.8, No.10, (May 1998), pp. 563-572.

Hornstein, I., Alcover, A., & Katzav, S. (2004). Vav proteins, masters of the world of cytoskeleton organization. *Cellular Signalling* Vol.16, No.1, (January 2004), pp. 1-11.

Houlard, M., Arudchandran, R., Regnier-Ricard, F., Germani, A., Gisselbrecht, S., Blank, U., Rivera, J., & Varin-Blank, N. (2002). Vav1 is a component of transcriptionally active complexes.*The Journal of Experimental Medicine*, Vol.195, No.9, (May 2002), pp. 1115-1127.

Hsu, H.C., Tsai, W.H., Chen, P.G., Hsu, M.L., Ho, C.K., & Wang, S.Y. (1999). In vitro effect of granulocyte-colony stimulating factor and all-trans retinoic acid on the expression of inflammatory cytokines and adhesion molecules in acute promyelocytic leukemic cells. *European Journal of Haematology*, Vol.63, No.1, (July 1999), pp.11-18.

Janmey, P.A., Xian, W., & Flanagan, L.A. (1999). Controlling cytoskeleton structure by phosphoinositide-protein interactions: phosphoinositide binding protein domains and effects of lipid packing. *Chemistry and Physics of Lipids*, Vol.101, No.1, (August 1999), pp. 93-107.

Jasek, E., Mirecka, J., & Litwin, J.A. (2008). Effect of differentiating agents (all-trans retinoic acid and phorbol 12-myristate 13-acetate) on drug sensitivity of HL60 and NB4 cells in vitro. *Folia Histochemica et Cytobiologica*, Vol.46, No.3, (December 2008), pp.323-330, ISSN, 0239-8508.

Kastner P., & Chan, S. (2008). PU.1: a crucial and versatile player in hematopoiesis and leukemia. *The International Journal of Biochemistry and Cell Biology*, Vol.40, No.1, (n.d.), pp. 22-27.

Katzav, S. (2004). Vav1: an oncogene that regulates specific transcriptional activation of T cells. *Blood*, Vol.103, No.7, (April 2004), pp. 2443-2451.

Katzav, S. (2009). Vav1: a hematopoietic signal transduction molecule involved in human malignancies. *The International Journal of Biochemistry & Cell Biology*, Vol.41, No.6, (June 2009), pp. 1245-1248.

Khatau, S.B., Hale, C.M., Stewart-Hutchinson, P.J., Patel, M.S., Stewart, C.L., Searson, P.C., Hodzic, D., & Wirtz, D. (2009). A perinuclear actin cap regulates nuclear shape. *Proceedings of the National Academy of Sciences of the United States of America*, Vol.106, No.45, (November 2009), pp. 19017-19122.

Kim, C., Marchal, C.C., Penninger, J. & Dinauer M.C. (2003). The hemopoietic Rho/Rac guanine nucleotide exchange factor Vav1 regulates N-formyl-methionyl-leucyl-phenylalanine-activated neutrophil functions. *Journal of Immunology*, Vol.171, No.8, (October 2003), pp. 4425-4430.

Kogan, S.C. (2009). Curing APL: differentiation or destruction? *Cancer Cell*, Vol.15, No.1, (January 2009), pp. 7-8.

Kong, Y.Y., Fischer, K.D., Bachmann, M.F., Mariathasan, S., Kozieradzki, I., Nghiem, M.P., Bouchard, D., Bernstein, A., Ohashi, P.S. & Penninger, J.M. (1998). Vav regulates peptide-specific apoptosis in thymocytes. *The Journal of Experimental Medicine*,Vol.188, No.11, (December 1998), pp. 2099-2111.

Lamkin T.J., Chin, V., Varvayanis, S., Smith, J.L., Sramkoski, R.M., Jacobberger, J.W., & Yen, A. (2006). Retinoic acid-induced CD38 expression in HL-60 myeloblastic leukemia cells regulates cell differentiation or viability depending on expression levels. *Journal of Cellular Biochemistry*, Vol.97, No.6, (April 2006), pp. 1328-1338.

Lanotte M., Martin-Thouvenin, V., Najman, S. Balerini, P., Valensi, F., & Berger, R. (1991). NB4, a maturation inducible cell line with t(15;17) marker isolated from a human acute promyelocytic leukemia (M3). *Blood*, Vol.77, No.5, (March 1991), pp. 1080-1086.

Law, D. A., Nannizzi-Alaimo, L., Ministri, K., Hughes, P. E., Forsyth, J.,Turner, M., Shattil, S. J., Ginsberg, M. H., Tybulewicz, V. L. J., & Phillips,D. R. (1999). Genetic and pharmacological analyses of Syk function in aII-b3 signaling in platelets. *Blood*, Vol.93, No.8, (April 1999), pp. 2645-2652.

Lazer, G., Pe'er, L., Farago, M., Machida, K., Mayer, B.J., & Katzav, S. (2010). Tyrosine residues at the carboxyl terminus of Vav1 play an important role in regulation of its biological activity. *The Journal of Biological Chemistry*, Vol.285, No.30, (July 2010), pp. 23075-23085.

Li, G.H., Fan, Y.Z., Liu, X.W., Zhang, B.F., Yin, D.D., He, F., Huang, S.Y., Kang, Z.J., Xu, H., Liu, Q., Wu, Y.L., Niu, X.L., Zhang, L., Liu, L., Hao, M.W., Han, H., & Liang, Y.M. (2010). Notch signaling maintains proliferation and survival of the HL60 human promyelocytic leukemia cell line and promotes the phosphorylation of the Rb protein. *Molecular and Cellular Biochemistry*, Vol.340, No. 1-2, (July 2010), pp. 7-14.

Liou, J.Y., Ghelani, D., Yeh, S., & Wu, K.K. (2007). Nonsteroidal anti-inflammatory drugs induce colorectal cancer cell apoptosis by suppressing 14-3-3epsilon. *Cancer Research*, Vol.67, No.7, (April 2007), pp. 3185-3191.

Liu, C.R., Ma, C.S., Ning, J.Y., You, J.F., Liao, S.L., & Zheng, J. (2004). Differential thymosin beta 10 expression levels and actin filament organization in tumor cell lines with different metastatic potential. *Chinese Medical Journal*, Vol.117, No.2, (February 2004), pp. 213- 218.

Lo-Coco F., & Ammatuna, E. (2006). The biology of acute promyelocytic leukemia and its impact on diagnosis and treatment. *Hematology*, (January 2006), pp. 156-161.

López-Pedrera, C., Villalba, J.M., Siendones, E., Barbarroja, N. Gómez-Díaz, C., Rodríguez-Ariza, A., Buendía, P., Torres, A., & Velasco, F. (2006). Proteomic analysis of acute myeloid leukemia: Identification of potential early biomarkers and therapeutic targets. *Proteomics*, Vol.6, No.S1, (April 2006), pp. 293-299.

Lupher, M.L., Jr., Rao, N., Eck, M.J., & Band, H. The Cbl protooncoprotein: a negative regulator of immune receptor signal transduction. *Immunology Today*, Vol.20, No.8, (August 1999), pp. 375-382.

Menard, R.E., & Mattingly, R.R. (2004). Gbetagamma subunits stimulate p21-activated kinase 1 (PAK1) through activation of PI3-kinase and Akt but act independently of Rac1/Cdc42. *FEBS Letters*, Vol.556, No.1-3, (January 2004), pp. 187-192.

Miletic, A.V., Sakata-Sogawa, K., Hiroshima, M., Hamann, M.J., Gomez, T. S., Ota, N., Kloeppel, T., Kanagawa, O., Tokunaga, M., Billadeau, D.D., & Swat, W. (2006). Vav1 acidic region tyrosine 174 is required for the formation of T cell receptor-induced microclusters and is essential in T cell development and activation. *The Journal of Biological Chemistry*, Vol.281, No.50, (December 2006), pp. 38257–38265.

Mueller, B.U., Pabst, T., Fos, J., Petkovic, V., Fey, M.F., Asou, N., Buergi, U., & Tenen, D.G. (2006). ATRA resolves the differentiation block in t(15;17) acute myeloid leukemia by restoring PU.1 expression. *Blood*, Vol.107, No.8, (April 2006), pp. 3330-3338.

Murao, S., Gemmell, M.A., Callaham, M.F., Anderson, N.L., & Huberman, E. (1983). Control of macrophage cell differentiation in human promyelocytic HL-60 leukemia cells by 1,25-dihydroxyvitamin D3 and phorbol-12-myristate-13-acetate. *Cancer Research*, Vol.43, No.10, (October 1983), pp. 4989-4996.

Nasr, R., Guillemin, M.C., Ferhi, O., Soilihi, H., Peres, L., Berthier, C., Rousselot, P., Robledo-Sarmiento, M., Lallemand-Breitenbach, V., Gourmel, B., Vitoux, D., Pandolfi, P.P., Rochette-Egly, C., Zhu, J., & de Thé, H. (2008). Eradication of acute promyelocytic leukemia-initiating cells through PML-RARA degradation. *Nature Medicine*, Vol.14, No.12, (December 2008), pp. 1333-1342.

Niggli, V., & Keller, H. (1997). The phosphatidylinositol 3-kinase inhibitor wortmannin markedly reduces chemotactic peptide-induced locomotion and increases in cytoskeletal actin in human neutrophils. *European Journal of Pharmacology*, Vol.335, No.1, (September 1997), pp. 43–52.

Ohishi, K., Katayama, N., Shiku, H., Varnum-Finney, B., & Bernstein, I.D. (2003). Notch signalling in hematopoiesis. *Seminars in Cell & Developmental Biology*, Vol.14, No.2, (April 2003), pp. 143– 150.

Ottinger, E., Botfield, M.C., & Shoelson, S.E. (1998). Tandem SH2 domains confer high specificity in tyrosine kinase signaling. *The Journal of Biological Chemistry*, Vol.273, No.2, (January 1998), pp. 729–735.

Pahl H.L., Scheibe, R.J., Zhang, D.E., Chen, H.M., Galson, D.L., Maki, R.A., & Tenen, D.G. (1993). The proto-oncogene PU.1 regulates expression of the myeloid-specific CD11b promoter. *The Journal of Biological Chemistry*, Vol.268, No.7, (March 1993), pp. 5014-5020.

Pauker, M.H., & Barda-Saad, M. (2011). Studies of novel interactions between Nck and VAV SH3 domains. *Communicative & Integrative Biology*, Vol.4, No.2, (March/April 2011), pp. 175-177.

Phillipson, M., Heit, B., Parsons, S.A., Petri, B., Mullaly, S.C., Colarusso, P., Gower, R.M., Neely, G., Simon, S.I., & Kubes, P. (2009). Vav1 is essential for mechanotactic crawling and migration of neutrophils out of the inflamed microvasculature. *Journal of Immunology*, Vol.182, No.11, (June 2009), pp. 6870-6878.

Pivniouk, V.I., Martin, T.R., Lu-Kuo, J.M., Katz, H.R., Oettgen, H.C., & Geha, R.S. (1999). SLP-76 deficiency impairs signaling via the high-affinity IgE receptor in mast cells. *The Journal of Clinical Investigation*, Vol.103, No.12, (June 1999), pp. 1737-1743.

Qin, S., & Yamamura, H. (1997). Up-regulation of Syk activity during HL60 cell differentiation into granulocyte but not into monocyte/macrophage-lineage. *Biochemical and Biophysical Ressearch Communications*, Vol.236, No.3, (July 1997), pp. 697-701.

Rho, S.B., Chun, T., Lee, S.H., Park, K., & Lee, J.H. (2004). The interaction between E-tropomodulin and thymosin beta-10 rescues tumor cells from thymosin beta-10 mediated apoptosis by restoring actin architecture. *FEBS Letters*, Vol.557, No.1-3, (January 2004), pp. 57–63.

Romero, F., Dargemont, C., Pozo, F., Reeves, W.H., Camonis, J., Gisselbrecht, S., & Fischer S. (1996). p95vav associates with the nuclear protein Ku-70. *Molecular and Cellular Biology*, Vol.16, No.1, (January 1996), pp. 37-44.

Romero, F., Germani, A., Puvion, E., Camonis, J., Varin-Blank, N., Gisselbrecht, S., & Fischer, S. (1998). Vav binding to heterogeneous nuclear ribonucleoprotein (hnRNP) C. Evidence for Vav-hnRNP interactions in an RNA-dependent manner. *The Journal of Biological Chemistry*, Vol.273, No.10, (March 1998), pp. 5923-5931.

Sanchez, J.A., & Wangh, L.J. (1999). New insights into the mechanisms of nuclear segmentation in human neutrophils. *Journal of Cellular Biochemistry*, Vol.73, No.1, (April 1999), pp. 1-10.

Sanchez-Aguilera, A., Lee, Y.J., Lo Celso, C., Ferraro, F., Brumme, K., Mondal, S., Kim, C., Dorrance, A., Luo, H.R., Scadden, D.T, & Williams D.A. (2011). Guanine nucleotide exchange factor Vav1 regulates perivascular homing and bone marrow retention of hematopoietic stem and progenitor cells. *Proceedings of the National Academy of Sciences of the United States of America*, Vol.108, No.23, (June 2011), pp. 9607-9612.

Sanford, J.R., Ellis, J., & Cáceres, J.F. (2005). Multiple roles of arginine/serine-rich splicing factors in RNA processing. *Biochemical Society Transactions*, Vol.33, No.3, (June 2005), pp. 443-446.

Schneider H., &. Rudd, C.E. (2008). CD28 and Grb-2, relative to Gads or Grap, preferentially co-operate with Vav1 in the activation of NFAT/AP-1 transcription. *Biochemical and Biophysical Ressearch Communications*, Vol.369, No.2, (May 2008), pp. 616-621.

Schymeinsky, J., Sindrilaru, A., Frommhold, D., Sperandio, M., Gerstl, R., Then, C., Mócsai, A., Scharffetter-Kochanek, K., & Walzog, B. (2006). The Vav binding site of the non-receptor tyrosine kinase Syk at Tyr 348 is critical for beta2 integrin (CD11/CD18)-mediated neutrophil migration. *Blood*, Vol.108, No.12, (December 2006), pp. 3919-3927.

Seow C.J., Chue, S.C., & Wong, W.S. (2002). Piceatannol, a Syk-selective tyrosine kinase inhibitor, attenuated antigen challenge of guinea pig airways in vitro. *European Journal of Pharmacology*, Vol.443, No.1-3, (May 2002), pp. 189-196.

Shi, Y., Tohyama, Y., Kadono, T., He, J., Miah, S.M., Hazama, R., Tanaka, C., Tohyama, K., & Yamamura, H. (2006). Protein-tyrosine kinase Syk is required for pathogen engulfment in complement-mediated phagocytosis. *Blood*, Vol.107, No.11, (June 2006), pp. 4554-4562.

Song, X., & Norman, A.W. (1998). 1Alpha,25-dihydroxyvitamin D3 and phorbol ester mediate the expression of alkaline phosphatase in NB4 acute promyelocytic leukemia cells. *Leukemia Research*, Vol.22, No.1, (January 1998), pp. 69-76.

Stephens, L., Ellson, C., & Hawkins, P. (2002). Roles of PI3Ks in leukocyte chemotaxis and phagocytosis. *Current Opinion in Cell Biology*, Vol.14, No.2, (April 2002), pp. 203–213.

Stricker, J., Falzone, T., & Gardel, M.L. (2010). Mechanics of the F-actin cytoskeleton. *Journal of Biomechanics*, Vol.43, No.1, (January 2010), pp. 9-14.

Takenawa, T., & Itoh, T. (2001). Phosphoinositides, key molecules for regulation of actin cytoskeletal organization and membrane traffic from the plasma membrane. *Biochimica et Biophysica Acta,* Vol.1533, No.3, (October 2001), pp. 190-106.

Tallman, M. (2007). Treatment of relapsed or refractory acute promyelocytic leukemia. *Best Practice & Research Clinical Haematology,* Vol.20, No.1, (March 2007), pp. 57-65.

Tuosto, L., Michel, F., & Acuto, O. (1996). p95vav associates with tyrosine-phosphorylated SLP-76 in antigen-stimulated T cells. *The Journal of Experimental Medicine,* Vol.184, No.3, (September 1996), pp. 1161–1166.

Tybulewicz, V.L. (2005). Vav-family proteins in T-cell signalling. *Current Opinion in Immunology,* Vol.17, No.3, (June 2005), 267-274.

Vedham, V., Phee, H., & Coggeshall, K.M. (2005). Vav activation and function as a rac guanine nucleotide exchange factor in macrophage colony-stimulating factor-induced macrophage chemotaxis. *Molecular and Cellular Biology,* Vol.25, No.10, (May 2005), pp. 4211-4220.

Visani, G., Tosi, P., Ottaviani, E., Zaccaria, A., Baccini, C., Manfroi, S., Pastano, R., Remiddi, C., Morelli, A., Molinari, A.L., Zanchini, R., & Tura, S. (1996). All-trans retinoic acid and in vitro cytokine production by acute promyelocytic leukemia cells. *European Journal of Haematology,* Vol.57, No.4, (October 1996), pp. 301–306.

Von Mikecz, A. (2006). The nuclear ubiquitin-proteasome system. *Journal of Cell Science,* Vol.119, No.10, (May 2006), pp. 1977-1984.

Wan, J., Wang, J., Cheng, H., Yu, Y. Xing, G., Oiu, Z., Qian, X., & He, F.(2001). Proteomic analysis of apoptosis initiation induced by all-trans retinoic acid in human acute promyelocytic leukemia cells. *Electrophoresis,* Vol.22, No.14, (August 2001), pp. 3026-3037.

Wang, D., Jensen, R., Gendeh, G., Williams, K. & Pallavicini, M.G. (2004). Proteome and transcriptome analysis of retinoic acid-induced differentiation of human acute promyelocytic leukemia cells, NB4. *Journal of Proteome Research,* Vol.3, No.3, (May-June 2004), pp. 627-635.

Wang, F., Herzmark, P., Weiner, O.D., Srinivasan, S., Servant, G., & Bourne, H.R. (2002). Lipid products of PI3Ks maintain persistent cell polarity and directed motility in neutrophils. *Nature Cell Biology,* Vol.4, No.7, (July 2002), pp. 513–518.

Wells, C.M., Bhavsar, P.J., Evans, I.R., Vigorito, E., Turner, M., Tybulewicz, V., & Ridley A.J. (2005). Vav1 and Vav2 play different roles in macrophage migration and cytoskeletal organization. *Experimental Cell Research,* Vol.1, No.2, (November 2005), pp. 303-310.

Yang, L., Zhao, H., Li, S.W., Ahrens, K., Collins, C., Eckenrode, S., Ruan, Q.G., McIndoe, R.A., & She, J.X. (2003). Gene expression profiling during all-trans retinoic acid-induced cell differentiation of acute promyelocytic leukemia cells. *The Journal of Molecular Diagnostics,* Vol.5, No.4, (November 2003), pp. 212-221.

Yu, B., Martins, R.S., Li, P., Amarasinghe, G.K., Umetani, J., Fernandez-Zapico, M.E., Billadeau,D.D., Machius, M., Tomchick, D.R., Rosen, M.K. (2010). Structural and Energetic Mechanisms of Cooperative Autoinhibition and Activation of Vav1. *Cell,* Vol.140, (January 22), pp. 246–256.

Zhang, R., Tsai, F.Y., & Orkin, S.H. (1994). Hematopoietic development of vav-/- mouse embryonic stem cells. *Proceedings of the National Academy of Sciences of the United States of America* Vol.91, No.26, (December 1994), pp. 12755-12759.

Zou, L., Wu, Y., Pei, L., Zhong, D., Gen, M., Zhao, T., Wu, J., Ni, B., Mou, Z., Han, J., Chen, Y., Zhi, Y. (2005). Identification of leukemia-associated antigens in chronic myeloid leukemia by proteomic analysis. *Leukemia Research,* Vol.29, No.12, (December 2005), pp. 1387-1391.

p15INK4b, a Tumor Suppressor in Acute Myeloid Leukemia

Joanna Fares[1,2], Linda Wolff[1] and Juraj Bies[1]
[1]Laboratory of Cellular Oncology, National Cancer Institute, NIH, Bethesda, Maryland,
[2]Georgetown University, Department of Biochemistry and Molecular Biology,
Washington DC,
USA

1. Introduction

p15INK4b expression is lost in a striking 80% of all patients suffering from acute myeloid leukemia (AML). Specific inactivation of the gene by aberrant promoter hypermethylation is also detected in about 50% of patients diagnosed with myelodysplastic syndromes (MDS) and almost 60% of patients with myeloproliferative disorders (MPD). More importantly, a strong correlation between the methylation levels of *p15INK4b* and poor prognosis is now well established in these patients. Hypermethylation levels also provide a marker for subsequent transformation and progression of the disease to a more aggressive phenotype. These clinical observations establish the repression of *p15INK4b* expression by promoter hypermethylation as the most prevalent genetic abnormality in myeloid leukemia. The *p15INK4b* gene (also referred to as *CDKN2B* and *MTS2*) encodes a 15kDa cyclin dependent kinase inhibitor (CDKI). Specific and preferential epigenetic targeting of *p15INK4b* for silencing over other CDKIs such as *p16INK4a* and *p21WAF/CIP* in AML, MDS and MPD patients strongly supports a role for this protein as a tumor suppressor in hematological malignancies of the myeloid lineage.

This chapter provides a review of the literature outlining the high prevalence of *p15INK4b* loss of expression in human myeloid malignancies, as well as the latest research carried out in mice which supports a role for p15Ink4b as a tumor suppressor. It also focuses on the well established function of p15INK4b in the control of the cell cycle, as well as its role during early and late myeloid cells development. Finally, this chapter discusses the multiple mechanisms by which *p15INK4b* is silenced and presents a few examples of clinical studies of drugs that target *p15INK4b* for re-expression. These include treatments for reversing aberrant DNA methylation, and are currently being tested and used for the therapy of MDS and AML.

2. Role of p15INK4b in myeloid malignancies

2.1 Inactivation in human AML and MDS

p15INK4b silencing by promoter hypermethylation occurs almost exclusively in cancers of the hematopoietic system, and is observed in acute leukemias of myeloid (AML) and lymphoid (ALL) origins (Drexler, 1998). Aberrant hypermethylation occurs at the gene's

CpG islands which extend throughout the promoter region, exon 1 and part of intron 1 (Herman et al., 1996). DNA methylation is the addition of methyl groups on cytosine bases on the DNA molecules of mammalian cells which affects gene expression (Deaton et al., 2011). Methylation is carried out by the enzymes DNA methyltransferases (DNMT) which catalyze the reaction converting cytosine to 5-methylcytosine (Bird et al., 2002). In the earlier studies DNA methylation was assessed by southern blotting and methylation-specific PCR technique and more recently by more sensitive assays including bisulfate pyrosequencing and genome-wide sequencing methods (Deaton et al., 2011).

Despite the broad clinical diversity of AML, with more than a hundred cytogenetic alterations described (Vardiman et al., 2002; Trost et al., 2006), aberrant methylation of *p15INK4b* has been reported in up to 80% of patients with primary and secondary AML. Hypermethylation levels have been shown to correlate with a reduction in the mRNA and the protein expression levels of p15INK4b (Cameron et al., 1999; Matsuno et al., 2005). Furthermore, density of the methylation has been shown to vary greatly between and within AML patients and its levels closely correlate with the degree of transcriptional repression (Aggerholm et al., 1999, Cameron et al., 1999). AML classification into ten different subtypes was originally defined by the French-American-British (FAB) cooperative group (Bennett et al., 1976, 1985). Numerous studies have been conducted to assess the methylation levels of *p15INK4b* on samples of patients with AML across the different FAB subtypes (Herman et al., 1996, 1997; Aggerholm et al., 1999; Guo et al., 2000; Chim et al., 2001a, 2001b; Christiansen et al., 2003; Garcia-Manero et al., 2003; Teofili et al., 2003; Shimamoto et al., 2005). In patients with adult and childhood AML, hypermethylation of *p15INK4b* in cells isolated from bone marrow and peripheral blood is observed in nearly all morphological FAB subtypes. Higher frequencies are generally observed in the M1, M2, M3 and M4 subtypes than in the M5, M6 or M7 subtypes and are found to occur in the vast majority of the patients' leukemic cells (Aggerholm et al., 1999; Wong et al., 2000; Shimamoto et al., 2005; Tsellou et al., 2005). In patients with therapy-induced AML (t-AML), aberrant methylation of *p15INK4b* (in over 90% of patients) is found to be independent from the patient's type of previous therapy which ranges from alkylating agents, topoisomerase II inhibitors to radiotherapy (Christiansen et al., 2003).

A similar pattern of aberrant methylation is also well documented in patients with MDS (Uchida et al., 1997; Quesnel et al., 1998; Aoki et al., 2000; Tien et al., 2001; Christiansen et al., 2003; Teofili et al., 2003). The FAB classification system for MDS is mainly based on the percentage of blast cells in the bone marrow and the peripheral blood and the degree of cytopenia (Bennet et al., 1982). Methylation levels have also been shown to increase during follow-up and in conversion to overt AML (Tien et al., 2001, Christiansen et al., 2003). Importantly, aberrant DNA methylation of *p15INK4b* was found to be one of the most dominant molecular events in MDS progression to AML (Jiang et al., 2009). Similar to AML, cytogenetics of MDS is also a crucial factor in the prognosis and development of the disease (Haase et al., 2007). The World Health Organization (WHO) classification system for myeloid neoplasms was developed and takes into consideration both morphology and cytogenetic abnormalities (Harris et al., 2000). In MDS patients, methylation of *p15INK4b* is associated with an increased percentage of immature myeloblasts in the bone marrow (Christiansen et al., 2003). The presence of DNA hypermethylation at the *p15INK4b* promoter is found predominantly in high risk MDS patients with increased levels being reported in the subtypes characterized by advanced stages of the disease such as refractory anemia with excess blasts (RAEB). Reduced levels are reported in patients with the early stages of MDS such as refractory anemia (RA) and refractory anemia with ringed sideroblasts (RARS) (Uchida et al., 1997; Christiansen et al., 2003). However, more recently, it was found that even in patients with the RARS subtype, which falls within the lower risk of MDS, *p15INK4b* was found to be the most frequently methylated gene (>20% of cases) of 25 known tumor suppressors that were evaluated in the study (Valencia et al., 2011). Although most studies have been conducted in MDS in adults, comparable levels of aberrant methylation patterns have been observed in pediatric MDS patients as well (Hasegawa et al., 2005), and a similar correlation with the disease subtypes has been established (Rodrigues et al., 2010).

In chronic myelomonocytic leukemia (CMML), aberrant methylation of *p15INK4b* is found in about 60% of cases and is associated with a high proportion of blastic transformation (Tessema et al., 2003). CMML is a disease that was originally categorized under myelodysplastic disorders, but is now classified by the WHO as a disorder that bridges MDS with myeloproliferative features (Harris et al., 1999). In these patients, genomic sequencing techniques have revealed that hypermethylation spans a wide area in the 5' region of the gene and is correlated with reduced expression of the mRNA levels. High variability between and within individual patients, consistent with observations in AML patients, were also reported (Tessema et al., 2003, Aggerholm et al., 1999, Cameron et al., 1999). In the pediatric form of the disease, juvenile myelomonocytic leukemia (JMML), *p15INK4b* hypermethylation is found to be a less frequent, however, still significant event (17% of cases) (Hasegawa et al., 2005).

With regards to cytogenetic abnormalities, *p15INK4b* methylation levels have been found to occur at higher frequencies in AML/MDS patients with an unfavorable karyotype (Wong et al., 2000; Galm et al., 2005; Shimamoto et al., 2005; Markus et al., 2007). Cases with unmethylated or low levels of hypermethylated *p15INK4b* were associated with normal karyotype or with those karyotypic abnormalities that are associated with a favorable prognosis (Wong et al., 2000; Markus et al., 2007). Studies have consistently reported an increased tendency for *p15INK4b* hypermethylation in unfavorable cytogenetics (Shimamoto et al., 2005). These results suggest interplay between *p15INK4b* loss of expression and the frequent chromosomal translocations, inversions and deletions observed in AML and MDS. The mechanisms underlying *p15INK4b* hypermethylation are not completely understood, but a few theories involving maintaining and de-novo DNA methylation through action of DNA methyltransferases (DNMT), as well as histone modification pathways have been suggested to play a role (Paul et al., 2010). Specifically in t-AML and therapy-induced MDS (t-MDS), deletion or loss of chromosome arm 7q, which is the most common cytogenetic abnormality in those categories, has been found to be closely associated with hypermethylation of *p15INK4b* (Christiansen et al., 2003).

p15INK4b is now used as an independent prognosticator in AML and MDS (Chim et al., 2001b; Teofili et al., 2003; Christiansen et al., 2003; Shimamoto et al., 2005; Chim et al., 2006). In the many categories of the diseases, aberrant *p15INK4b* methylation levels have been associated with a generally poor prognosis. In studies that monitor patients across all AML FAB subtypes, patients without *p15INK4b* hypermethylation at diagnosis had increased complete remission rates which also correlated with increased survival times (Shimamoto et al., 2005; Deneberg et al., 2010). Consistent with these observations, in APL patients, abnormal *p15INK4b* methylation was associated with a shorter disease-free survival (DFS) period and a higher incidence of relapse during the 5-year follow up period (Teofili et al.,

2003). In the relapsed patients, the *p15INK4b* hypermethylation levels remained persistent following treatment. In contrast, the patients without detectable hypermethylation displayed prolonged survival (Chim et al., 2001b). Additionally, as previously stated, patients with MDS with high methylation levels at diagnosis had a significantly higher chance of the disease progressing to AML (Tien et al., 2001; Jiang et al., 2009). It was also reported that in early stage of MDS, the *p15INK4b* hypermethylation is a negative risk factor for patients, closely correlating with leukemic transformation (Aggerholm et al., 2006). The same correlation has been shown in patients with t-MDS, in which methylation resulted in significantly shorter survival (Christiansen et al., 2003). A recent study showed that the high levels of methylation in lower risk MDS categories suggest a poor prognosis in those patients as well (Valencia et al, 2011). In JMML p15INK4b hypermethylation was associated with reduced overall survival rates and higher relapse of the disease following hematopoietic stem cell transplantation (Olk-Batz et al., 2011). All these results suggest that lack of *p15INK4b* expression, mediated by promoter hypermethylation, not only affects the prognosis in patients with AML and MDS, but can be used to predict the outcome of the diseases.

The studies described above confirm that aberrant hypermethylation levels of *p15INK4b* have important prognostic implications for clinical monitoring in MDS and assessment of risk of progression into AML. However, its potential use as a biomarker in leukemia excluded estimation of minimal residual disease in patients who have achieved clinical remission, and its implications in terms of subsequent relapse. A study aiming at addressing this issue, evaluated *p15INK4b* methylation levels in AML patients in complete clinical remission (Agrawal et al., 2007). The study reported that even in remission, leukemia patients that harbored a significant amount of methylation in the bone marrow cells had a higher risk for leukemia relapse. Moreover, the time of disease-free survival was found to be significantly reduced in correlation with the amount of residual hypermethylation of the *p15Ink4b* gene. Concurrently, low levels of *p15INK4b* methylation during complete remission were associated with reduced relapse rates during the 12 month follow-up. It was suggested that analysis of *p15INK4b* methylation levels during clinical remission can be potentially used as a prognosticator for the occurrence of relapse (Agrawal et al., 2007).

In recent years, it has been suggested in a number of studies that DNA methylation of *p15INK4b* could also help predict response to therapy (Grovdal et al., 2007; Shen et al., 2009). Grövdal et al. (2007) studied DNA methylation patterns in older patients with high risk MDS and AML following MDS. Patients were treated with conventional induction therapy. Methylation levels of *p15INK4b*, *E-cadherin*, and *HIC1* (hypermethylated in cancer 1), were assessed prior to initiation of treatment. Abnormal levels of methylation of *p15INK4b* alone did not correlate with decreased complete remission (CR), but all patients with all three genes methylated did not achieve CR. Another study, in which patients with MDS and AML were treated with the DNA methyltransferase inhibitor 5-azacytidine (5-aza-C), reported consistent results with these observations (Raj et al., 2007; Tran et al., 2011). Patients with levels exceeding 24% methylation in the *p15Ink4b* promoter region did not respond to treatment (Raj et al., 2007). The possibility of using methylation of *p15INK4b* as an indicator for treatment outcome is still under investigation. However, results suggest that studying *p15INK4b* methylation density in conjunction with other altered genes at diagnosis and monitoring its levels following treatment might have predictive information with respect to the patient's response to treatment.

Although hypermethylation is the most common mode of inactivation of *p15INK4b* in myeloid neoplasms, other silencing mechanisms have also been described. In AML with chromosome 16 inversion (*inv16*), the overall *p15INK4b* methylation levels are found to be very low and almost comparable to levels in normal patients. However, expression of the gene is severely suppressed. In this type of AML, the inversion (16) results in a fusion protein between the core binding factor (CBFβ) and the smooth myosin heavy chain gene (SMMHC). This chimeric transcription factor CBFβ-SMMHC binds directly to the promoter of *p15INK4b* and represses its expression (Markus et al., 2007). These results further emphasize an important role of *p15INK4b* silencing in leukemogenesis of the myeloid lineage, and suggest, that in the absence of a repressive epigenetic event, other mechanisms may result in inhibition of *p15INK4b* expression (Markus et al., 2007).

2.2 Inactivation in other types of human leukemias

In B and T cell acute lymphoblastic leukemias (B-ALL, T-ALL), *p15INK4b* hypermethylation as well as deletion of the entire 9p21 locus which includes *p15INK4b*, *p16INK4a* and *ARF* genes has been reported (Roussel, 1999; Ruas et al., 1998). Homozygous deletions of *p16INK4a* and *p15INK4b* are found in approximately 30% of childhood acute lymphoblastic leukemia at first presentation, with striking rates in T-ALL (60 to 80%), and lower rates in B-cell precursor ALL (5 to 20%) (Drexler HG, 1998; Chim et al., 2001a). Further studies have analyzed methylation levels of the two genes in these disease categories specifically in terms of overall survival and absence of relapse at 6 years of follow-up. *p15INK4b* and *p16INK4a* methylation levels were found to occur at similar rates (35%) in adults and children with mature B-ALL (Graf-Einsiedel et al., 2002). Deletion of the entire locus was observed in 12% and 30% of children and adults, respectively. Interestingly, results show that deletion is associated with poor overall survival (OS) in adults only, but not in children (Van Zutven et al., 2005; Mirebeau et al., 2006; Kim et al., 2009). Furthermore, it did not affect the type of relapse or DFS time in children. In untreated adult patients with precursor B-ALL, high methylation levels of *p15INK4b* (found in 43% of patients) were significantly associated with decreased DFS at 4 years (Hoshino et al., 2002). Recent methylation profiles in 95 children with ALL supported older studies showing that methylation of *p15INK4b* occurred predominantly in T-ALL as opposed to B-ALL, and *p15INK4b* is one of the most commonly methylated genes among the 14 genes analyzed (Takeuchi et al., 2011). A clear correlation between increased methylation and prognoses in T-ALL has not been established.

2.3 p15Ink4b as a tumor suppressor in mice

To define the role of p15INK4b as a tumor suppressor in AML, mouse models have been developed and characterized (Latres et al., 2000; Wolff et al., 2003a, 2004; Bies et al., 2010). These have provided strong experimental evidence to support the hypothesis that loss of p15INK4b function plays an important role in the development of myeloid leukemia.

A p15Ink4b-/- mouse model was first described by Latres et al. (2000). Mice were generated by genetic targeting with elimination of the second coding exon of the p15Ink4b gene. Knockout mice were viable, fertile, and did not exhibit any behavioral abnormalities. Mouse embryonic fibroblasts were found to have a higher proliferation rate and plating efficiency when compared to their wild type counterparts. More importantly, they were more susceptible to transformation with *c-myc* and *ras* oncogenes, confirming the reported results that p15Ink4b participates in the tumor suppressor activity triggered after inappropriate oncogenic *ras* activation of the Raf-Mek-Erk pathway (Malumbres et al., 2000). However, with respect to AML, deleting p15Ink4b did not result in leukemogenesis in these mice. Of note, extramedullary hematopoiesis and lymphoid hyperplasia in the spleen were observed in mice aged less than 9 months and resulted in death of over 75% of the mice at an older age. Taken together, these experimental results were the first to suggest that p15Ink4b might be playing a tumor suppressor role in AML (Latres et al., 2000).

A role for p15Ink4b in myeloid neoplasia in mice was first supported by the finding that retrovirus-induced AML had hypermethylation of the CpG promoter region of the *p15Ink4b* gene. Based upon this, further mouse models were developed to determine if loss of p15Ink4b increases susceptibility to myeloid leukemia when additional oncogenic events were provided by retroviral insertional mutagenesis. For these studies, a specific retrovirus with a broad tropism and the capability of inducing a high incidence of myeloid leukemia was constructed (Wolff et al., 2003b and 2004). It consists of a recombinant virus incorporating Moloney murine leukemia virus (Mo-MuLV) sequences, and regulatory LTR sequences of retrovirus 4070A. The recombinant virus, named MOL4070LTR, combines the capacity of 4070A to accelerate myeloid disease with the wide tropism of Mo-MuLV, and successfully produced myeloid disease when inoculated intraperitoneally into wild-type FVB and BALB/c mice as neonates (Wolff et al., 2003b). The *p15Ink4b* knockout mice were developed using the same targeting vector as described by Latres et al. (2000), and MOL4070LTR was inoculated into neonates. While there was no incidence of disease in control wild-type mice (p15Ink4b$^{+/+}$), a significant percentage of heterozygous mice (p15Ink4b$^{+/-}$) developed myeloid leukemia within a year. Surprisingly, a smaller percentage of homozygous knockout mice (p15Ink4b$^{-/-}$) developed myeloid tumors (Wolff et al., 2003a). Further experiments demonstrated that in heterozygous p15Ink4b$^{+/-}$ mice, the second remaining *p15Ink4b* allele was actually hypermethylated, with a reduction of its mRNA expression. This data supported the fact that p15Ink4b functions as a tumor suppressor for myeloid leukemia, however, it was difficult to explain why mice heterozygous for the null allele were more susceptible than homozygous null mice. One explanation might be that in the homozygous null mice, *p15Ink4b* is lost in all the tissues and loss of expression in one tissue may have compensating effects on loss in another tissue.

A new mouse system in which deletion of the gene is restricted to the myeloid lineage was developed to mimic more closely myeloid lineage disease in man (Bies et al., 2010). The mouse strain utilizes a Cre-loxP system for conditional deletion of the *p15Ink4b* gene through action of Cre recombinase exclusively expressed in blood cells of the myeloid lineage (Clausen et al., 1999). In this model, Cre recombinase specifically recognizes loxP sites to mediate efficient excision of exon 2 of the *p15Ink4b* gene in myeloid cells. In order to monitor disease development in mice with targeted *p15Ink4b* deletion (p15Ink4b$^{fl/fl}$ LysMcre), white cell counts were performed in circulating blood from targeted and wild-type animals from different age groups. Interestingly, p15Ink4b$^{fl/fl}$LysMcre mice showed a significant increase in the number of circulating monocytes compared to control mice (p15Ink4b$^{wt/wt}$LysMcre), whereas neutrophils, lymphocytes, platelets and red blood cell counts were not affected. Monocytosis remained in targeted mice beyond 8 months of age, while wild-type mice showed a marked decrease in monocytes resulting in an even greater significance in the statistical comparisons (Figure 3A). Expansion of myelomonocytic cells in the bone marrow (BM) of p15Ink4b$^{fl/fl}$LysMcre mice was also observed. Analysis of BM cells for the cell surface markers Gr-1, Mac-1 and c-Kit revealed that BM cells from p15Ink4b$^{fl/fl}$LysMcre mice had a significant increase in both mature myeloid (Gr-1$^+$/Mac-1$^+$) and monocytic (Gr-1$^{-/lo}$/Mac-1$^+$) cells. This increase correlated with a significantly higher proportion of immature myeloid (Mac-1$^{+/lo}$/c-Kit$^+$) cells in the BM. Inactivation of *p15Ink4b* in myeloid cells promoted a mild preleukemic myeloproliferative-like disease (Bies et al., 2010). A small percentage of the targeted mice spontaneously progressed to a form of leukemia featuring an increased number of mature circulating myeloid cells in the peripheral blood, as well as an increase in the number of progenitors in the BM. The disease observed in mice most closely resembled an advanced form of CMML (Bies et al., 2010). However, the disease did not progress to an acute form of leukemia over the period of 15 months in any of the mice. These results were in agreement with studies carried on in the embryonal p15Ink4b$^{-/-}$ mice, and suggested that inactivation of the *p15Ink4b* gene without an additional genetic/epigenetic hit is not sufficient to cause acute leukemia. Retrovirus-induced mutagenesis in p15Ink4b$^{fl/fl}$LysMcre mice was used to identify genetic changes that

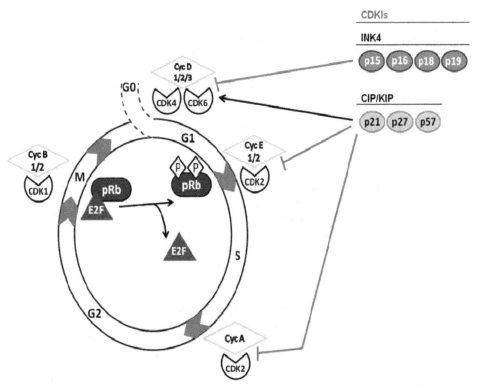

Fig. 1. Cell cycle regulation by the CDKI families. CDKs are switched on and off at different times during the cell cycle; the cyclins Ds-dependent kinases 4 and 6, and CDK2/cyclin E, CDK2/cyclin A regulate G1 progression and entry into the S phase. CDK1/cyclin B regulates entry and exit from mitosis. The CDK/cyclin complexes phosphorylate pRb to allow for the transcription of genes under the control of E2Fs which include factors necessary for cell cycle progression. CIP/KIP family members of CDKI can be either activators or inhibitors of cyclin/CDK assembly (Sherr & Roberts, 1999).

could cooperate with the loss of p15Ink4b in leukemia development. Mice inoculated with the MOL4070LTR retrovirus were monitored for 15 months for signs of disease. Control mice developed leukemia with low penetrance, whereas the incidence of retrovirus-induced leukemia was statistically highly significant for the p15Ink4b[fl/fl]LysMcre animals. Additionally, phenotypic analyses of tumor cells demonstrated a strong bias towards the development of AML in the knockout animals. Myeloid–specific inactivation of *p15Ink4b* results in retrovirus-induced development of tumors mostly monocytic (F4/80[+], F4/80[+]/Mac1[+]) and myelomonocytic (F4/80[+]/Mac1[+]/Gr-1[+]), whereas there was an equal distribution of lymphoid and monocytic tumors in the control mice (Figure 3B). Results generated using this model complement the embryonal *p15nk4b[-/-]* studies and demonstrate an active role for *p15Ink4b* silencing in promoting the establishment of preleukemic conditions. These results also provided strong experimental evidence that p15Ink4b functions as a tumor suppressor for myeloid leukemia development (Bies et al., 2010).

3. Conventional and novel functions of p15INK4b

3.1 p15INK4B as a regulator of the cell cycle

p15INK4b belongs to the INK4 family of cyclin-dependent kinases inhibitors (CDKIs). The family comprises three other members – p16INK4a, p18INK4c and p19INK4d and is one of two families of CDKIs that have been identified and defined based on their structure and CDK specificities. INK4 proteins all show a high and exclusive specificity towards the activity of cyclin-dependent kinase 4 (CDK 4) and cyclin-dependent kinase 6 (CDK6) during the early and mid-G1 phase of the cell cycle (Sherr & Roberts, 1999). The cell cycle is comprised of 4 phases, G1, S, G2 (also referred to as interphase), and M phase (mitosis). Entrance of cells from the quiescent G0/G1 phase into cycle is governed by the actions of kinases CDK4/CDK6 and CDK2 that are activated by cyclins Ds and Es, respectively (Figure 1).

During the transition to S phase, CDKs hyperphosphorylate pRb causing its dissociation from the nuclear transcription factors E2Fs. E2Fs regulate the transcription of genes which are required for the completion of the cell cycle and include cyclins A and E, thymidine synthetase and PCNA (Korenjak & Brehm, 2005). Throughout the S, G2 and M phases, pRb is kept in a hyperphosphorylated state by an orchestrated mechanism that involves sequential activities of multiple cyclins/CDKs (Sherr & Roberts, 1999). INK4 proteins inhibit CDKs/cyclin Ds complexes and, therefore, function in G1-S checkpoint control. When INK4 proteins block formation of these complexes, the pRb is in a hypophosphorylated, active state and interacts with E2F to inhibit its function (Korenjak & Brehm, 2005). Structural studies have demonstrated that INK4 proteins perform their inhibitory activity by allosteric competition with cyclins Ds to bind CDK4 and CDK6. CDK4/6-INK4s protein complexes have reduced affinity toward the D-type cyclins (Jeffrey et al., 2000; Yuan et al 2000).

p15INK4b and *p16INK4a* are tandemly linked on human chromosome 9p21 within a 40kb DNA region, whereas *p18INK4c* and *p19INK4d* are located in the chromosomal regions 1p32.3 and 19p13.2, respectively. The 9p21 chromosomal locus is referred to as the INK4/ARF locus has been tightly linked to the formation of many types of tumors (Nobori et al., 1994). In addition to *p15INK4b* and *p16INK4a*, it also encodes a third gene called *p14ARF*, originally identified as an alternative transcript of *p16INK4a* (Figure 2). *p14ARF* is transcribed from exon 1β and exons 2 and 3 of *p16INK4a*, but using a different reading frame (Figure 2). The p14ARF protein (p19Arf in mouse) is immunologically and functionally unrelated to the p16INK4a protein; they are not considered to be isoforms and do not share sequence homology or overlapping roles in the cell (Ozenne et al., 2010; Sherr CJ, 2006). Furthermore, p14ARF bears little or no structural similarities with the INK4 family members, and is unable to bind or inhibit CDKs. It is not considered to be part of the INK4 family of inhibitors, but it still participates in the negative regulation of the cell cycle by antagonizing the effects of MDM2, a ubiquitin ligase that targets the tumor suppressor protein p53 for degradation by the 26S proteasome (Ruas et al., 1998).

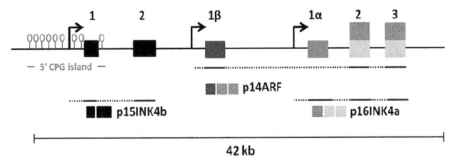

Fig. 2. 9p21 chromosomal locus showing the promoters and exons that are involved in the transcription of *p15INK4b*, *p14ARF* and *p16INK4a* genes. The CpG island is depicted for the *p15INK4b* gene only and extends throughout the promoter region, exon 1 and part of intron 1 (Herman et al., 1996).

INK4 family members are highly conserved among species, with over 90% identity between the human and the corresponding mouse proteins. In human, the four proteins share roughly 40% sequence homology with each other and have a very closely related structure, characterized by the presence of ankyrin motif tandem repeats. Four ankyrin repeats are found in p15INK4b and p16INK4a, and five repeats in p18INK4c and p19INK4d (Yuan et al., 2000). Ankyrin motif repeats consist of a helix-loop-helix structure that promotes protein-protein interaction (Li et al., 1999). Structural studies involving programmed mutations and generation of chimeric proteins have revealed that the third ankyrin repeat is necessary for the interaction with CDK4 and CDK6, and is responsible for the inhibitory activity of these CDKIs. Crystallography work on the CDK6 bound p16INK4a, p18INK4c and p19INK4d suggested that the INK4 proteins bind to one side of the catalytic cleft, opposite to the cyclin binding site, and that binding and recognition are mediated mostly via hydrogen bonds (Brotherton et al., 1998; Noh et al., 1999; Russo et al., 1998). INK4 proteins were found not to interfere with the cyclin binding site which is consistent with the presence of INK4s/cyclin Ds/CDK4 or CDK6 ternary complexes. When bound in the absence of cyclin D, they cause a conformation switch in CDK4 and CDK6 which distorts the cyclin and the ATP-binding sites leading to rapid recycling of unbound D-type cyclins by the ubiquitin-dependent 26S proteasome. The specificity towards CDK 4 and CDK6 was found to be due primarily to the critical residues involved in the hydrogen bonds with INK4 proteins which are conserved exclusively in CDK4 and CDK6, but not in the other CDKs (Russo et al., 1998). Interestingly, several of the residues necessary for recognition and binding have been reported to be mutated in cancer (Li et al., 1999).

The structural similarities observed between the INK4 proteins are consistent with the shared biological and biochemical properties of these molecules. However, the expression pattern of each of the human INK4 proteins appears to be highly specific to the cell type and tissue localization, as well as the differentiation stage of the cells (Shwaller et al., 1997; Thullberg et al., 2000). For instance, in normal hematopoietic cells, the expression of p15INK4b is shown to be lineage restricted, and is mainly detected in monocytes and lymphocytes, but not in any of the erythroid precursors (Teofili et al., 1998). Myeloid-restricted expression of *p15INK4b* is observed in peripheral blood and bone marrow and its levels are reported to be increased during megakaryocyte and monocyte/macrophage differentiation (Furukawa et al., 2000; Teofili et al., 2001; Haviernik et al., 2003).

p15INK4b, in particular, is an important downstream effector of anti-proliferative signaling by the transforming growth factor- β1 (TGF-β1) (Hannon & Beach, 1994). In different human and mouse cell lines, treatment with this negative growth factor, as well as interleukin 6 (IL-6) or Interferon β (IFN- β) leads to G0/G1 cell cycle arrest (Schmidt et al., 2004; Haviernik et al., 2003). Treatment with TGF-β1 induces a significant increase in the transcription levels of *p15INK4b*, but also induces a major increase in p15INK4b protein stability (Sandhu et al., 1997). Following treatment with TGF-β1, p15INK4b-CDK4/6 complexes are more abundant compared to the Cyclin D-Cdk4 complexes indicating strong inhibitor activity (Sandhu et al., 1997). In contrast to *p15INK4b*, whose expression is absent in hematopoietic stem cells, but increases as the cells mature along the myeloid lineage, *p16INK4a* is highly expressed in hematopoietic stem cells, and down-regulated with differentiation of all lineages (Furukawa et al., 2000). *p18INK4c* is found to be the most homogeneously and abundantly expressed member of the family, whereas *p19INK4d* is the most restricted, and its expression is limited to lymphoid cell, epithelial cells, seminiferous tubes and adrenal gland cells (Thullberg et al., 2000). The differential expression patterns of the INK4 proteins, suggest non-overlapping physiological functions.

Despite their common function in regulation of the cell cycle, the four members are found to be differentially involved in tumorigenesis. Mouse knock-out models along with genetic screenings of human tumors and gene expression profiling of cell lines have been used to help elucidate the role of these cell cycle inhibitors in the establishment and progression of cancer (Cánepa et al., 2007). In concordance with the molecular analysis of human tumor tissues, mice deficient in different Ink4 proteins display an increased susceptibility to the development of various types of tumors with variable penetrance. *p16INK4a* is a family member that has a prominent role in carcinomas of the pancreas and the bladder, glioblastomas, leukemias and melanomas among others. Its expression is lost by several mechanisms including point mutations, small deletion and epigenetic modifications which have been reported in thousands of human cancers (Serrano et al., 1996; Krimpenfort et al., 2001). On the other hand, as previously described, *p15INK4b* is noted to be silenced primarily by an epigenetic mechanism in human cancers, and loss of its expression through hypermethylation of its promoter region is well documented in hematologic neoplasms in particular (Drexler HG, 1998; Roussel, 1999). In these types of cancers, inactivation of *p15INK4b* has been reported in the absence of aberrant modification or deletion of *p16INK4a*. In contrast with p15INK4b and p16INK4a, p18INK4c was originally found to play a more limited role as a human tumor suppressor, and p19INK4d is not thought to be involved in the pathogenesis of cancer (Thullberg et al., 2000). *p18Ink4c*-null mice are viable but display an unusual phenotype with pronounced gigantism, lymphomas and more importantly pituitary hyperplasia (Franklin et al., 1998). Later examination of these mice revealed that p18Ink4c is a haploinsufficient tumor suppressor for spontaneous and carcinogen-induced pituitary tumors and lymphomas (Bai et al., 2003). Loss of p16Ink4a expression was shown to be a necessary event in conjunction with loss of p18Ink4c for the mice to develop aggressive advanced stages of pituitary carcinoma (Morishita et al., 2004). Furthermore, it is now clear that p18INK4c is a tumor suppressor in human glioblastoma multiform and hepatocellular carcinoma (Solomon, 2008a and 2008b). Interestingly, studies in mice deficient for p19Ink4d have not revealed increased susceptibility to any cancer or other proliferative diseases, suggesting a limited or nonexistent role in carcinogenesis (Buchold et al. 2007, Zindy et al, 2000).

Although these cell cycle regulators exhibit overlapping and surely compensatory activities mainly due to their structural similarities (Krimpenfort et al., 2007), their temporal and tissue-restricted expression patterns as well as their differential involvement in the pathogenesis of human cancers clearly suggest that they can harbor specific and distinct functions during development.

3.2 Function as a regulator of cell fate during early myelopoiesis

The strikingly high prevalence of *p15INK4b* loss of expression during the development of myeloid disease in human patients has triggered scientists to explore alternate functions for this CDKI. As a cell cycle regulator, p15INK4b was suggested to be one of the players determining the fine balances in differentiation and proliferation of myeloid cells. To test this hypothesis, the previously described p15Ink4b germline knockout mice as well as murine transplant models were used. Results revealed a novel role for the protein during early and late stages of myeloid cells development (Rosu-Myles et al., 2007, 2008).

Myelopoiesis is the process by which an undifferentiated progenitor cell gives rise to mature differentiated functional myeloid cells. The process takes place in the bone marrow and is driven by a pool of hematopoietic cytokines that have different binding specificities to cell surface markers in a stage and lineage dependent manner. Committed progenitors with a restricted myeloid lineage fate arise from earlier common myeloid progenitor cells (CMP), who themselves originate from hematopoietic stem cells (HSC) (Akashi et al. 2000).

In p15Ink4b knockout mice (p15Ink4b-/-), loss of p15Ink4b was found to favor the differentiation of CMPs into granulocyte macrophage progenitors (GMP) which results in an imbalance between the erythroid and myeloid compartments (Rosu-Myles et al 2007). This defect was in the bipotent differentiation capacity of the CMP, and did not affect the frequency of early long-term HSCs, or their ability to self-renew and proliferate. Therefore, this finding differs from the traditional role of p15Ink4b in regulating the cell cycle. As shown in Figure 3A, the increased number of myeloid progenitors was found to occur at the expense of differentiation of CMPs towards the erythroid progenitors .Furthermore, competitive repopulating assays have shown that the defect is intrinsic to the cells. Loss of p15Ink4b provided a competitive advantage over the wild-type cells within the myeloid compartment (Rosu-Myles et al., 2007).

Interestingly, an earlier study carried out in p18Ink4c-/- mice, had shown that this CDKI also impacts cell fate but targets a different cell type. Deletion of p18Ink4c was found to result in a long-term engraftment advantage in HSCs. The observed effects were not due to increased proliferation capacity of the cells, but rather to an enhanced potential of self-renewal of these cells as opposed to differentiation. This lead to an efficient expansion of HSCs as well as hematopoietic progenitor pools, which fully retained their multi-lineage differentiation potential (Yuan et al., 2004).

3.3 Function in cell cycle arrest in late myeloid cell development

In addition to its hypothesized role in cell fate decision of early myeloid progenitors, p15Ink4b is implicated during the late stages of myelopoiesis. In this case its role appears to be the induction of cell-cycle arrest. p15Ink4b expression has been shown to increase specifically during myeloid differentiation in vivo both in human bone marrow and peripheral blood cells (Teofili et al. 2000); and in vitro, in murine M1 myeloblastic cells which undergo monocytic differentiation following treatment with IL-6 (Schmidt et al 2004).

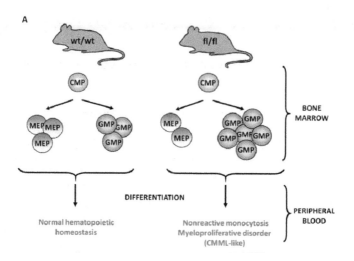

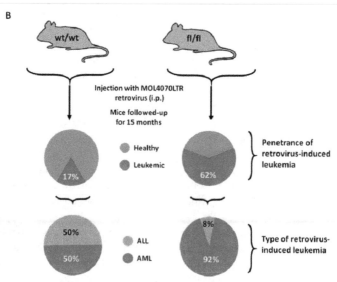

Fig. 3. The loss of p15Ink4b in myeloid lineage results in: A. Imbalance in the myeloid progenitor pools and nonreactive monocytosis; B. Increased incidence of the retrovirus-induced leukemia with preference toward the myeloid phenotype.

The M1 leukemia cell line, does not express p53, proliferates autonomously and is often used as a model for monocytic differentiation. When terminal differentiation is induced in these cells, upregulation of p15Ink4b expression is accompanied by inhibition of Cdk4 kinase activity as well as by a decrease in levels of phosphorylated Rb (Bergh et al., 1999). Furthermore, over-expression of p15Ink4b in M1 cells causes cell cycle arrest in the G1 phase, providing additional evidence for the implication of the protein in maturation and cell cycle inhibition of late stage progenitors (Haviernik et al., 2003). This function is further supported by studies in human CD34+ hematopoietic progenitor cells. When expression of p15INK4b is triggered, higher levels of the protein are associated with transcriptional upregulation of genes known to induce myeloid differentiation, such as the colony stimulating factor 1 receptor gene (c-fms), the myeloperoxidase gene (mpo) and lactoferrin (lf), among others (Furukawa et al 2000). Overexpression of p15INK4b is also linked with a dramatic decrease in early blast progenitor populations and an increase in the numbers of cells that adopt a myeloid morphology (Teofili et al., 2000).

This data suggests that p15INK4b has functions during both the early and late stages of myelopoiesis; in early progenitors, p15Ink4b influences cell fate by altering the balance between myeloid and erythroid progenitors, whereas during late myelopoiesis, p15INK4b appears to be causing withdrawal from the cell-cycle in response to cytokines.

4. Targeting p15INK4b for re-expression in AML and MDS

The reversible nature of epigenetic alterations makes them very attractive therapeutic targets for AML and MDS. In the case of *p15INK4b*, these epigenetic alterations consist of DNA methylation as well as chromatin remodeling by post-transcriptional histone modifications. Studying the association of *p15INK4b* promoter DNA methylation with histone modifications revealed important insight into the interplay of these two types of epigenetic mechanisms (Paul et al., 2010). Histones undergo post-transcriptional modifications that target primarily the N-terminal tail regions, and involve the attachment of phospho, acetyl, methyl, ribosyl, and small ubiquitin-like modifier or ubiquitin groups on the side chains of the different amino acids residues of histone molecules (Biancotto et al., 2010). Acetylation and de-acetylation of lysine residues are catalyzed by two groups of enzymes with opposing actions: histone acetyltransferases (HAT) and histone deacetylases (HDAC) (Jenuwein & Allis, 2001), whereas histone methyltransferases (HMT), and histone demethylases (HDM) control the balance of histone methylations. Similar to DNA methylation, histone modifications are fully biochemically reversible, result in changes in the protein structure and affect the affinity of histone tails to DNA molecules (Varier & Timmers, 2011). Paul et al. (2010) found that in AML cell lines with aberrant *p15INK4b* DNA hypermethylation, the histone 3 trimethylated at lysine 4 (H3K4me3), which is a transcriptional activation mark, was at lower levels than in AML cell lines without hypermethylation. Interestingly, irrespective of the methylation status of *p15INK4b*, this study also reported the presence of the repressive mark H3K27me3 (histone 3 trimethylated at lysine 27) at the 9p21 locus. Human AML blasts with hypermethylation of *p15INK4b* were similarly found to have H3K27me3, but lacked H3K4me3 at the gene.

The tight collaboration of the different epigenetic alterations in silencing the *p15INK4b* gene makes combinatorial therapeutics a promising approach for its reexpression. Importantly, removal of methyl groups from hypermethylated CpG clusters associated with the gene promoter reverses the inhibitory effects and restores normal gene expression (Jones &

Baylin, 2002). The DNMT inhibitor 5-azacytidine (5-aza-C) and its analogue 5-aza-deoxycytidine (5-aza-dC, Decitabine) are powerful hypomethylating agents that are used in the therapy of high-risk MDS and AML. It has been demonstrated that they can lead to the reversal of hypermethylation and subsequent reexpression of the *p15INK4b* gene in patients with MDS (Daskalakis et al., 2002; Farinha et al., 2004; Gore et al., 2006; Santos et al., 2010). It was shown that treatment of patient blasts with hypomethylating agent Decitabine also affects histone modifications. Paul et al. (2010) provided evidence that the levels of H3K4me3 increased with retention of H3K27me3, thus inducing a state of bivalency. The use of other HMT inhibitors such as 3-Deazaneplanocin A (DZNep) have been reported to successfully decrease global DNA methylation levels, but not to induce re-expression of specific genes including *p15INK4b* (Flotho et al., 2009; Miranda et al., 2009).

HDAC inhibitors such as Trichostatin A (TSA) have been used for targeting of histone acetylations. In the case of AML samples with *p15INK4b* hypermethylation, it was shown that TSA treatment alone is insufficient to increase p15INK4b expression levels (Scott et al., 2007; Paul et al., 2010). However, studies that incorporated the use of both HDAC and DNMT inhibitors have proven successful at inducing higher levels of p15INK4b expression (Cameron et al., 1999; Scott et al., 2007; Paul et al., 2010).

5. Conclusion

p15INK4b is a CDK inhibitor whose expression is lost in a very high proportion of patients with MDS and AML. This implicates an important role for the loss of the protein expression in the development of myeloid disease in humans. Its role in myeloid leukemogenesis as a tumor suppressor is now confirmed by research carried out in several mouse models. In addition to its role in inhibiting CDKs to arrest the cell cycle during late myeloid development, it is now known to affect cell fate decisions during early myelopoiesis. In myeloid progenitors, loss of p15Ink4b results in an imbalance in the progenitor pools, and favors the expansion of GMPs at the expense of MEPs. Importantly, when deleted in the cells of the myeloid lineage only, mice develop nonreactive monocytosis and are strongly predisposed to succumb to retrovirus-induced leukemia, especially of myeloid origin. These results validate a tight link between loss of p15INK4b and human myeloid neoplasia. Clinical observations that associate *p15INK4b* demethylation and re-expression with improved prognosis and survival, further stress the importance of this gene in AML and MDS treatment.

6. References

Aggerholm A, Guldberg P, Hokland M & Hokland P (1999). Extensive intra- and inter-individual heterogeneity of p15INK4B methylation in acute myeloid leukemia. *Cancer Research,* Vol.59, No.2, (January 2009), pp. 436-441, ISSN 0008-5472

Aggerholm A, Holm MS, Guldberg P, Olesen LH & Hokland P (2006). Promoter hypermethylation of p15INK4B, HIC1, CDH1, and ER is frequent in myelodysplastic syndrome and predicts poor prognosis in early-stage patients. *European Journal of Hematology,* Vol.76, No.1, (January 2006), pp. 23-32, ISSN 0902-4441

Agrawal S, Unterberg M, Koschmieder S, zur Stadt U, Verbeek W, Büchner T, Berdel WE, Serve H & Müller-Tidow C (2007). DNA methylation of tumor suppressor genes in clinical remission predicts the relapse risk in acute myeloid leukemia. *Cancer Research*, Vol.67, No.3, (February 2007), pp. 1370-1377, ISSN 0008-5472

Akashi K, Traver D, Miyamoto T & Weissman IL (2000). A clonogenic common myeloid progenitor that gives rise to all myeloid lineages. *Nature*, Vol.404, No.6774, (March 2000), pp. 193-197, ISSN 0028-0836

Aoki E, Uchida T, Ohashi H, Nagai H, Murase T, Ichikawa A, Yamao K, Hotta T, Kinoshita T, Saito H & Murate T(2000). Methylation status of the p15INK4B gene in hematopoietic progenitors and peripheral blood cells in myelodysplastic syndromes. *Leukemia*, Vol.14, No.4, pp. 586-593, ISSN 0887-6924

Bai F, Pei XH, Godfrey VL & Xiong Y. (2003) Haploinsufficiency of p18(INK4c) sensitizes mice to carcinogen-induced tumorigenesis. *Molecular and Cellular Biology*, Vol.23, No.4, (February 2003), pp. 1269–1277, ISSN 0270-7306

Bennett JM, Catovsky D, Daniel MT, Flandrin G, Galton DA, Gralnick HR & Sultan C (1976). Proposals for the classification of the acute leukaemias, French-American-British (FAB) co-operative group. *British Journal of Haematology* Vol.33, No.4, (August 1976), pp. 451-458, ISSN 0007-1048

Bennett JM, Catovsky D, Daniel MT, Flandrin G, Galton DA, Gralnick HR & Sultan C (1982). Proposals for the classification of the myelodysplastic syndromes. *British Journal of Haematology*, Vol.51, No.2, (June 1982), pp. 189-199, ISSN 0007-1048

Bennett JM, Catovsky D, Daniel MT, Flandrin G, Galton DA, Gralnick HR & Sultan C (1985). Proposed revised criteria for the classification of acute myeloid leukemia. A report of the French-American-British Cooperative Group. *Annals of Internal Medicine*, Vol. 103, No.4, (October 1985), pp. 620-625, ISSN 0003-4819

Bergh G, Ehinger M, Olsson I, Jacobsen SE & Gullberg U (1999). Involvement of the retinoblastoma protein in monocytic and neutrophilic lineage commitment of human bone marrow progenitor cells. *Blood*, Vol.94, No.6, (September 1999), pp. 1971-1978, ISSN 0006-4971

Biancotto C, Frigè G & Minucci S (2010). Histone modification therapy of cancer. *Advances in Genetics*, Vol.70, pp. 341-386, ISSN 0065-2660

Bies J, Sramko M, Fares J, Rosu-Myles M, Zhang S, Koller R & Wolff L (2010). Myeloid-specific inactivation of p15Ink4b results in monocytosis and predisposition to myeloid leukemia. *Blood*, Vol.116, No.6, (August 2010), pp. 979-987, ISSN 0006-4971

Bird A (2002). DNA methylation patterns and epigenetic memory. *Genes and Development*, Vol.16, No.1, (January 2002), pp. 6-21, ISSN 0890-9369

Brotherton DH, Dhanaraj V, Wick S, Brizuela L, Domaille PJ, Volyanik E, Xu X, Parisini E, Smith BO, Archer SJ, Serrano M, Brenner SL, Blundell TL & Laue ED (1998). Crystal structure of the complex of the cyclin D-dependent kinase Cdk6 bound to the cell cycle inhibitor p19INK4d. *Nature*, Vol.395, No.6699, (September 1998), pp. 244–250, ISSN 0028-0836

Buchold GM, Magyar PL & O'Brien DA (2007). Mice lacking cyclin-dependent kinase inhibitor p19Ink4d show strain-specific effects on male reproduction. *Molecular Reproduction and Development*, Vol.74, No.8, (August 2007), pp. 1008-1020, ISSN 1040-452X

Cameron EE, Baylin SB & Herman JG (1999). p15(INK4B) CpG island methylation in primary acute leukemia is heterogeneous and suggests density as a critical factor for transcriptional silencing. *Blood*, Vol.94, No.7, (October 1999), pp. 2445-2451, ISSN 0006-4971

Cánepa ET, Scassa ME, Ceruti JM, Marazita MC, Carcagno AL, Sirkin PF & Ogara MF (2007). INK4 proteins, a family of mammalian CDK inhibitors with novel biological functions. *IUBMB Life*, Vol.59, No.7, (July 2007), pp. 419-426, ISSN 1521-6543

Chim CS, Liang R, Tam CY & Kwong YL (2001). Methylation of p15 and p16 genes in acute promyelocytic leukemia: potential diagnostic and prognostic significance. *Journal of Clinical Oncology*, Vol.19, No.7, (April 2001), pp. 2033-2040, ISSN 0732-183X

Chim CS, Tam CY, Liang R & Kwong YL (2001). Methylation of p15 and p16 genes in adult acute leukemia: lack of prognostic significance. *Cancer*, Vol.91, No.12, (June 2001), pp. 2222-2229, ISSN 0008-543X

Chim CS & Kwong YL (2006). Adverse prognostic impact of CDKN2B hyper-methylation in acute promyelocytic leukemia. *Leukemia and Lymphoma*, Vol.47, No.5, (May 2006), pp. 815-825, ISSN 1042-8194

Christiansen DH, Andersen MK & Pedersen-Bjergaard J (2003). Methylation of p15INK4B is common, is associated with deletion of genes on chromosome arm 7q and predicts a poor prognosis in therapy-related myelodysplasia and acute myeloid leukemia. *Leukemia*, Vol.17, No.9, (September 2003), pp. 1813-1819, ISSN 0887-6924

Clausen BE, Burkhardt C, Reith W, Renkawitz R & Forster I (1999). Conditional gene targeting in macrophages and granulocytes using LysMcre mice. *Transgenic Research*, Vol.8, No.4, (August 1999), pp. 265-277, ISSN 0962-8819

Daskalakis M, Nguyen TT, Nguyen C, Guldberg P, Köhler G, Wijermans P, Jones PA & Lübbert M (2002). Demethylation of a hypermethylated P15/INK4B gene in patients with myelodysplastic syndrome by 5-Aza-2'-deoxycytidine (decitabine) treatment. *Blood*, Vol.100, No.8, (October 2002), pp. 2957-2964. ISSN 0006-4971

Deaton AM & Bird A (2011). CpG islands and the regulation of transcription. *Genes and Development*, Vol.25, No.10, (May 2011), pp. 1010-1022, ISSN 0890-9369

Deneberg S, Grövdal M, Karimi M, Jansson M, Nahi H, Corbacioglu A, Gaidzik V, Döhner K, Paul C, Ekström TJ, Hellström-Lindberg E & Lehmann S (2010). Gene-specific and global methylation patterns predict outcome in patients with acute myeloid leukemia. *Leukemia*, Vol.24, No.5, (May 2010), pp. 932-941, ISSN 0887-6924

Drexler HG (1998). Review of alterations of the cyclin-dependent kinase inhibitor INK4 family genes p15, p16, p18 and p19 in human leukemia-lymphoma cells. *Leukemia*, Vol.12, No.6, (June 1998), pp. 845-859, ISSN 0887-6924

Farinha NJ, Shaker S, Lemaire M, Momparler L, Bernstein M & Momparler RL (2004). Activation of expression of p15, p73 and E-cadherin in leukemic cells by different concentrations of 5-aza-2'-deoxycytidine (Decitabine). *Anticancer Research*, Vol.24, No.1, (January 2004), pp. 75-78, ISSN 0250-7005

Flotho C, Claus R, Batz C, Schneider M, Sandrock I, Ihde S, Plass C, Niemeyer CM & Lübbert M (2009). The DNA methyltransferase inhibitors azacitidine, decitabine and zebularine exert differential effects on cancer gene expression in acute myeloid leukemia cells. *Leukemia*, Vol.23, No.6, (June 2009), pp. 1019-1028, ISSN 0887-6924

Franklin, D.S., Godfrey, V.L., Lee, H., Kovalev, G.I., Schoonhoven, R., Chen-Kiang, S., Su, L. & Xiong, Y (1998). CDK inhibitors p18(INK4c) and p27(Kip1) mediate two separate pathways to collaboratively suppress pituitary tumorigenesis. *Genes and Development*, Vol.12, No.18, (September 1998), pp. 2899–2911, ISSN 0890-9369

Furukawa Y, Kikuchi J, Nakamura M, Iwase S, Yamada H & Matsuda M (2000) Lineage-specific regulation of cell cycle control gene expression during haematopoietic cell differentiation. *British Journal of Haematology*, Vol.110, No.3, (September 2000), pp. 663-673, ISSN 0007-1048

Galm O, Wilop S, Lüders C, Jost E, Gehbauer G, Herman JG & Osieka R (2005). Clinical implications of aberrant DNA methylation patterns in acute myelogenous leukemia. *Annals of Hematology*, Vol.84, No.1, (December 2005), pp. 39-46, ISSN 0939-5555

Garcia-Manero G (2003). Prognostic implications of epigenetic silencing of p15INK4B in acute promyelocytic leukemia. *Leukemia*, Vol.17, No.5, (May 2003), pp. 839-840, ISSN 0887-6924

Gore SD, Baylin S, Sugar E, Carraway H, Miller CB, Carducci M, Grever M, Galm O, Dauses T, Karp JE, Rudek MA, Zhao M, Smith BD, Manning J, Jiemjit A, Dover G, Mays A, Zwiebel J, Murgo A, Weng LJ & Herman JG (2006). Combined DNA methyltransferase and histone deacetylase inhibition in the treatment of myeloid neoplasms. *Cancer Research*, Vol.66, No.12, (June 2006), pp. 6361-6369, ISSN 0008-5472

Guo SX, Taki T, Ohnishi H, Piao HY, Tabuchi K, Bessho F, Hanada R, Yanagisawa M & Hayashi Y (2000). Hypermethylation of p16 and p15 genes and RB protein expression in acute leukemia. *Leukemia Research*, Vol.24, No.1, (January 2000), pp. 39-46, ISSN 0145-2126

Graf Einsiedel H, Taube T, Hartmann R, Wellmann S, Seifert G, Henze G & Seeger K. (2002). Deletion analysis of p16(INKa) and p15(INKb) in relapsed childhood acute lymphoblastic leukemia. *Blood*, Vol.99, No.12 (June 2002), pp. 4629-4631, ISSN 0006-4971

Grövdal M, Khan R, Aggerholm A, Antunovic P, Astermark J, Bernell P, Engström LM, Kjeldsen L, Linder O, Nilsson L, Olsson A, Wallvik J, Tangen JM, Oberg G, Jacobsen SE, Hokland P, Porwit A & Hellström-Lindberg E (2007). Negative effect of DNA hypermethylation on the outcome of intensive chemotherapy in older patients with high-risk myelodysplastic syndromes and acute myeloid leukemia following myelodysplastic syndrome. *Clinical Cancer Research*, Vol.13, No.23, (December 2007), pp. 7107-7112, ISSN 1078-0432

Haase D, Germing U, Schanz J, Pfeilstöcker M, Nösslinger T, Hildebrandt B, Kundgen A, Lübbert M, Kunzmann R, Giagounidis AA, Aul C, Trümper L, Krieger O, Stauder R, Müller TH, Wimazal F, Valent P, Fonatsch C & Steidl C (2007). New insights into the prognostic impact of the karyotype in MDS and correlation with subtypes: evidence from a core dataset of 2124 patients. *Blood*, Vol.110, No.13, (December 2007), pp. 4385-4395, ISSN 0006-4971

Hannon GJ & Beach D (1994). p15INK4B is a potential effector of TGF-beta-induced cell cycle arrest. *Nature*, Vol.371, No.6494, (September 1994), pp. 257-261, ISSN 0028-0836

Harris NL, Jaffe ES, Diebold J, Flandrin G, Muller-Hermelink HK, Vardiman J, Lister TA & Bloomfield CD (1999). World Health Organization classification of neoplastic diseases of the hematopoietic and lymphoid tissues: report of the Clinical Advisory Committee meeting-Airlie House, Virginia, November 1997. *Journal of Clinical Oncology*, Vol.17, No.12, (December 1999), pp. 3835-3849, ISSN 0732-183X

Harris NL, Jaffe ES, Diebold J, Flandrin G, Muller-Hermelink HK, Vardiman J, Lister TA & Bloomfield CD (2000). The World Health Organization classification of hematological malignancies report of the Clinical Advisory Committee Meeting, Airlie House, Virginia, November 1997. *Modern Pathology*, Vol.13, No.2, (February 2000), pp.193-207, ISSN 0893-3952

Hasegawa D, Manabe A, Kubota T, Kawasaki H, Hirose I, Ohtsuka Y, Tsuruta T, Ebihara Y, Goto Y, Zhao XY, Sakashita K, Koike K, Isomura M, Kojima S, Hoshika A, Tsuji K & Nakahata T (2005). Methylation status of the p15 and p16 genes in paediatric myelodysplastic syndrome and juvenile myelomonocytic leukaemia. *British Journal of Haematology*, Vol.128, No.6, (March 2005), pp.805-812, ISSN 0007-1048

Haviernik P, Schmidt M, Hu X & Wolff L (2003).Consistent inactivation of p19(Arf) but not p15(Ink4b) in murine myeloid cells transformed in vivo by deregulated c-Myc. *Oncogene*, Vol.22, No.11, (March 2003), pp. 1600-1610, ISSN 0950-9232

Herman JG, Jen J, Merlo A & Baylin SB (1996). Hypermethylation-associated inactivation indicates a tumor suppressor role for p15INK4B. *Cancer Research*, Vol.56, No.4, (February 1996), pp. 722-727, ISSN 0008-5472

Herman JG, Civin CI, Issa JP, Collector MI, Sharkis SJ & Baylin SB (1997). Distinct patterns of inactivation of p15INK4B and p16INK4A characterize the major types of hematological malignancies. *Cancer Research*, Vol.57, No.5, (March 1997), pp. 837-841, ISSN 0008-5472

Hoshino K, Asou N, Okubo T, Suzushima H, Kiyokawa T, Kawano F & Mitsuya H (2002). The absence of the p15INK4B gene alterations in adult patients with precursor B-cell acute lymphoblastic leukaemia is a favourable prognostic factor. *British Journal of Haematology*, Vol.117, No.3, (June 2002), pp. 531-540, ISSN 0007-1048

Jeffrey PD, Tong L & Pavletich NP (2000). Structural basis of inhibition of CDK-cyclin complexes by INK4 inhibitors. *Genes and Development*, Vol.14, No.24, (December 2000), pp. 3115-3125, ISSN 0890-9369

Jenuwein T & Allis CD (2001). Translating the histone code. *Science*, Vol.293, No.5532, (August 2001), pp. 1074-1080, ISSN 0036-8075

Jiang Y, Dunbar A, Gondek LP, Mohan S, Rataul M, O'Keefe C, Sekeres M, Saunthararajah Y & Maciejewski JP (2009). Aberrant DNA methylation is a dominant mechanism in MDS progression to AML. *Blood*, Vol.113, No.6, (February 2009), pp.1315-1325, ISSN 0006-4971

Jones PA & Baylin SB. (2002). The fundamental role of epigenetic events in cancer. *Nature Reviews Genetics*, Vol.3, No.6, (June 2002), pp. 415-428 ISSN 1471-0056

Kim M, Yim SH, Cho NS, Kang SH, Ko DH, Oh B, Kim TY, Min HJ, She CJ, Kang HJ, Shin HY, Ahn HS, Yoon SS, Kim BK, Shin HR, Han KS, Cho HI & Lee DS (2009). Homozygous deletion of CDKN2A (p16, p14) and CDKN2B (p15) genes is a poor prognostic factor in adult but not in childhood B-lineage acute lymphoblastic leukemia: a comparative deletion and hypermethylation study. *Cancer Genetics and Cytogenetics*, Vol.195, No.1, (November 2009), pp. 59-65, ISSN 0165-4608

Korenjak M & Brehm A (2005). E2F-Rb complexes regulating transcription of genes important for differentiation and development. *Current Opinion in Genetics and Development*, Vol.15, No.5, (October 2005), pp. 520-527, ISSN 0959-437X

Krimpenfort P, Quon KC, Mooi WJ, Loonstra A & Berns A (2001). Loss of p16INK4A confers susceptibility to metastatic melanoma in mice. *Nature*, Vol.413, No.6851, (September 2001), pp. 83-86, ISSN 0028-0836

Krimpenfort P, Ijpenberg A, Song JY, van der Valk M, Nawijn M, Zevenhoven J & Berns A (2007). p15Ink4b is a critical tumor suppressor in the absence of p16INK4A. *Nature*, Vol.448, No.7156, (August 2007), pp.943-946, ISSN 0028-0836

Latres E, Malumbres M, Sotillo R, Martín J, Ortega S, Martín-Caballero J, Flores JM, Cordón-Cardo C & Barbacid M (2000). Limited overlapping roles of p15(INK4b) and p18(INK4c) cell cycle inhibitors in proliferation and tumorigenesis. *EMBO Journal*, Vol.19, No.13, (July 2000), pp. 3496-3506, ISSN 0261-4189

Li J, Byeon IJ, Ericson K, Poi MJ, O'Maille P, Selby T & Tsai MD (1999). Tumor suppressor INK4: determination of the solution structure of p18INK4c and demonstration of the functional significance of loops in p18INK4c and p16INK4A. *Biochemistry*, Vol.38, No.10, (March 1999), pp.2930-2940, ISSN 0006-2960

Malumbres M, Pérez De Castro I, Hernández MI, Jiménez M, Corral T & Pellicer A (2000). Cellular response to oncogenic ras involves induction of the Cdk4 and Cdk6 inhibitor p15(INK4b). *Molecular and Cellular Biology*, Vol.20, No.8, (April 2000), pp. 2915-2925, ISSN 0270-7306

Markus J, Garin MT, Bies J, Galili N, Raza A, Thirman MJ, Le Beau MM, Rowley JD, Liu PP & Wolff L (2007). Methylation-independent silencing of the tumor suppressor INK4b (p15) by CBFbeta-SMMHC in acute myelogenous leukemia with inv(16). *Cancer Research*, Vol.67, No.3, (February 2007), pp. 992-1000, ISSN 0008-5472

Matsuno N, Hoshino K, Nanri T, Kawakita T, Suzushima H, Kawano F, Mitsuya H & Asou N (2005). p15 mRNA expression detected by real-time quantitative reverse transcriptase-polymerase chain reaction correlates with the methylation density of the gene in adult acute leukemia. *Leukemia Research*, Vol.29, No.5, (May 2005), pp. 557-564, ISSN 0145-2126

Mirebeau D, Acquaviva C, Suciu S, Bertin R, Dastugue N, Robert A, Boutard P, Méchinaud F, Plouvier E, Otten J, Vilmer E & Cavé H (2006). The prognostic significance of CDKN2A, CDKN2B and MTAP inactivation in B-lineage acute lymphoblastic leukemia of childhood. Results of the EORTC studies 58881 and 58951. *Haematologica*, Vol.91, No.7, (July 2006), pp. 881-885, ISSN 0390-6078

Miranda TB, Cortez CC, Yoo CB, Liang G, Abe M, Kelly TK, Marquez VE & Jones PA (2009). DZNep is a global histone methylation inhibitor that reactivates developmental genes not silenced by DNA methylation. *Molecular Cancer Therapeutics*, Vol.8, No.6, (June 2009), pp. 1579-1588, ISSN 1535-7163

Morishita A, Masaki T, Yoshiji H, Nakai S, Ogi T, Miyauchi Y, Yoshida S, Funaki T, Uchida N, Kita Y, Funakoshi F, Usuki H, Okada S, Izuishi K, Watanabe S, Kurokohchi K & Kuriyama S (2004). Reduced expression of cell cycle regulator p18(INK4C) in human hepatocellular carcinoma. *Hepatology*, Vol.40, No.3, (September 2004), pp. 677-686, ISSN 0270-9139

Nobori T, Miura K, Wu DJ, Lois A, Takabayashi K & Carson DA (1994). Deletions of the cyclin-dependent kinase-4 inhibitor gene in multiple human cancers. *Nature*, Vol.368, No.6473, (April 1994), pp. 753-756, ISSN 0028-0836

Noh SJ, Li Y, Xiong Y & Guan KL (1999). Identification of functional elements of p18INK4C essential for binding and inhibition of cyclin-dependent kinase (CDK) 4 and CDK6. *Cancer Research*, Vol.59, No.3, (February 1999), pp. 558-564, ISSN 0008-5472

Olk-Batz C, Poetsch AR, Nöllke P, Claus R, Zucknick M, Sandrock I, Witte T, Strahm B, Hasle H, Zecca M, Stary J, Bergstraesser E, De Moerloose B, Trebo M, van den Heuvel-Eibrink MM, Wojcik D, Locatelli F, Plass C, Niemeyer CM, Flotho C & the European Working Group of Myelodysplastic Syndromes in Childhood (EWOG-MDS) (2011). Aberrant DNA methylation characterizes juvenile myelomonocytic leukemia with poor outcome. *Blood*, Vol.117, No.18, (May 2011), pp. 4871-4880, ISSN 0006-4971

Ozenne P, Eymin B, Brambilla E & Gazzeri S (2010). The ARF tumor suppressor: structure, functions and status in cancer. *International Journal of Cancer*, Vol.127, No.10, (November 2010), pp. 2239-2947, ISSN 0020-7136

Paul TA, Bies J, Small D & Wolff L (2010). Signatures of polycomb repression and reduced H3K4 trimethylation are associated with p15INK4b DNA methylation in AML. *Blood*, Vol.115, No.15, (April 2010), pp. 3098-3108, ISSN 0006-4971

Quesnel B, Guillerm G, Vereecque R, Wattel E, Preudhomme C, Bauters F, Vanrumbeke M & Fenaux P (1998) Methylation of the p15(INK4b) gene in myelodysplastic syndromes is frequent and acquired during disease progression. *Blood*, Vol.91, No.8, (April 1998), pp. 2985–2990, ISSN 0006-4971

Raj K, John A, Ho A, Chronis C, Khan S, Samuel J, Pomplun S, Thomas NS & Mufti GJ (2007). CDKN2B methylation status and isolated chromosome 7 abnormalities predict responses to treatment with 5-azacytidine. *Leukemia*, Vol.21, No.9, (September 2007), pp. 1937-1944, ISSN 0887-6924

Rodrigues EF, Santos-Rebouças CB, Gonçalves Pimentel MM, Mencalha AL, Dobbin J, Da Costa ES, Fernandez Cde S, Bouzas LF, Abdelhay E & De Souza Fernandez T (2010). Epigenetic alterations of p15(INK4B) and p16(INK4A) genes in pediatric primary myelodysplastic syndrome. *Leukemia and Lymphoma*, Vol.51, No.10, (October 2010), pp. 1887-1894, ISSN 1042-8194

Rosu-Myles M, Taylor BJ & Wolff L (2007). Loss of the tumor suppressor p15Ink4b enhances myeloid progenitor formation from common myeloid progenitors. *Experimental Hematology*, Vol.35, No.3, (March 2007), pp. 394-406, ISSN 0301-472X

Rosu-Myles M & Wolff L (2008). p15Ink4b: dual function in myelopoiesis and inactivation in myeloid disease. *Blood Cells, Molecules and Diseases*, Vol.40, No.3, (May 2008), pp. 406-409, ISSN 1079-9796

Roussel, M.F (1999). The INK4 family of cell cycle inhibitors in cancer. *Oncogene*, Vol.18, No.38, (September 1999), pp. 5311–5317, ISSN 0950-9232

Ruas M & Peters G. (1998). The p16INK4A/CDKN2A tumor suppressor and its relatives. *Biochimica et Biophysica Acta (BBA) - Reviews on Cancer*, Vol.1378, No.2, (October 1998), pp. 115-77, ISSN 0304-419X

Russo AA, Tong L, Lee JO, Jeffrey PD & Pavletich NP (1998). Structural basis for inhibition of the cyclin-dependent kinase Cdk6 by the tumour suppressor p16INK4A. *Nature,* Vol.395, No.6699, (September 1998), pp. 237-243, ISSN 0028-0836

Sandhu C, Garbe J, Bhattacharya N, Daksis J, Pan CH, Yaswen P, Koh J, Slingerland JM & Stampfer MR (1997).Transforming growth factor beta stabilizes p15INK4B protein, increases p15INK4B-cdk4 complexes, and inhibits cyclin D1-cdk4 association in human mammary epithelial cells. *Molecular and Cellular Biology,* Vol.17, No.5, (May 1997), pp. 2458-2467, ISSN 0270-7306

Santos FP, Kantarjian H, Garcia-Manero G, Issa JP & Ravandi F (2010).Decitabine in the treatment of myelodysplastic syndromes. *Expert Review of Anticancer Therapy,* Vol.10, No.1, (January 2010), pp. 9-22, ISSN 1473-7140

Schmidt M, Bies J, Tamura T, Ozato K & Wolff L (2004). The interferon regulatory factor ICSBP/IRF-8 in combination with PU.1 up-regulates expression of tumor suppressor p15(Ink4b) in murine myeloid cells. *Blood,* Vol.103, No.11, (June 2004), pp. 4142-4149, ISSN 0006-4971

Schwaller J, Pabst T, Koeffler HP, Niklaus G, Loetscher P, Fey MF & Tobler A (1997). Expression and regulation of G1 cell-cycle inhibitors (p16INK4A, p15INK4B, p18INK4C, p19INK4D) in human acute myeloid leukemia and normal myeloid cells. *Leukemia,* Vol.11, No.1, (January 1997), pp. 54-63, ISSN 0887-6924

Scott SA, Lakshimikuttysamma A, Sheridan DP, Sanche SE, Geyer CR & DeCoteau JF (2007). Zebularine inhibits human acute myeloid leukemia cell growth in vitro in association with p15INK4B demethylation and reexpression. *Experimental Hematology,* Vol.35, No.2, (February 2007), pp. 263-273, ISSN 0301-472X

Serrano, M., Lee, H., Chin, L., Cordon-Cardo, C., Beach, D. & DePinho, R.A (1996). Role of the INK4A locus in tumor suppression and cell mortality. *Cell,* Vol.85, No.1, (April 1996), pp. 27–37, ISSN 0092-8674

Shen L, Kantarjian H, Guo Y, Lin E, Shan J, Huang X, Berry D, Ahmed S, Zhu W, Pierce S, Kondo Y, Oki Y, Jelinek J, Saba H, Estey E & Issa JP (2009). DNA methylation predicts survival and response to therapy in patients with myelodysplastic syndromes. *Journal of Clinical Oncology,* Vol.28, No.4, (February 2009), pp. 605-613, ISSN 0732-183X

Sherr CJ & Roberts JM. (1999). CDK inhibitors: positive and negative regulators of G1-phase progression. *Genes and Development,* Vol.13, No.12, (June 1999), pp. 1501-1512, ISSN 0890-9369

Sherr CJ (2006). Divorcing ARF and p53: an unsettled case. *Nature Reviews Cancer,* Vol.6, No.9, (September 2006), pp. 663-673, ISSN 1474-175X

Shimamoto T, Ohyashiki JH & Ohyashiki K (2005). Methylation of p15(INK4b) and E-cadherin genes is independently correlated with poor prognosis in acute myeloid leukemia. *Leukemia Research,* Vol.29, No.6, (June 2005), pp. 653-659, ISSN 0145-2126

Solomon DA, Kim JS, Jean W & Waldman T (2008). Conspirators in a capital crime: co-deletion of p18INK4c and p16INK4A/p14ARF/p15INK4b in glioblastoma multiforme. *Cancer Research,* Vol.68, No.21, (November 2008), pp. 8657-8560, ISSN 0008-5472

Solomon DA, Kim JS, Jenkins S, Ressom H, Huang M, Coppa N, Mabanta L, Bigner D, Yan H, Jean W & Waldman T. (2008). Identification of p18 INK4c as a tumor suppressor gene in glioblastoma multiforme. *Cancer Research*, Vol.68, No.8, (April 2008), pp. 2564-2569, ISSN 0008-5472

Takeuchi S, Matsushita M, Zimmermann M, Ikezoe T, Komatsu N, Seriu T, Schrappe M, Bartram CR & Koeffler HP (2011). Clinical significance of aberrant DNA methylation in childhood acute lymphoblastic leukemia. *Leukemia Research*, n.d. ISSN 0145-2126

Teofili L, Rutella S, Chiusolo P, La Barbera EO, Rumi C, Ranelletti FO, Maggiano N, Leone G & Larocca LM (1998). Expression of p15INK4B in normal hematopoiesis. *Experimental Hematology*, Vol.26, No.12, (November 1998), pp. 1133-1139, ISSN 0301-472X

Teofili L, Morosetti R, Martini M, Urbano R, Putzulu R, Rutella S, Pierelli L, Leone G & Larocca LM (2000). Expression of cyclin-dependent kinase inhibitor p15INK4B during normal and leukemic myeloid differentiation. *Experimental Hematology*, Vol.28, No.5, (May 2000), pp. 519-526, ISSN 0301-472X

Teofili L, Martini M, Di Mario A, Rutella S, Urbano R, Luongo M, Leone G & Larocca LM (2001). Expression of p15(ink4b) gene during megakaryocytic differentiation of normal and myelodysplastic hematopoietic progenitors. *Blood*, Vol.98, No.2, (July 2001), pp. 495-497, ISSN 0006-4971

Teofili L, Martini M, Luongo M, Diverio D, Capelli G, Breccia M, Lo Coco F, Leone G & Larocca LM (2003). Hypermethylation of GpG islands in the promoter region of p15(INK4b) in acute promyelocytic leukemia represses p15(INK4b) expression and correlates with poor prognosis. *Leukemia*, Vol.17, No.5, (May 2003), pp. 919–924, ISSN 0887-6924

Tessema M, Länger F, Dingemann J, Ganser A, Kreipe H & Lehmann U (2003). Aberrant methylation and impaired expression of the p15(INK4b) cell cycle regulatory gene in chronic myelomonocytic leukemia (CMML). *Leukemia*, Vol.17, No.5, (May 2003), pp. 910-918, ISSN 0887-6924

Thullberg M, Bartkova J, Khan S, Hansen K, Rönnstrand L, Lukas J, Strauss M & Bartek J (2000). Distinct versus redundant properties among members of the INK4 family of cyclin-dependent kinase inhibitors. *FEBS Letters*, Vol.470, No.2, (March 2000), pp. 161-166, ISSN 0014-5793

Tien HF, Tang JH, Tsay W, Liu MC, Lee FY, Wang CH, Chen YC & Shen MC (2001). Methylation of the p15(INK4B) gene in myelodysplastic syndrome: It can be detected early at diagnosis or during disease progression and is highly associated with leukaemic transformation. *British Journal of Hematology*, Vol.112, No.1, (January 2001), pp. 148–154, ISSN 0007-1048

Tran HT, Kim HN, Lee IK, Kim YK, Ahn JS, Yang DH, Lee JJ & Kim HJ (2011). DNA methylation changes following 5-azacitidine treatment in patients with myelodysplastic syndrome. *Journal of Korean Medical Science*, Vol.26, No.2, (February 2011), pp. 207-213, ISSN 1011-8934

Trost D, Hildebrandt B, Beier M, Müller N, Germing U & Royer-Pokora B (2006). Molecular cytogenetic profiling of complex karyotypes in primary myelodysplastic syndromes and acute myeloid leukemia. *Cancer Genetics and Cytogenetics*, Vol.165, No.1, (February 2006), pp. 51-63, ISSN 0165-4608

Tsellou E, Troungos C, Moschovi M, Athanasiadou-Piperopoulou F, Polychronopoulou S, Kosmidis H, Kalmanti M, Hatzakis A, Dessypris N, Kalofoutis A & Petridou E (2005). Hypermethylation of CpG islands in the promoter region of the p15INK4B gene in childhood acute leukaemia. *European Journal of Cancer*, Vol.41, No.4, (March 2005), pp. 584-589, ISSN 0959-8049

Uchida T, Kinoshita T, Nagai H, Nakahara Y, Saito H, Hotta T & Murate T (1997). Hypermethylation of the p15INK4B gene in myelodysplastic syndromes. *Blood*, Vol.90, No.4, (August 1997), pp. 1403-1409, ISSN 0006-4971

Valencia A, Cervera J, Such E, Ibañez M, Gómez I, Luna I, Senent L, Oltra S, Sanz MA & Sanz GF (2011). Aberrant methylation of tumor suppressor genes in patients with refractory anemia with ring sideroblasts. *Leukemia Research*, Vol.35, No.4, (April 2011), pp. 479-483, ISSN 0145-2126

Van Zutven LJ, van Drunen E, de Bont JM, Wattel MM, Den Boer ML, Pieters R, Hagemeijer A, Slater RM & Beverloo HB (2005). CDKN2 deletions have no prognostic value in childhood precursor-B acute lymphoblastic leukaemia. *Leukemia*, Vol.19, No.7, (July 2005), pp. 1281-1284, ISSN 0887-6924

Vardiman JW, Harris NL & Brunning RD (2002). The World Health Organization (WHO) classification of the myeloid neoplasms. *Blood*, Vol.100, No.7, (October 2002), pp. 2292-2302, ISSN 0006-4971

Varier RA & Timmers HT (2011). Histone lysine methylation and demethylation pathways in cancer. *Biochimica et Biophysica Acta (BBA) - Reviews on Cancer*, Vol.1815, No.1, (January 2011), pp. 75-89, ISSN 0304-419X

Wolff L, Garin MT, Koller R, Bies J, Liao W, Malumbres M, Tessarollo L, Powell D & Perella C (2003) Hypermethylation of the Ink4b locus in murine myeloid leukemia and increased susceptibility to leukemia in p15(Ink4b)-deficient mice. *Oncogene*, Vol.22, No.58, (December 2003), pp. 9265-9274, ISSN 0950-9232

Wolff L, Koller R, Hu X & Anver MR (2003). A Moloney murine leukemia virus-based retrovirus with 4070A long terminal repeat sequences induces a high incidence of myeloid as well as lymphoid neoplasms. *Journal of Virology*, Vol.7, No.8, (April 2003), pp. 4965-4971, ISSN 0022-538X

Wolff L, Garin MT, Koller R, Bies J, Tessarollo L, Anver MR, Powell D & Perella C (2004) A novel retrovirus provides the cooperating oncogenic event(s) required to demonstrate the tumor suppressor activity of p15Ink4b in myeloid cells in vivo. *Blood Cells, Molecules and Diseases*, Vol.32, No.1, (January 2004), pp. 226-231, ISSN 1079-9796

Wong IH, Ng MH, Huang DP & Lee JC (2000). Aberrant p15 promoter methylation in adult and childhood acute leukemias of nearly all morphologic subtypes: potential prognostic implications. *Blood*, Vol.95, No.6, (March 2000), pp. 1942–1949, ISSN 0006-4971

Yuan C, Selby TL, Li J, Byeon IJ & Tsai MD (2000). Tumor suppressor INK4: refinement of p16INK4A structure and determination of p15INK4b structure by comparative modeling and NMR data. *Protein Science*, Vol.9, No.6, (June 2000), pp. 1120-1128, ISSN 0961-8368

Yuan Y, Shen H, Franklin DS, Scadden DT & Cheng T (2004). In vivo self-renewing divisions of haematopoietic stem cells are increased in the absence of the early G1-phase inhibitor, p18INK4C. *Nature Cell Biology*, Vol.6, No.5, (May 2004), pp. 436-442, ISSN 1465-7392

Zindy F, Quelle DE, Roussel MF & Sherr CJ (1997). Expression of the p16INK4A tumor suppressor versus other INK4 family members during mouse development and aging. *Oncogene*, Vol.15, No.2, (July 1997) pp. 203-211, ISSN 0950-9232

Zindy F., van Deursen J., Grosveld G., Sherr C.J. & Roussel M.F (2000). INK4d-deficient mice are fertile despite testicular atrophy. *Molecular and Cellular Biology*, Vol.20, No.1, (January 2000), pp. 372–378, ISSN 0270-7306

3

Analysis of Leukemogenic Gene Products in Hematopoietic Progenitor Cells

Julia Schanda[1], Reinhard Henschler[2],
Manuel Grez[1] and Christian Wichmann[1]
[1]Georg-Speyer-Haus, Institute for Biomedical Research, Frankfurt am Main
[2]Institute of Transfusion Medicine, German Red Cross Blood Center, Frankfurt am Main
Germany

1. Introduction

One major limitation in the development of effective and targeted cancer therapies is the incomplete understanding of the molecular mechanisms driving malignant cell growth and the resistance of residual 'cancer stem cells' to standard therapies, such as chemotherapy and radiation. Consequently, numerous attempts have been made to elucidate the molecular circuits initiating and perpetuating malignant cell transformation.

Among the different cancer entities, leukemias harbor only a few mutations and therefore represent a good model system for the study of oncogenesis. The cloning and subsequent analysis of leukemia-associated gene products have strongly facilitated the understanding of their biological function and the development of appropriate model systems. In early experiments, leukemia-associated oncogenes were ectopically expressed in fibroblasts, a cell type which is not optimal for modeling leukemia initiation and progression. Later, the development of cell separation methods for murine and human hematopoietic precursor cells allowed for the isolation of specific target cells, in large quantities and with high cell population purity (Belvedere et al., 1999). Together with the utilization of retroviral expression vectors, which enable stable integration and expression of a transgene of choice, these cell isolation procedures represent a significant methodological improvement for leukemia modeling approaches in the hematopoietic tissue. With these technologies in hand, the genetic lesions of leukemia can be better modeled in the appropriate cell compartment. By performing cell biology experiments and tumor sample deep sequencing it became clear that both solid tumors and hematological malignancies depend on multiple oncogenic alterations to ultimately result in cellular transformation (Hanahan & Weinberg, 2000, 2011; Kinzler & Vogelstein, 1996). Additionally, the overall number of mutated genes in solid tumors was found to be higher than in leukemias. These observations resulted in the formulation of the multi-hit model of tumorigenesis. Initiating mutations induce stem cell expansion and survival, thereby allowing for the occurrence of additional genetic alterations that result in the progression of malignant transformation. The later stages of this process are characterized by uncontrolled proliferation with overgrowth of the ´healthy´ cell compartment and metastasis, in the case of solid tumors. This multi-hit cancer model has been well described for colon cancer by Kenneth W. Kinzler and Bert Vogelstein (Kinzler &

Vogelstein, 1996). Similarly, it has been suggested for hematopoietic malignancies, that only a concerted signaling network resulting from the activity of several activated oncogenes leads to full transformation of preleukemic cell clones. However, the exact chronological order of these genetic events and the causality of their mutual cooperation are hardly understood (Schuringa et al., 2010).

Myeloid leukemia represents a well-depicted tumor entity in terms of molecular pathogenesis. It is characterized by an uncontrolled proliferation behavior based on the aberrant self-renewal capacity of the myeloid progenitor cell compartment including the erythroid, monocytic and granulocytic lineages. Depending on the morphology and genetics of the cells and its clinical progression, myeloid leukemia is classified as either acute myeloid leukemia (AML) or chronic myeloid leukemia (CML). AML is distinguished by the rapid proliferation of immature myeloid progenitor cells, which overgrow the normal hematopoietic cells. AML is the most common acute leukemia, which predominantly affects adults. Its incidence strongly increases with age, with a median age at diagnosis of 65 years, suggesting that several oncogenic events are required for the onset and progression of the disease (Estey & Dohner, 2006). If left untreated, the disease proceeds rapidly and is typically fatal within weeks or months. To date, numerous AML-specific fusion genes and mutations have been described (Look, 1997). Chromosomal translocations and mutations involving the AML1 gene are amongst the most common alterations found in AML (Schnittger et al., 2011). AML1 is an essential transcription factor that controls the myeloid cell differentiation of progenitor cells into mature blood cells. Both point mutations and chromosomal translocations, such as t(8;21) and t(3;21), disrupt the physiological function of AML1 and hinder the normal maturation process of the progenitor cells (Niebuhr et al., 2008). IIn addition, mutations of the receptor tyrosine kinase, c-kit, are frequently detected in these cells and seem to be associated with poor prognosis due to their correlation with higher relapse rates after chemotherapy (Boissel et al., 2006; Paschka et al., 2006). Mutations of the nucleophosmin (NPM1) gene are also frequently observed in AML. This gene is involved in multiple cellular processes including protein shuttling between the nucleus and cytoplasm, RNA biogenesis, cell cycle control and transcriptional regulation. It is also described as a cellular stress sensor associated with the p53-dependent apoptosis pathway (Grisendi et al., 2006). Commonly identified NPM1 mutations render this protein mislocalized to the cytoplasm. The oncogenic mechanisms behind this phenomenon are currently under intense investigation (Falini et al., 2010; Falini et al., 2007). Among the mutated kinases in AML, mutations of the FLT3 cytokine receptor gene are common and are associated with poor prognosis (Gilliland & Griffin, 2002; Meshinchi et al., 2001). Hyperactive FLT3 induces a strong intracellular signal transduction response, mainly by activating STAT5, a latent transcription factor important for self-renewal and proliferation of hematopoietic progenitors. For this leukemia entity, FLT3-inhibitors blocking its kinase activity are currently being tested in clinical trials (Wiernik, 2010). Isocitrate dehydrogenases, IDH1 and IDH2, represent genes that were recently identified to be frequently mutated in AML with adverse prognosis in cytogenetically normal leukemias (Mardis et al., 2009; Paschka et al., 2010). Mutations in IDH genes have also been found in human brain tumors, including gliomas. Interestingly, the accumulation of an intracellular metabolite, 2-hydroxyglutarate, was discovered in these tumor cells (Dang et al., 2009). This so-called 'oncometabolite' alters the genome-wide histone and DNA methylation patterns, thereby exerting oncogenic activity (Xu et al., 2011).

Chronic myeloid leukemia is characterized by the increased proliferation rate of mature granulocytes and their precursors. The course of disease can be divided into three phases:

the chronic phase, the accelerated phase and the acute phase with typical features of AML (Sawyers, 1999). The t(9;22) chromosomal translocation, also called the Philadelphia chromosome, which generates the fusion protein BCR/ABL, is frequently observed in CML patient samples. The BCR-portion of the fusion protein triggers multimerization of the ABL portion, thereby locking the ABL kinase into a hyperactive state. BCR/ABL multimers induce constitutive intracellular proliferation and survival signaling, thereby triggering the development of leukemia (Hoelbl et al., 2010; Melo & Barnes, 2007). Over the last years, a breakthrough in the treatment of CML was achieved with the development of the ABL-kinase inhibitor, imatinib (Sawyers et al., 2002). BCR/ABL positive CML patients are now treated with one of several targeted, first-line therapies, including imatinib, dasatinib, and nilotinib, which have dramatically increased patient survival rates to nearly 90% since the advent of these therapies. These kinase inhibitors specifically inhibit the oncogenic tyrosine kinase activity of BCR/ABL. For the first time, an inhibitor has been developed that targets a driving oncogene with high efficiency, which is currently used in many clinical trials (Garcia-Manero et al., 2003). Later, it was found that imatinib also targets c-kit, a receptor tyrosine kinase frequently mutated in gastrointestinal stromal tumors (GIST), thereby widening the application spectrum of imatinib to include solid tumors (Demetri, 2002). Currently, large efforts are being made in the development of specific inhibitors for other oncoproteins. The elucidation of the molecular mechanisms controlling the process of leukemic transformation represents a prerequisite for the development of targeted oncogene inhibitors designed to improve current therapeutic strategies for myeloid leukemias.

For both acute and chronic myeloid leukemia, 'leukemia stem cells' are most likely the origin of disease and are probably responsible for recurrence after chemotherapy (Trumpp & Wiestler, 2008). These leukemia stem cells share common features with normal stem cells. They are described as dormant or slowly cycling cells with an increased self-renewal capacity and a resistance to chemotherapeutic drugs. It has been proposed that they reside in the bone marrow niches and can fully regenerate the leukemia after standard chemotherapy. Perturbed self-renewal programs of leukemia stem cells represent a major problem for leukemia therapy. Even in BCR/ABL positive CML, for which a specific oncogene inhibitor is available, CML stem cells are resistant to imatinib treatment (Holyoake et al., 1999). Therefore, lifelong treatment of CML patients with tyrosine kinase inhibitors is necessary (Corbin et al., 2011; Diamond & Melo, 2011).

Most of the current understandings of leukemogenic fusion genes and mutations have resulted from overexpression experiments using either cell line models or primary murine and human hematopoietic stem cells, both in vitro and in vivo. In these studies, leukemic gene products were usually expressed with the help of retroviral expression vectors resulting in ectopic and stable expression. This represents a convenient experimental strategy to model leukemia in mammalian hematopoietic stem and progenitor cells. The following sections will recapitulate the different retroviral expression vector systems used for modeling leukemia development and will summarize exemplary results acquired from studies of both the murine and human progenitor cell systems.

2. Retroviral vector systems and expression cassettes

When modeling leukemia in the mammalian hematopoietic system, there are two major strategies used to express a leukemia-associated gene product. The creation of knock-in or transgenic mice enables robust transgene expression *in vivo*. However, transgene expression is usually not restricted to a certain tissue and permanent oncogene expression often causes delirious side effects, e.g. embryonic lethality, thereby impeding accurate analysis. Alternatively, genes can be delivered by retroviral vectors directly into the hematopoietic system via bone marrow transplantation of hematopoietic progenitors, transduced with the gene of interest (GOI). Gene marking of few cells also more precisely resembles leukemia development from a single cell clone. In addition, this method provides the advantage of rapid testing of numerous gene expression constructs in contrast to the time-consuming gene-manipulation of mice. Therefore, gamma-retroviral and lentiviral expression vector systems represent attractive and efficient techniques for the stable expression of a gene of interest in hematopoietic progenitor cells. Retroviruses are enveloped RNA viruses. Viral RNA is linear, single-stranded and approximately 7-12 kb in size. The common characteristic of retroviruses is their strategy of replication: the viral RNA is reverse transcribed into linear double-stranded DNA followed by its integration into the genome of the cell (Coffin et al., 2007). The most commonly used delivery system is the gamma-retroviral vector system. These vectors are derived from the Moloney murine leukemia virus (Mo-MLV) genome (Kohn et al., 1987). The murine stem cell virus (MSCV) expression vector is one of the most frequently employed vector systems, as it enables stable and high transgene expression in virtually all cell types (Hawley et al., 1994). This vector is available with several marker genes, such as the enhanced green fluorescent protein (eGFP) and derivatives thereof, which are co-expressed via the internal ribosomal entry site (IRES) elements. One of the disadvantages of gamma-retroviral vectors is their inability to target non-dividing cells. Successful cell transduction is completely dependent on the breakdown of the nuclear membrane during mitosis (Roe et al., 1993). In contrast, lentiviral vectors, which are mostly derived from the HIV-1 genome, are able to integrate into both dividing and non-dividing cells (Lewis et al., 1992; Lewis & Emerman, 1994). Compared with gamma-retroviral vectors, lentiviral vectors have the capacity to incorporate larger transgenes, up to 10 kilobases, although vector titers decrease when using larger inserts (Matrai et al., 2010). The integration of retroviral vectors into the cell genome results in the stable and permanent expression of the transgene, which is transferred to all daughter cells during cell division. Therefore, retrovirally transduced oncogene expressing cells resemble cancer cells in that they pass their oncogenic alterations down to all progeny. However, during integration into the genome there is a risk of insertional mutagenesis (Baum, 2007). This must be kept in mind while analyzing the potential oncogenic effects of a transgene delivered by retroviral vectors. In general, gamma-retro as well as lentiviral vectors integrate into transcriptional units. Gamma-retroviruses tend to integrate either upstream or downstream of the start of transcriptional units (Wu et al., 2003), while lentiviral vectors integrate randomly within a transcriptional unit (Naldini et al., 2006). During retroviral integration into the genome of a cell, there is a risk of proto-oncogene activation close to the integration site of the vector driven by either the enhancer element or the promoter sequences present in the U3 region of the viral long terminal repeats (LTRs). Deletion of the U3 region within the LTRs and the insertion of an internal enhancer/promoter result in the formation of self-inactivating (SIN) vectors with the reduced risk of cellular oncogene activation (Yu et al., 1986). Retroviral particle production and transduction procedures represent convenient routine methods, which can be carried out in any laboratory with the appropriate laboratory biosafety level. For safety reasons, genes required for the assembly of the viral particles, *gag*, *pol* and *env*, are expressed from separate, so-called 'helper plasmids'. In contrast to the expression vector, which codes for the gene of interest, the helper plasmids do not contain coding sequences for the packaging signal. Therefore, transcribed RNAs from the helper plasmids are not incorporated into the virus particle. With these replication defective retroviral particles, only a single round of transduction is possible. Thus, the risk of generating replication competent virus particles during production is greatly reduced. Retroviral transduction efficacy can be improved by concentrating the viral particles via ultracentrifugation (Kanbe & Zhang, 2004; Naldini et al., 1996). Gamma-retroviral particles can be preloaded onto RetroNectin-coated surfaces. RetroNectin, a recombinant peptide consisting of a mixture of fragments of the fibronectin molecule, co-localizes the viral particles and target cells into close proximity, thereby strongly increasing the efficiency of transduction (Hanenberg et al., 1996). A standard protocol for routine gamma-retroviral particle production and transduction of suspension cells is provided in Table 1. Expression of the gene of interest is usually coupled to the expression of a marker gene. This allows for immediate determination of the viral transduction efficacy as well as for the identification of transduced cells for the measurement of proliferation, differentiation and cell death. EGFP is the most commonly used marker protein, which exhibits a bright green fluorescence after laser excitation at 488 nm. Enrichment of vector-transduced fluorescent-labeled cells can be performed by fluorescence activated cell sorting (FACS). The usage of drug-selectable marker genes, such as neomycin and puromycin, represents another method used to obtain pure populations of transduced cells. Cellular expression of more than one transgene by retroviral vectors can be accomplished by a variety of strategies (Figure 1).

The inclusion of an internal promoter allows for the expression of a second transgene when one transgene is expressed from the vector 5´-LTR. However, this approach also carries the risk of promoter interference with the vector LTR during retroviral particle production, thereby reducing vector titers and expression levels of the GOI (de Felipe et al., 1999). Another commonly employed strategy is the expression of two separate genes from one single transcript using the IRES element derived from the picornavirus (Gallardo et al., 1997). The IRES element allows for the initiation of mRNA translation in a 5′ cap-independent manner (Mountford & Smith, 1995). However, expression levels of the two genes usually differ significantly. Typically, the gene located downstream is expressed at a level ten times lower than that of the other gene (Mizuguchi et al., 2000). The gene of interest and the marker gene can be fused to increase their stability and to allow for expression from one promoter. However, fusing two transgenes can result in functional restriction of the proteins caused by the fusion. Therefore, a short, flexible linker should be used to connect the proteins (Robinson & Sauer, 1998). Repeats of small side chain amino acids, such as glycine, serine and alanine, are well suited for the creation of linker sequences. The expression of two separate transgenes in equimolar amounts can be accomplished using 'self-cleaving' 2A peptides, originating from the foot-and-mouth disease virus (Ryan et al., 1991). The 2A peptide sequence disrupts the peptide bond formation via a ribosomal skip mechanism, which releases the polypeptide from the translational complex and allows the production of the downstream translation product (Donnelly et al., 2001).

Step 1: Retroviral vector production	• For retroviral vector particle production subconfluent (80%) adherent cell lines (e.g. HEK293T, HeLA) are co-transfected with the retroviral expression construct and the appropriate helper plasmids • 6 hours (or overnight) after transfection, exchange the appropriate medium for the target cells • 24 hours later, harvest the viral supernatant: centrifuge the viral supernatant at 1.500 rpm to pellet cell debris and filtrate the supernatant (0.22 µm filter) • Virus supernatant is ready for transduction or can be stored at – 80°C for several months
Step 2: Preparation of RetroNectin- coated plates	• One day before transduction (at least 6 hours), add 500 µl RetroNectin (RN) solution (50 µg/ml) to each well of a 24-well plate (non-tissue culture treated) and incubate overnight at room temperature • The next day, discard the RN solution (reusable up to 8 times), add 1 ml stop solution (1xPBS+2% BSA) and incubate for 30 minutes at room temperature • Discard the stop solution, rinse 1x with HBSS solution and 1x with 1xPBS • Coated plates are ready for virus preload (RN coated plates can be stored in 4°C with PBS)
Step 3: Preload of viral particles	• Quickly defrost the virus supernatant and dilute as necessary • Discard the 1xPBS and add the viral supernatant with the appropriate multiplicities of infection (MOI) • Centrifuge at 3000 rpm at 4°C for 20-25 minutes • Discard the viral supernatant and repeat the preload *at least* 3 times, each with the appropriate volume (minimum: 500 µl)
Step 4: Transduction of target cells	• Remove the remaining viral supernatant before adding the cells • Count the cells and dilute the cells to a concentration of 7.5×10^5 cells/ml in the appropriate culture medium • Add 500 µl (minimum) cell suspension to each well and incubate at 37°C and 5% CO_2 for at least 8 hours (or overnight) • Optional: The addition of protamine sulfate (4 µg/ml) might increase the transduction efficiency • Prepare a second RN coated 24-well plate and repeat the preload and transduction procedure for a second, third or fourth transduction (max. 2 transductions per day) • 8 hours after the final transduction, exchange the medium and transfer the transduced cells into a fresh tissue-coated 24-well plate without RN • Optional: Wash the plate 3x with 1x PBS to collect the remaining cells from the plate

Table 1. Vector particle production and transduction standard protocol for suspension cells with gamma-retroviral vectors.

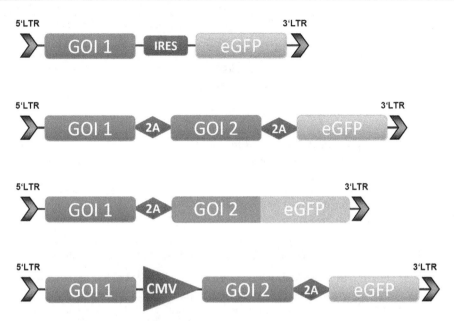

Fig. 1. Retroviral co-expression vector constructs, including eGFP as a marker gene. The depicted co-expression vectors are based on a standard 5'-LTR driven retroviral expression vector (top). 2A elements allow for co-expression of several GOI at equimolar levels. For intracellular stabilization, the GOI can be fused to eGFP. An internal promoter, e.g. the CMV promoter, drives GOI 2 expression independently of GOI 1. LTR, long terminal repeats; GOI, gene of interest; IRES, internal ribosomal entry site; 2A, 2A peptide sequence; eGFP, enhanced green fluorescent protein; CMV, cytomegalovirus.

In the context of the MSCV-based retroviral vectors, it has been shown that coupling four transgenes via three different 2A peptide cleavage sequences can generate four separate proteins both *in vitro* and *in vivo*. One restriction with this system is that the small remaining 2A-tag at the N-terminal end of the protein may potentially affect protein function (Szymczak et al., 2004). Therefore, proper cleavage and function of the individual proteins should be carefully verified. Table 2 summarizes the advantages and disadvantages of the different expression cassettes used for the co-expression of two genes of interest.

The 'lentiviral gene ontology' (LeGO) vectors represent a useful collection of state-of-the-art expression vectors for functional gene analysis. These vectors contain the retroviral enhancer/promoter of the spleen focus-forming virus, which has a broad and high expression pattern. LeGO expression vectors are available with a wide spectrum of different fluorescent markers, e.g. Cerulean, eGFP, tdTomato and mCherry, which are expressed in combination with the gene of interest via IRES elements. LeGO vectors that contain fluorescent marker genes linked via 2A peptides to different drug-selectable genes, e.g. blasticidin, hygromycin, neomycin, puromycin or zeocin, are also available. Furthermore, the expression cassettes of these LeGO vectors are flanked by loxP sites, which allows for displacement of the transgene after introduction of the CRE recombinase (Weber, 2007; Weber et al., 2008; Weber et al., 2010).

	IRES	2A	2nd promoter (internal)	Co-transduction
Advantage	Expression of 2 separate transgenes	Equal expression levels of the 2 genes	Expression of 2 separate transgenes	Independent expression; results in single and double transduced cells
Disadvantage	10x lower expression of the downstream gene	Remaining 2A tag at the end of the N-terminal protein	Low titer of viral particles	Low rate of double transduced cells; increases risk of insertional mutagenesis
Literature	*Gallardo et al., 1997 Mizuguchi et al., 2000*	*Szymczak et al., 2004*	*Felipe et al., 1999*	*Rizo et al., 2010*

Table 2. Overview of expression cassette elements for co-expression of two genes of interest.

To accurately characterize oncogene activity it is important to have the ability to selectively induce and terminate oncogene expression. This is particularly important if the delivered gene product is toxic at high concentrations. The regulation of gene expression can be achieved by using the tetracycline-controlled transactivator (tTA)-responsive promoter (Tet-system), a prokaryotic inducible promoter system that is also applicable to mammalian cells (Gossen & Bujard, 1992). The Tet system comprises two components: one component that drives expression of the transactivator (tTA) and a second component that contains the (tTA)-responsive promoter element for transgene expression. In the first developed 'tet-off' system, the transactivator binds to the promoter in the absence of tetracycline. The addition of tetracycline inhibits its binding, thereby resulting in inhibition of transgene expression (Gossen et al., 1995). To avoid constant tetracycline supplementation, a reverse system ('tet-on' system) allows for transgene expression only in the presence of doxycycline, a tetracycline derivate (Gossen et al., 1995). Traditionally, transactivator and promoter components had to be introduced by two separate transduction steps to obtain inducible gene expression. The development of an 'all-in-one' vector system circumvents this complication. In this system, all components required for tet-regulated transgene expression have been inserted as a bidirectional expression cassette (Heinz et al., 2011). Another means of intracellular oncogene dosage control is the regulation at the protein level. With this type of expression control, the gene of interest can be fused to a small destabilizing domain, thereby mediating the intracellular destruction of the protein by targeting it for proteasomal degradation. Degradation of the fusion protein can be specifically blocked by cell membrane-permeable small molecules, which bind to and inhibit the destabilizing domain mediated degradation, thereby resulting in the accumulation of the expressed transgene (Banaszynski et al., 2006).

3. Murine progenitor cells

Murine hematopoietic stem and progenitor cells have been well characterized. To study these cell types, progenitor cells can be simply isolated from the bone marrow. After femora and tibia preparation, bone marrow cells can be harvested by flushing the bones. Further purification of hematopoietic progenitor cells is typically carried out by 'lineage depletion'. Using this method, differentiated 'lineage positive' cells, such as monocytes and macrophages, T- and B- cells, erythrocytes and granulocytes, are separated from their committed precursors, the 'lineage negative' fraction. Freshly isolated, complete bone marrow suspension cells are incubated with a mixture of magnetically labeled antibodies against cell surface markers for mature blood cells, typically B220, CD4, CD8, Gr-1, Mac-1 and Ter-119. Separation of the lineage negative progenitor cell fraction is performed by passing the labeled and non-labeled cells through magnetic columns (Challen et al., 2009). Amongst all vertebrates, the murine hematopoietic system is the best characterized. For the subdivision of stem and progenitor cell populations, the LSK- and SLAM-markers have become widely accepted. LSK (lin-, Sca1+, c-kit+) cells lack the markers of mature blood cells and simultaneously express high levels of the stem cell markers, Sca1 and c-kit. As little as one hundred LSK cells have been shown to be sufficient for the long-term multilineage repopulation of lethally irradiated recipient mice (Okada et al., 1992). The LSK cell compartment can be further separated into hematopoietic stem cells (HSCs) and multipotent progenitors (MPPs) depending on their diverse expression pattern of the family of 'signaling lymphocyte activation molecule' (SLAM) receptors (Kiel et al., 2005). The SLAM cell surface marker, CD150, is exclusively expressed on HSCs, whereas CD244 is expressed by transiently reconstituting MPPs. CD34 and Flt3 expression patterns further allow for the discrimination between long term-HSC (LT-HSCs; CD34-/Flt3-) and short term HSCs (ST-HSCs; CD34+/Flt3+) (Adolfsson et al., 2001; Osawa et al., 1996). ST-HSCs have a reduced self-renewal capacity for a restricted time compared with the life-long self-renewal capacity of LT-HSCs (Adolfsson et al., 2001; Morrison & Weissman, 1994; Yang et al., 2005). Because the murine hematopoietic system has been well characterized, with precisely classified and characterized stem and progenitor cell compartments, and simple precursor cell purification procedures have been established and optimized, murine hematopoietic progenitor cells are well suited for the functional analysis of oncogenic fusion genes and mutations associated with leukemia development.

The cell transforming activity of a given leukemia-associated oncogene can be measured by performing an *in vitro* colony forming unit (CFU) assay. This assay allows for the quantification of colony forming progenitors and their iterative replating capacity. Hematopoietic progenitor cells expressing the gene of interest are plated in methylcellulose at low density. In general, normal progenitor cells only form colonies in the first round of plating. However, oncogene-expressing cells are able to confer serial replating capacity for several rounds of plating. For example, cells expressing the t(8;21) translocation product, AML1/ETO, are able to confer serial replating for up to 13 rounds of plating (Rhoades et al., 2000). Transgene expressing murine progenitor cells can also be cultivated in liquid suspension cultures. Here, cytokines such as IL3, IL6 and SCF must be supplemented continuously. Under these *ex vivo* cultivation parameters specific for cell differentiation, proliferation and apoptosis can be measured under various cell culture conditions, such as serum or cytokine deprivation and hypoxic conditions, which imitate the hypoxic niches of the bone marrow.

Gene modified precursor cells can be further examined *in vivo* in a mouse transplantation model. In this case, immediately after retroviral gene transfer, lineage depleted bone marrow cells stably expressing the oncogene of interest are transplanted into lethally irradiated syngeneic recipient mice. The transplantation is performed by injection of gene-modified cells into the tail vein or the retro-orbital sinus of recipient mice (Larochelle et al., 1995). For successful hematopoietic rescue, transplanted cells must reach the appropriate milieu in the bone marrow niches, which supports their proliferation and differentiation; this cell migration process is referred to as 'homing' (Szilvassy et al., 1999). To analyze disease progression in mice following the transplantation of progenitor cells body weight and blood profile values must be documented carefully over time. If transplanted mice develop any symptoms of leukemia, e.g. sudden body weight reduction, increasing peripheral leukocyte counts or poor general health conditions, they should be sacrificed and analyzed. Blood cells isolated from the periphery, spleen and bone marrow compartment can be studied separately. Flow cytometric analysis conveniently allows for the detection of oncogene expressing blood cells by discerning the expression of the fluorescence marker proteins. Gene marked cells can be examined for cellular differentiation (CD differentiation marker), the proliferation/cell cycle profile and apoptosis by AnnexinV-staining, for example. FACS based methods allow for the parallel analysis of transduced and non-transduced cells, using the latter as the internal experimental control. Transgene expression of leukemic cells must be analyzed by RT-PCR and western immunoblotting, which assesses mRNA and protein levels, respectively. There are highly specific antibodies that can detect epitope-tagged oncoproteins, e.g. Ha- or Flag-tagged proteins, even at very low expression levels (Terpe, 2003). To exclude the potential oncogenic effects of vector-mediated insertional mutagenesis, clonality and integration site analysis must be performed carefully. The oncogene activity of the expressed transgene can be accurately validated by analyzing the downstream signal transduction pathways of the cell. For example, phosphorylated STAT5 and CRKL are regarded as downstream indicators of oncogenic BCR/ABL signaling. Bone marrow and spleen, which are the target organs of leukemic origin, and peripheral blood must be analyzed for the presence of immature blast cells. This can be carried out by conventional blood smear and flow cytometric analysis. For organ histology, samples of each organ, including the spleen, liver, lymph nodes and thymus, are transferred into paraffin, sectioned and examined. Hematoxylin and eosin are the most commonly used staining solutions in histology for light microscopical analysis. A final validation of the leukemia must be demonstrated by re-transplantating the leukemic blood cells into secondary lethally irradiated recipient mice. In these secondary transplanted mice, leukemia onset should appear much earlier than in primary recipients. In 2002, Kogan et al published the 'Bethesda proposals for the classification of hematopoietic neoplasms in mice' (Kogan et al., 2002). As with the World Health Organization (WHO) classification of human disorders, theses proposals utilize morphologic, immunophenotypic, clinical, biological and genetic characteristics to classify neoplasms.

Both methods, the colony-forming assay and the mouse transplantation model are commonly used techniques for the investigation of the transforming potential of oncogenes in leukemia (Figure 2).

The following examples illustrate both the genetic and biochemical approaches utilizing murine hematopoietic progenitor cells for leukemia modeling.

The acute promyelocytic leukemia (APL) associated t(15;17) translocation product, PML/RARα, is one of the most studied fusion proteins associated with AML (Puccetti & Ruthardt, 2004). In the clinical setting, APL patients not only respond well to 'all trans retinoic acid' (ATRA) therapy, which has been well documented (Huang et al., 1988), but also benefit from treatment with arsenic trioxide (Chen et al., 1997), which exerts a profound anti-cancer effect by inducing the degradation of the PML/RARα oncoprotein. Retroviral expression of PML/RARα in murine progenitor cells efficiently induces leukemia development in transplanted lethally irradiated recipient mice (Minucci et al., 2002). The efficacy of arsenic trioxide and ATRA has been recapitulated in PML/RARα mouse models displaying the impressive anti-leukemia effects of both substances (Rego et al., 2000). Furthermore, in transplantation models based on ATRA-resistant APL cell lines, treatment with arsenic trioxide significantly decreases tumor formation (Kinjo et al., 2000). Zhang et al have further showed that arsenic trioxide functions by directly binding to PML/RARα. The researchers identified cysteine residues within the PML portion that are directly bound by arsenic trioxide, which triggered SUMOylation and subsequent degradation of the oncoprotein (Zhang et al., 2010).

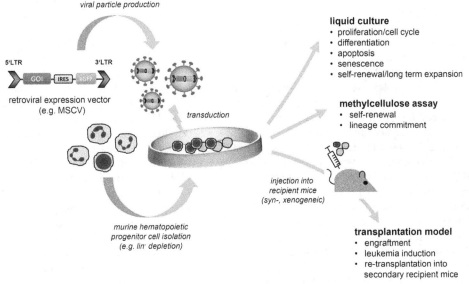

Fig. 2. Functional analysis of gene-modified murine/human hematopoietic progenitor cells. Experimental procedures include cloning of the retroviral expression vector, viral particle production, hematopoietic progenitor cell isolation, transduction and functional analysis in methylcellulose assays, liquid cultures and murine syngeneic or xenogeneic mouse transplantation models. GOI, gene of interest; MSCV, murine stem cell virus; LTR, long terminal repeats; lin-, lineage negative.

Other reports have described that oncogene expression experiments involving murine progenitor cells supported the clinical finding reporting a highly leukemogenic splice variant of the familiar AML1/ETO fusion gene resulting from the translocation t(8;21). Several groups have shown that the full length AML1/ETO protein does not lead to the development of leukemia when transplanting LSK bone marrow cells expressing AML1/ETO into syngeneic mice (de Guzman et al., 2002). However, in similar transplantation experiments performed by Yan and colleagues, one mouse developed leukemia 14 weeks after bone marrow transplantation. Further analysis showed that a C-terminal truncated AML1/ETO protein was expressed in this mouse due to a one-base pair insertion into the full length AML1/ETO gene. Subsequently, the cloning and creation of mice expressing the truncated protein by transplantation of transduced progenitor cells again revealed a rapid leukemia development (Yan et al., 2004). Consequently, these results led to the investigation and identification of a naturally occurring splice variant of AML1/ETO in t(8;21) patients by sophisticated gene expression analysis of patient material. This splice variant, termed AML1/ETO9A, is almost structurally identical to the truncated form expressed in the leukemic mouse. Expression of this newly discovered splice isoform in mice also induced rapid leukemia development (Yan et al., 2006). In conclusion, these oncogene expression experiments using murine progenitor cells led to the clinical identification of a potent oncogenic AML1/ETO splice variant. Further experiments must be performed to understand whether the AML1/ETO splice isoform is the driving oncogene in human t(8;21) leukemia cells.

The usage of oncogene expressing vectors has also facilitated the understanding of the protein domain structure-function relationship. Biophysical and biochemical experiments have been used to identify highly conserved domains within several oncoproteins, which might represent valuable target structures for molecular intervention. This has been demonstrated with the AML1/ETO fusion protein. Here, a central region, the *nervy* homology region 2 (NHR2), was found to play an essential role in the leukemogenic activity of the fusion protein. Analysis of the crystal structure revealed a tetrameric formation that is essential for the serial colony formation capacity of murine progenitor cells in methylcellulose assays (Liu et al., 2006). By performing additional bioinformatic molecular modeling analyses, five amino acids were identified within the large NHR2 tetramer-interface that are important for oligomer formation. Substitution of these critical residues led to the conversion of tetramers into dimers with the complete loss of the transforming abilities of AML1/ETO. Transplantation of retroviral infected murine bone marrow cells expressing the AML1/ETO protein harboring these five substitutions showed that these amino acids play a critical role in transformation, as the mice failed to develop leukemia. Interestingly, the identified amino acids are clustered in one region at the top of the NHR2 dimer surface, thereby representing a potential target site for molecular intervention (Wichmann et al., 2010). These findings, which reveal the molecular determinants of oncogene activity, are the result of a productive combination of bioinformatics, biochemical and cell-biological analyses. Furthermore, proof of concept of oncogene targeting was demonstrated using a synthetic oligomerization domain. This domain was integrated into the AML1/ETO fusion gene, thereby replacing the NHR2 tetramer domain. Specific inhibitors that disrupt the oligomerization of this synthetic domain within AML1/ETO completely blocked the replating capacity of retrovirally transduced AML1/ETO expressing murine progenitor cells (Kwok et al., 2009).

By expressing leukemia fusion genes in murine cells, one can assess exactly which gene product from a balanced translocation, which often generates two different reciprocal fusion genes, is responsible for driving the leukemic activity. Bursen and colleagues have reported interesting findings regarding the function of the reciprocal fusion proteins, AF4/MLL and MLL/AF4, which are generated by the chromosomal translocation t(4;11) in high-risk infant acute mixed lineage leukemia. They analyzed the leukemia-inducing capacity of these two fusion genes in mice by transplantation of retrovirally transduced Lin-/Sca1+ cells expressing either one or both of the reciprocal fusion genes. They could show that expression of AF4/MLL alone was sufficient to promote leukemia development, while the reciprocal translocation, MLL/AF4, completely lacked leukemogenic potential (Bursen et al., 2010).

4. The human CD34+ progenitor cell system

Human blood progenitor cells are characterized by the high expression levels of the cell surface marker CD34 and the absence of CD38 expression (CD34+/CD38-). CD34 is a member of the single-pass transmembrane sialomucin protein family, which is expressed in early hematopoietic and vascular-associated tissues; however, little is known about its exact biological function (Furness & McNagny, 2006). There are a variety of ways to obtain hematopoietic CD34+ cells from the human body. The cells can be isolated from the peripheral blood by leukapheresis after stimulation and mobilization of the bone marrow precursors with G-CSF (granulocytic colony stimulating factor). Bone marrow aspiration represents the classical but invasive isolation method, which also allows for the isolation of large numbers of CD34+ cells. A third option involves the usage of placental derived cord blood cells of which the quality/stemness and engraftment potential are superior to that of adult CD34+ stem cells (Hao et al., 1995). The efficient enrichment of human hematopoietic CD34+ cells can be achieved by immunomagnetic cell sorting, which represents a standard and convenient method in laboratory work (Clarke & Davies, 2001). Magnetic labeled CD34-antibodies are used to recover high-purity populations of CD34+ cells by passing cells through magnetic columns. Isolated CD34+ cells can then be used for clinical and experimental purposes. For transgene expression studies, the cells can be manipulated by retroviral transduction immediately after recovery or after a short pre-cultivation in a cytokine cocktail, which usually contains IL-3, IL6 and SCF for cell cycle activation. Like the murine system, transduced human CD34+ cells can be propagated *in vitro* in methylcellulose assays for colony formation as well as in long-term liquid cultures used to assess self-renewal and proliferation/expansion capacities (Figure 1). Furthermore, human CD34+ cells expressing leukemic gene products can be transplanted into severe combined immunodeficient (NOD/SCID) mice (xenotransplants). Additionally, the NOG (NOD/Shi-scid/IL-2Ry^{null}) mice accept heterologous transplanted cells more easily than any other type of immunodeficient nude or NOD/SCID mice. Therefore, the NOG mouse system is a highly efficient recipient model for the engraftment, proliferation and differentiation of human cells (Ito et al., 2002).

The transformation of human cells requires additional genetic alterations when compared with their murine counterparts (Hahn et al., 1999; Rangarajan & Weinberg, 2003). This is reflected by the observation that singular expression of several oncogenes induces leukemia in the murine system but fails to transform human CD34+ cells in the NOD/SCID humanized leukemia mouse model. Further evidence of this concept has been demonstrated by gene expression analysis of healthy individuals. Here, oncogenes such as BCR/ABL and AML1/ETO have been frequently detected in individuals completely lacking any sign of disease (Song et al., 2011). As CD34+ cells represent the human hematopoietic stem/progenitor cell population, these cells can be regarded as appropriate target cells used to study the biological effects of oncogenes in human leukemia development.

The following passages provide an overview of recent experiments addressing the leukemogenic activity of several myeloid leukemia associated oncogenes expressed alone or in combination in human hematopoietic CD34+ progenitor cells. In all cases, genes were delivered using gamma-retroviral vectors co-expressing the marker genes eGFP or dNGFR (truncated nerve growth factor receptor), which allowed for the convenient detection of gene-modified cells by FACS analysis.

Grignani et al have reported that ectopic expression of PML/RARα in human CD34+ *ex vivo* cultures rapidly induced the cellular differentiation of progenitor cells towards the promyelocytic stage, followed by a block in further terminal differentiation into granulocytes, which resembled typical features of primary human acute promyelocytic leukemia (Grignani et al., 2000). In cytokine deprived liquid cultures, PML/RARα expressing cells survived and continued to expand, whereas control cells stopped proliferation and died by apoptosis. The terminal differentiation block induced by PML/RARα could be overcome by treatment with ATRA, a drug that has dramatically improved the overall survival of APL patients. They further demonstrated that a mutation of the N-CoR repressor binding interface within the PML portion of the fusion protein completely disrupted the observed biological effects, thereby suggesting that N-CoR triggered transcriptional repression is an essential prerequisite for PML/RARα oncogene activity in human hematopoietic progenitor cells.

Among the AML oncogenes, hyperactive tyrosine kinases play a major role in disease development and have gathered much attention since the kinase inhibitor imatinib has been proven to be highly beneficial for BCR/ABL positive CML patients (Druker et al., 1996; Sawyers et al., 2002; Brandts et al., 2007). Chung and colleagues retrovirally expressed a related constitutive active tyrosine kinase, FLT3-ITD, which is frequently found in AML patient samples associated with poor prognosis (Gilliland & Griffin, 2002). Stable expression of FLT3-ITD conferred a strong short-term proliferative signal in human CD34+ cells with enhanced erythropoiesis for two weeks after transduction *ex vivo*. The cells were blocked in terminal differentiation and colony formation was enhanced when compared with control cells. These effects could be partially substituted by expression of a constitutive active STAT5 mutant, a major downstream target of the hyperactive FLT3-ITD kinase. Moreover, FLT3-ITD triggered effects that could be blocked via inhibition with the FLT3-inhibitor tyrphostin (Chung et al., 2005). Despite these significant effects, FLT3-ITD transgene-expressing CD34+ cells are neither able to expand further in *ex vivo* cultures nor able to induce leukemia in the NOD/SCID mouse transplantation model.

Stable ectopic expression of several leukemogenic fusion genes resulting from chromosomal translocations leads to enhanced *ex vivo* CD34+ cell expansion for up to several months (Abdul-Nabi et al., 2010). This has previously been shown for the t(8;21) associated fusion protein AML1/ETO, which is capable of expanding human CD34+ cells *ex vivo* for several months with a cumulative cell expansion of more than 10^{15}-fold. Retroviral expression of AML1/ETO resulted in a sustained proliferation potential using a cytokine cocktail that included IL3, IL6, SCF, FLT3, GM-CSF, TPO and EPO, all at low concentrations. The cells display the typical differentiation block as observed in myeloid blast cells and grow out from a mixed culture of transduced and non-transduced cells. Even after several weeks in *ex vivo* culture, the cells are capable of colony formation in methylcellulose assays and, more importantly, of engraftment into immunodeficient NOD/SCID mice (Mulloy et al., 2003; Mulloy et al., 2002). Phenotypically, a subpopulation of the cells continues to express CD34, while the majority of the cells express the myeloid specific markers CD13 and CD33, in the absence of erythroid markers. Continuous expansion of the cells completely depends on the CD34+ subgroup. Erythroid differentiation was shown to be blocked by the AML1/ETO fusion protein via direct inhibition of GATA1 transcription factor activity (Choi et al., 2006). However, expression of AML1/ETO does not lead to leukemia development in transplanted immunodeficient NOD/SCID mice, suggesting that additional genetic hits must occur for full-blown AML development. Similar results were obtained from analysis of the inv(16) fusion protein CBFB/MYH11. Expression of this fusion gene also caused enhanced proliferation and expansion of CD34+ cells over several months with retention of the engraftment potential in NOD/SCID mice. However, as also observed with AML1/ETO, transplanted mice do not develop leukemia (Wunderlich et al., 2006). Therefore, both oncogenes confer a preleukemic status and subsequent alterations are required for the transition to overt leukemia.

To decipher the genetic signature of AML, Abdul-Nabi and colleagues have assessed various AML-associated fusion proteins for their ability to enhance CD34+ cell expansion *ex vivo* and subsequently analyzed their gene expression profiles (Abdul-Nabi et al., 2010). In this study, experiments were also performed with gamma-retroviral vectors expressing the fusion genes AML1/ETO, PML/RARα, MLL/AF9 and NUP98/HOXA9 together with eGFP. To identify key target genes responsible for the expansion of CD34+ cells the authors performed gene array analysis of FACS-sorted eGFP+ cells expressing the indicated oncogenes, which identifies the induced and repressed target genes during the *ex vivo* selection process. One interesting candidate gene that was shown to be specifically upregulated due to both AML1/ETO and PML/RARα expression was the p53-inhibiting molecule MDM2. The authors could further show that activation of the gatekeeper protein p53, by blocking the MDM2-p53 protein-protein interaction with the small molecule compound Nutlin-3, was sufficient to completely block AML1/ETO induced selection and expansion of CD34+ progenitor cells. Therefore, Nutlin-3 is proposed to function as an inhibitor for AML1/ETO positive leukemias by reactivating p53 and consecutively eliminating the leukemic cells via the induction of apoptosis. Two independent groups have shown that retroviral expression of the NUP98/HOXA9 fusion gene, which is found in myelodysplastic syndrome (MDS) and AML patients, resulted in a similar outgrowth of transgene expressing cells with maintenance of self-renewal potential *ex vivo* and increased engraftment capacity in NOD/SCID mice (Chung et al., 2006; Takeda et al., 2006). This outgrowth was accompanied by high levels of HOX gene expression, a typical feature for this leukemia entity.

Regardless of their remarkable *ex vivo* cell expansion properties, the AML associated gene products described above, PML/RARα, FLT3-ITD, NUP98/HOXA9 and AML1/ETO, were not able to independently induce leukemia in transplanted NOD/SCID mice. Therefore, it is likely that additional genetic alterations are required for full cellular transformation in AML. In this regard it was shown that oncogenic RAS signaling, triggered by N-Ras^{G12D} overexpression, does increase AML1/ETO engraftment capacity in NOD/SCID mice but is still not sufficient to overcome the leukemia onset defect in the NOD/SCID mouse model (Chou et al., 2011).

Interestingly, MLL rearrangements are typically found in aggressive infant or therapy related leukemias (Aplan, 2006). In contrast to AML derived gene products, ectopic expression of either MLL/AF9 or MLL/ENL mixed-lineage leukemia fusion genes, as a single genetic event, results in the development of myeloid or lymphoid leukemias in the NOD/SCID mouse model approximately 100 days after transplantation (Barabe et al., 2007; Wei et al., 2008). Morphological analysis has revealed that AML and B-ALL leukemias are associated with both MLL rearrangements. Remarkably, *ex vivo* expanded cells gave rise to leukemia in NOD/SCID mice, even after 70 days of *in vitro* culture prior to transplantation in sublethally irradiated mice. The reasons for the striking differences between AML and

MLL fusion genes in their ability to induce leukemia onset in NOD/SCID mice are completely unknown. A direct comparison of deregulated genes may reveal which additional pathways are activated in MLL leukemic human CD34+ cells.

Recently, a report was published describing a true oncogenic cooperativeness in human CD34+ cell expansion and leukemia induction in NOD/SCID mice (Rizo et al., 2010). The authors convincingly have shown that retroviral co-expression of the CML associated oncogene, BCR/ABL, and the polycomb ring finger oncogene, BMI1, leads to leukemia induction within 4-5 months after transplantation. The isolated human leukemia cells were re-transplantable into secondary recipient mice, which induced leukemia with a shortened latency. *In vitro*, the co-expression of both oncogenes in human CD34+ cells allowed for the establishment of myeloid and lymphoid long-term cultures with self-renewing properties. This report also describes a series of valuable cell culture methods for *in vitro* analysis of CD34+ cell proliferation and self-renewal. Finally, the authors have demonstrated that retroviral introduction of BMI1 into primary leukemia cells from CML chronic-phase patients elevated the proliferative capacity and self-renewal properties of the leukemia cells, while shRNA knockdown of BMI1 in blast crisis CML cells completely blocked their proliferation potential. These results highlight BMI1 as an attractive molecular target for blast crisis CML cells, which is especially important given the rates of BCR/ABL positive leukemic stem cell resistance to kinase inhibitors such as imatinib (Corbin et al., 2011). However, the exact molecular mechanisms of BCR/ABL and BMI1 oncogenic co-operation have to be addressed in further studies.

In conclusion, human CD34+ blood progenitor cells represent a powerful cell biology tool used for the analysis of leukemogenic gene product activity. Methods of isolation and purification of CD34+ cells have significantly improved and are broadly available for researchers. The cells can be propagated *ex vivo* and oncogene activity can be analyzed for a wide range of biological parameters, including differentiation, proliferation, self-renewal, senescence and apoptosis, using standard cell biology methods. CD34+ suspension cells can be cultured *ex vivo* as liquid cultures or on stromal layer cells. With the possibility to transplant these cells into sublethally irradiated NOD/SCID mice this is an ideal model system to study the function of human leukemia-associated oncogenes.

5. Conclusions

Powerful retroviral expression vectors and standardized enrichment technologies, which are used for the isolation of hematopoietic precursor cells from the murine and human bone marrow compartment, efficiently enabled the accurate modeling of leukemia initiation and progression in the appropriate cell compartment. Currently available expression vectors allow for the simultaneous expression of several genes, including oncogenes, marker genes for detection and selection genes used to isolate modified cells, which represent practical tools for modeling leukemia progression in hematopoietic cells. Among the introduced strategies, the humanized mouse model based on human CD34+ precursor cell transplantation into NOD/SCID mice represents a credible model system to study human leukemia. As described here, the expression of single oncogenes such as BCR/ABL and AML1/ETO, which are primarily found in older patients, does not lead to leukemia development, implying that disease develops as a result of secondary mutations. In contrast, the expression of several MLL fusion proteins, which are typically found in younger patients, was found to be sufficient to trigger leukemia development with high penetrance.

In total, these approaches will lead to a better understanding of the genetic alterations that are required for the onset of cellular transformation. Furthermore, these studies have the potential to propel the development of effective drugs designed to eradicate leukemia cells.

6. Acknowledgement

The authors are supported by research grants from the NGFN Cancer Network (grant 01GS0450, TP-10), the Deutsche Krebshilfe (grant 102362, TP-7), the LEOWE OSF (TP-C3) and the LOEWE CGT (startup grant CW). The Georg-Speyer-Haus is supported by the Bundesministerium für Gesundheit and the Hessisches Ministerium für Wissenschaft und Kunst.

7. References

Abdul-Nabi, A.M.; Yassin, E.R.; Varghese, N.; Deshmukh, H. & Yaseen, N.R. (2010). In vitro transformation of primary human CD34+ cells by AML fusion oncogenes: early gene expression profiling reveals possible drug target in AML. *PLoS One*, Vol. 5, No. 8, pp. e12464

Adolfsson, J.; Borge, O.J.; Bryder, D.; Theilgaard-Monch, K.; Astrand-Grundstrom, I.; Sitnicka, E.; Sasaki, Y. & Jacobsen, S.E.W. (2001). Upregulation of flt3 expression within the bone marrow Lin(-)Sca1(+)c-kit(+) stem cell compartment is accompanied by loss of self-renewal capacity. *Immunity*, Vol. 15, No. 4, pp. 659-669

Aplan, P.D. (2006). Chromosomal translocations involving the MLL gene: molecular mechanisms. *DNA Repair (Amst)*, Vol. 5, No. 9-10, pp. 1265-1272

Banaszynski, L.A.; Chen, L.C.; Maynard-Smith, L.A.; Ooi, A.G.L. & Wandless, T.J. (2006). A rapid, reversible, and tunable method to regulate protein function in living cells using synthetic small molecules. *Cell*, Vol. 126, No. 5, pp. 995-1004

Barabe, F.; Kennedy, J.A.; Hope, K.J. & Dick, J.E. (2007). Modeling the initiation and progression of human acute leukemia in mice. *Science*, Vol. 316, No. 5824, pp. 600-604

Baum, C. (2007). Insertional mutagenesis in gene therapy and stem cell biology. *Current Opinion in Hematology*, Vol. 14, No. 4, pp. 337-342

Belvedere, O.; Feruglio, C.; Malangone, W.; Bonora, M.L.; Donini, A.; Dorotea, L.; Tonutti, E.; Rinaldi, C.; Pittino, M.; Baccarani, M.; Del Frate, G.; Biffoni, F.; Sala, P.; Hilbert, D.M. & Degrassi, A. (1999). Phenotypic characterization of immunomagnetically purified umbilical cord blood CD34+ cells. *Blood Cells Mol Dis*, Vol. 25, No. 3-4, pp. 141-146

Boissel, N.; Leroy, H.; Brethon, B.; Philippe, N.; de Botton, S.; Auvrignon, A.; Raffoux, E.; Leblanc, T.; Thomas, X.; Hermine, O.; Quesnel, B.; Baruchel, A.; Leverger, G.; Dombret, H. & Preudhomme, C. (2006). Incidence and prognostic impact of c-Kit, FLT3, and Ras gene mutations in core binding factor acute myeloid leukemia (CBF-AML). *Leukemia*, Vol. 20, No. 6, pp. 965-970

Brandts, C.H.; Berdel, W.E. & Serve, H. (2007). Oncogenic signaling in acute myeloid leukemia. *Curr Drug Targets*, Vol. 8, No. 2, pp. 237-246

Bursen, A.; Schwabe, K.; Ruster, B.; Henschler, R.; Ruthardt, M.; Dingermann, T. & Marschalek, R. (2010). The AF4.MLL fusion protein is capable of inducing ALL in mice without requirement of MLL.AF4. *Blood*, Vol. 115, No. 17, pp. 3570-3579

Challen, G.A.; Boles, N.; Lin, K.K.Y. & Goodell, M.A. (2009). Mouse Hematopoietic Stem Cell Identification and Analysis. *Cytometry Part A*, Vol. 75A, No. 1, pp. 14-24

Chen, G.Q.; Shi, X.G.; Tang, W.; Xiong, S.M.; Zhu, J.; Cai, X.; Han, Z.G.; Ni, J.H.; Shi, G.Y.; Jia, P.M.; Liu, M.M.; He, K.L.; Niu, C.; Ma, J.; Zhang, P.; Zhang, T.D.; Paul, P.; Naoe, T.; Kitamura, K.; Miller, W.; Waxman, S.; Wang, Z.Y.; de The, H.; Chen, S.J. & Chen, Z. (1997). Use of arsenic trioxide (As2O3) in the treatment of acute promyelocytic leukemia (APL): I. As2O3 exerts dose-dependent dual effects on APL cells. Blood, Vol. 89, No. 9, pp. 3345-3353

Choi, Y.; Elagib, K.E.; Delehanty, L.L. & Goldfarb, A.N. (2006). Erythroid inhibition by the leukemic fusion AML1-ETO is associated with impaired acetylation of the major erythroid transcription factor GATA-1. Cancer Res, Vol. 66, No. 6, pp. 2990-2996

Chou, F.S.; Wunderlich, M.; Griesinger, A. & Mulloy, J.C. (2011). N-Ras(G12D) induces features of stepwise transformation in preleukemic human umbilical cord blood cultures expressing the AML1-ETO fusion gene. Blood, Vol. 117, No. 7, pp. 2237-2240

Chung, K.Y.; Morrone, G.; Schuringa, J.J.; Plasilova, M.; Shieh, J.H.; Zhang, Y.; Zhou, P. & Moore, M.A. (2006). Enforced expression of NUP98-HOXA9 in human CD34(+) cells enhances stem cell proliferation. Cancer Res, Vol. 66, No. 24, pp. 11781-11791

Chung, K.Y.; Morrone, G.; Schuringa, J.J.; Wong, B.; Dorn, D.C. & Moore, M.A. (2005). Enforced expression of an Flt3 internal tandem duplication in human CD34+ cells confers properties of self-renewal and enhanced erythropoiesis. Blood, Vol. 105, No. 1, pp. 77-84

Clarke, C. & Davies, S. (2001). Immunomagnetic cell separation. Methods Mol Med, Vol. 58, No. pp. 17-23

Coffin, J.M.; Hughes, S.H. & Varmus, H.E. (2007). Retroviruses, Cold Spring Harbor Laboratory Press, ISBN-10: 0-87969-571-4, New York, USA

Corbin, A.S.; Agarwal, A.; Loriaux, M.; Cortes, J.; Deininger, M.W. & Druker, B.J. (2011). Human chronic myeloid leukemia stem cells are insensitive to imatinib despite inhibition of BCR-ABL activity. J Clin Invest, Vol. 121, No. 1, pp. 396-409

Dang, L.; White, D.W.; Gross, S.; Bennett, B.D.; Bittinger, M.A.; Driggers, E.M.; Fantin, V.R.; Jang, H.G.; Jin, S.; Keenan, M.C.; Marks, K.M.; Prins, R.M.; Ward, P.S.; Yen, K.E.; Liau, L.M.; Rabinowitz, J.D.; Cantley, L.C.; Thompson, C.B.; Vander Heiden, M.G. & Su, S.M. (2009). Cancer-associated IDH1 mutations produce 2-hydroxyglutarate. Nature, Vol. 462, No. 7274, pp. 739-744

de Felipe, P.; Martin, V.; Cortes, M.L.; Ryan, M. & Izquierdo, M. (1999). Use of the 2A sequence from foot-and-mouth disease virus in the generation of retroviral vectors for gene therapy. Gene Therapy, Vol. 6, No. 2, pp. 198-208

de Guzman, C.G.; Warren, A.J.; Zhang, Z.; Gartland, L.; Erickson, P.; Drabkin, H.; Hiebert, S.W. & Klug, C.A. (2002). Hematopoietic stem cell expansion and distinct myeloid developmental abnormalities in a murine model of the AML1-ETO translocation. Molecular and Cellular Biology, Vol. 22, No. 15, pp. 5506-5517

Demetri, G.D. (2002). Targeting the molecular pathophysiology of gastrointestinal stromal tumors with imatinib. Mechanisms, successes, and challenges to rational drug development. Hematol Oncol Clin North Am, Vol. 16, No. 5, pp. 1115-1124

Diamond, J.M. & Melo, J.V. (2011). Mechanisms of resistance to BCR-ABL kinase inhibitors. Leuk Lymphoma, Vol. 52 Suppl 1, No. pp. 12-22

Donnelly, M.L.; Luke, G.; Mehrotra, A.; Li, X.; Hughes, L.E.; Gani, D. & Ryan, M.D. (2001). Analysis of the aphthovirus 2A/2B polyprotein 'cleavage' mechanism indicates not a proteolytic reaction, but a novel translational effect: a putative ribosomal 'skip'. Journal of General Virology, Vol. 82, No. Pt 5, pp. 1013-1025

Druker, B.J.; Tamura, S.; Buchdunger, E.; Ohno, S.; Segal, G.M.; Fanning, S.; Zimmermann, J. & Lydon, N.B. (1996). Effects of a selective inhibitor of the Abl tyrosine kinase on the growth of Bcr-Abl positive cells. *Nat Med*, Vol. 2, No. 5, pp. 561-566

Estey, E. & Dohner, H. (2006). Acute myeloid leukaemia. *Lancet*, Vol. 368, No. 9550, pp. 1894-1907

Falini, B.; Martelli, M.P.; Bolli, N.; Sportoletti, P.; Liso, A.; Tiacci, E. & Haferlach, T. (2010). Acute myeloid leukemia with mutated nucleophosmin (NPM1): is it a distinct entity? *Blood*, Vol. 117, No. 4, pp. 1109-1120

Falini, B.; Nicoletti, I.; Martelli, M.F. & Mecucci, C. (2007). Acute myeloid leukemia carrying cytoplasmic/mutated nucleophosmin (NPMc+ AML): biologic and clinical features. *Blood*, Vol. 109, No. 3, pp. 874-885

Furness, S.G. & McNagny, K. (2006). Beyond mere markers: functions for CD34 family of sialomucins in hematopoiesis. *Immunol Res*, Vol. 34, No. 1, pp. 13-32

Gallardo, H.F.; Tan, C. & Sadelain, M. (1997). The internal ribosomal entry site of the encephalomyocarditis virus enables reliable coexpression of two transgenes in human primary T lymphocytes. *Gene Therapy*, Vol. 4, No. 10, pp. 1115-1119

Garcia-Manero, G.; Faderl, S.; O'Brien, S.; Cortes, J.; Talpaz, M. & Kantarjian, H.M. (2003). Chronic myelogenous leukemia: a review and update of therapeutic strategies. *Cancer*, Vol. 98, No. 3, pp. 437-457

Gilliland, D.G. & Griffin, J.D. (2002). Role of FLT3 in leukemia. *Curr Opin Hematol*, Vol. 9, No. 4, pp. 274-281

Gossen, M. & Bujard, H. (1992). Tight Control of Gene-Expression in Mammalian-Cells by Tetracycline-Responsive Promoters. *Proceedings of the National Academy of Sciences of the United States of America*, Vol. 89, No. 12, pp. 5547-5551

Gossen, M.; Freundlieb, S.; Bender, G.; Muller, G.; Hillen, W. & Bujard, H. (1995). Transcriptional Activation by Tetracyclines in Mammalian-Cells. *Science*, Vol. 268, No. 5218, pp. 1766-1769

Grignani, F.; Valtieri, M.; Gabbianelli, M.; Gelmetti, V.; Botta, R.; Luchetti, L.; Masella, B.; Morsilli, O.; Pelosi, E.; Samoggia, P.; Pelicci, P.G. & Peschle, C. (2000). PML/RAR alpha fusion protein expression in normal human hematopoietic progenitors dictates myeloid commitment and the promyelocytic phenotype. *Blood*, Vol. 96, No. 4, pp. 1531-1537

Grisendi, S.; Mecucci, C.; Falini, B. & Pandolfi, P.P. (2006). Nucleophosmin and cancer. *Nat Rev Cancer*, Vol. 6, No. 7, pp. 493-505

Hahn, W.C.; Counter, C.M.; Lundberg, A.S.; Beijersbergen, R.L.; Brooks, M.W. & Weinberg, R.A. (1999). Creation of human tumour cells with defined genetic elements. *Nature*, Vol. 400, No. 6743, pp. 464-468

Hanahan, D. & Weinberg, R.A. (2000). The hallmarks of cancer. *Cell*, Vol. 100, No. 1, pp. 57-70

Hanahan, D. & Weinberg, R.A. (2011). Hallmarks of cancer: the next generation. *Cell*, Vol. 144, No. 5, pp. 646-674

Hanenberg, H.; Xiao, X.L.; Dilloo, D.; Hashino, K.; Kato, I. & Williams, D.A. (1996). Colocalization of retrovirus and target cells on specific fibronectin fragments increases genetic transduction of mammalian cells. *Nature Medicine*, Vol. 2, No. 8, pp. 876-882

Hao, Q.L.; Shah, A.J.; Thiemann, F.T.; Smogorzewska, E.M. & Crooks, G.M. (1995). A functional comparison of CD34 + CD38- cells in cord blood and bone marrow. *Blood*, Vol. 86, No. 10, pp. 3745-3753

Hawley, R.G.; Lieu, F.H.L.; Fong, A.Z.C. & Hawley, T.S. (1994). Versatile Retroviral Vectors for Potential Use in Gene-Therapy. *Gene Therapy*, Vol. 1, No. 2, pp. 136-138

Heinz, N.; Schambach, A.; Galla, M.; Maetzig, T.; Baum, C.; Loew, R. & Schiedlmeier, B. (2011). Retroviral and Transposon-Based Tet-Regulated All-In-One Vectors with Reduced Background Expression and Improved Dynamic Range. *Human Gene Therapy*, Vol. 22, No. 2, pp. 166-176

Hoelbl, A.; Schuster, C.; Kovacic, B.; Zhu, B.; Wickre, M.; Hoelzl, M.A.; Fajmann, S.; Grebien, F.; Warsch, W.; Stengl, G.; Hennighausen, L.; Poli, V.; Beug, H.; Moriggl, R. & Sexl, V. (2010). Stat5 is indispensable for the maintenance of bcr/abl-positive leukaemia. *EMBO Mol Med*, Vol. 2, No. 3, pp. 98-110

Holyoake, T.; Jiang, X.; Eaves, C. & Eaves, A. (1999). Isolation of a highly quiescent subpopulation of primitive leukemic cells in chronic myeloid leukemia. *Blood*,Vol. 94, No. 6, pp. 2056-2064

Huang, M.E.; Ye, Y.C.; Chen, S.R.; Chai, J.R.; Lu, J.X.; Zhoa, L.; Gu, L.J. & Wang, Z.Y. (1988). Use of all-trans retinoic acid in the treatment of acute promyelocytic leukemia. *Blood*, Vol. 72, No. 2, pp. 567-572

Ito, M.; Hiramatsu, H.; Kobayashi, K.; Suzue, K.; Kawahata, M.; Hioki, K.; Ueyama, Y.; Koyanagi, Y.; Sugamura, K.; Tsuji, K.; Heike, T. & Nakahata, T. (2002). NOD/SCID/gamma(c)(null) mouse: an excellent recipient mouse model for engraftment of human cells. *Blood*, Vol. 100, No. 9, pp. 3175-3182

Kanbe, E. & Zhang, D.E. (2004). A simple and quick method to concentrate MSCV retrovirus. *Blood Cells Molecules and Diseases*, Vol. 33, No. 1, pp. 64-67

Kiel, M.J.; Yilmaz, O.H.; Iwashita, T.; Terhorst, C. & Morrison, S.J. (2005). SLAM family receptors distinguish hematopoietic stem and progenitor cells and reveal endothelial niches for stem cells. *Cell*, Vol. 121, No. 7, pp. 1109-1121

Kinjo, K.; Kizaki, M.; Muto, A.; Fukuchi, Y.; Umezawa, A.; Yamato, K.; Nishihara, T.; Hata, J.; Ito, M.; Ueyama, Y. & Ikeda, Y. (2000). Arsenic trioxide (As2O3)-induced apoptosis and differentiation in retinoic acid-resistant acute promyelocytic leukemia model in hGM-CSF-producing transgenic SCID mice. *Leukemia*, Vol. 14, No. 3, pp. 431-438

Kinzler, K.W. & Vogelstein, B. (1996). Lessons from hereditary colorectal cancer. *Cell*, Vol. 87, No. 2, pp. 159-170

Kogan, S.C.; Ward, J.M.; Anver, M.R.; Berman, J.J.; Brayton, C.; Cardiff, R.D.; Carter, J.S.; de Coronado, S.; Downing, J.R.; Fredrickson, T.N.; Haines, D.C.; Harris, A.W.; Harris, N.L.; Hiai, H.; Jaffe, E.S.; MacLennan, I.C.; Pandolfi, P.P.; Pattengale, P.K.; Perkins, A.S.; Simpson, R.M.; Tuttle, M.S.; Wong, J.F. & Morse, H.C., 3rd. (2002). Bethesda proposals for classification of nonlymphoid hematopoietic neoplasms in mice. *Blood*, Vol. 100, No. 1, pp. 238-245

Kohn, D.B.; Kantoff, P.W.; Eglitis, M.A.; McLachlin, J.R.; Moen, R.C.; Karson, E.; Zwiebel, J.A.; Nienhuis, A.; Karlsson, S.; O'Reilly, R. & et al. (1987). Retroviral-mediated gene transfer into mammalian cells. *Blood Cells*, Vol. 13, No. 1-2, pp. 285-298

Kwok, C.; Zeisig, B.B.; Qiu, J.H.; Dong, S.O. & So, C.W.E. (2009). Transforming activity of AML1-ETO is independent of CBF beta and ETO interaction but requires formation of homo-oligomeric complexes. *Proceedings of the National Academy of Sciences of the United States of America*, Vol. 106, No. 8, pp. 2853-2858

Larochelle, A.; Vormoor, J.; Lapidot, T.; Sher, G.; Furukawa, T.; Li, Q.; Shultz, L.D.; Olivieri, N.F.; Stamatoyannopoulos, G. & Dick, J.E. (1995). Engraftment of immune-deficient mice with primitive hematopoietic cells from beta-thalassemia and sickle cell anemia patients: implications for evaluating human gene therapy protocols. *Hum Mol Genet*, Vol. 4, No. 2, pp. 163-172

Lewis, P.; Hensel, M. & Emerman, M. (1992). Human-Immunodeficiency-Virus Infection of Cells Arrested in the Cell-Cycle. *Embo Journal*, Vol. 11, No. 8, pp. 3053-3058

Lewis, P.F. & Emerman, M. (1994). Passage through Mitosis Is Required for Oncoretroviruses but Not for the Human-Immunodeficiency-Virus. *Journal of Virology*, Vol. 68, No. 1, pp. 510-516

Liu, Y.; Cheney, M.D.; Gaudet, J.J.; Chruszcz, M.; Lukasik, S.M.; Sugiyama, D.; Lary, J.; Cole, J.; Dauter, Z.; Minor, W.; Speck, N.A. & Bushweller, J.H. (2006). The tetramer structure of the Nervy homology two domain, NHR2, is critical for AML1/ETO's activity. *Cancer Cell*, Vol. 9, No. 4, pp. 249-260

Look, A.T. (1997). Oncogenic transcription factors in the human acute leukemias. *Science*, Vol. 278, No. 5340, pp. 1059-1064

Mardis, E.R.; Ding, L.; Dooling, D.J.; Larson, D.E.; McLellan, M.D.; Chen, K.; Koboldt, D.C.; Fulton, R.S.; Delehaunty, K.D.; McGrath, S.D.; Fulton, L.A.; Locke, D.P.; Magrini, V.J.; Abbott, R.M.; Vickery, T.L.; Reed, J.S.; Robinson, J.S.; Wylie, T.; Smith, S.M.; Carmichael, L.; Eldred, J.M.; Harris, C.C.; Walker, J.; Peck, J.B.; Du, F.; Dukes, A.F.; Sanderson, G.E.; Brummett, A.M.; Clark, E.; McMichael, J.F.; Meyer, R.J.; Schindler, J.K.; Pohl, C.S.; Wallis, J.W.; Shi, X.; Lin, L.; Schmidt, H.; Tang, Y.; Haipek, C.; Wiechert, M.E.; Ivy, J.V.; Kalicki, J.; Elliott, G.; Ries, R.E.; Payton, J.E.; Westervelt, P.; Tomasson, M.H.; Watson, M.A.; Baty, J.; Heath, S.; Shannon, W.D.; Nagarajan, R.; Link, D.C.; Walter, M.J.; Graubert, T.A.; DiPersio, J.F.; Wilson, R.K. & Ley, T.J.(2009). Recurring mutations found by sequencing an acute myeloid leukemia genome. *N Engl J Med*, Vol. 361, No. 11, pp. 1058-1066

Matrai, J.; Chuah, M.K.L. & VandenDriessche, T. (2010). Recent Advances in Lentiviral Vector Development and Applications (vol 18, pg 477, 2010). *Molecular Therapy*, Vol. 18, No. 5, pp. 1055-1055

Melo, J.V. & Barnes, D.J. (2007). Chronic myeloid leukaemia as a model of disease evolution in human cancer. *Nat Rev Cancer*, Vol. 7, No. 6, pp. 441-453

Meshinchi, S.; Woods, W.G.; Stirewalt, D.L.; Sweetser, D.A.; Buckley, J.D.; Tjoa, T.K.; Bernstein, I.D. & Radich, J.P. (2001). Prevalence and prognostic significance of Flt3 internal tandem duplication in pediatric acute myeloid leukemia. *Blood*, Vol. 97, No. 1, pp. 89-94

Minucci, S.; Monestiroli, S.; Giavara, S.; Ronzoni, S.; Marchesi, F.; Insinga, A.; Diverio, D.; Gasparini, P.; Capillo, M.; Colombo, E.; Matteucci, C.; Contegno, F.; Lo-Coco, F.; Scanziani, E.; Gobbi, A. & Pelicci, P.G. (2002). PML-RAR induces promyelocytic leukemias with high efficiency following retroviral gene transfer into purified murine hematopoietic progenitors. *Blood*, Vol. 100, No. 8, pp. 2989-2995

Mizuguchi, H.; Xu, Z.L.; Ishii-Watabe, A.; Uchida, E. & Hayakawa, T. (2000). IRES-dependent second gene expression is significantly lower than cap-dependent first gene expression in a bicistronic vector. *Molecular Therapy*, Vol. 1, No. 4, pp. 376-382

Morrison, S.J. & Weissman, I.L. (1994). The Long-Term Repopulating Subset of Hematopoietic Stem-Cells Is Deterministic and Isolatable by Phenotype. *Immunity*, Vol. 1, No. 8, pp. 661-673

Mountford, P.S. & Smith, A.G. (1995). Internal Ribosome Entry Sites and Dicistronic Rnas in Mammalian Transgenesis. *Trends in Genetics*, Vol. 11, No. 5, pp. 179-184

Mulloy, J.C.; Cammenga, J.; Berguido, F.J.; Wu, K.; Zhou, P.; Comenzo, R.L.; Jhanwar, S.; Moore, M.A. & Nimer, S.D. (2003). Maintaining the self-renewal and differentiation potential of human CD34+ hematopoietic cells using a single genetic element. *Blood*, Vol. 102, No. 13, pp. 4369-4376

Mulloy, J.C.; Cammenga, J.; MacKenzie, K.L.; Berguido, F.J.; Moore, M.A. & Nimer, S.D. (2002). The AML1-ETO fusion protein promotes the expansion of human hematopoietic stem cells. *Blood*, Vol. 99, No. 1, pp. 15-23

Naldini, L.; Blomer, U.; Gallay, P.; Ory, D.; Mulligan, R.; Gage, F.H.; Verma, I.M. & Trono, D. (1996). In vivo gene delivery and stable transduction of nondividing cells by a lentiviral vector. *Science*, Vol. 272, No. 5259, pp. 263-267

Naldini, L.; Montini, E.; Cesana, D.; Schmidt, M.; Sanvito, F.; Ponzoni, M.; Bartholomae, C.; Sergi, L.S.; Benedicenti, F.; Ambrosi, A.; Di Serio, C.; Doglioni, C. & von Kalle, C. (2006). Hematopoietic stem cell gene transfer in a tumor-prone mouse model uncovers low genotoxicity of lentiviral vector integration. *Nature Biotechnology*, Vol. 24, No. 6, pp. 687-696

Niebuhr, B.; Fischer, M.; Tager, M.; Cammenga, J. & Stocking, C. (2008). Gatekeeper function of the RUNX1 transcription factor in acute leukemia. *Blood Cells Mol Dis*, Vol. 40, No. 2, pp. 211-218

Okada, S.; Nakauchi, H.; Nagayoshi, K.; Nishikawa, S.; Miura, Y. & Suda, T. (1992). In vivo and in vitro stem cell function of c-kit- and Sca-1-positive murine hematopoietic cells. *Blood*, Vol. 80, No. 12, pp. 3044-3050

Osawa, M.; Hanada, K.; Hamada, H. & Nakauchi, H. (1996). Long-term lymphohematopoietic reconstitution by a single CD34-low/negative hematopoietic stem cell. *Science*, Vol. 273, No. 5272, pp. 242-245

Paschka, P.; Marcucci, G.; Ruppert, A.S.; Mrozek, K.; Chen, H.; Kittles, R.A.; Vukosavljevic, T.; Perrotti, D.; Vardiman, J.W.; Carroll, A.J.; Kolitz, J.E.; Larson, R.A. & Bloomfield, C.D. (2006). Adverse prognostic significance of KIT mutations in adult acute myeloid leukemia with inv(16) and t(8;21): a Cancer and Leukemia Group B Study. *J Clin Oncol*, Vol. 24, No. 24, pp. 3904-3911

Paschka, P.; Schlenk, R.F.; Gaidzik, V.I.; Habdank, M.; Kronke, J.; Bullinger, L.; Spath, D.; Kayser, S.; Zucknick, M.; Gotze, K.; Horst, H.A.; Germing, U.; Dohner, H. & Dohner, K. (2010). IDH1 and IDH2 mutations are frequent genetic alterations in acute myeloid leukemia and confer adverse prognosis in cytogenetically normal acute myeloid leukemia with NPM1 mutation without FLT3 internal tandem duplication. *J Clin Oncol*, Vol. 28, No. 22, pp. 3636-3643

Puccetti, E. & Ruthardt, M. (2004). Acute promyelocytic leukemia: PML/RARalpha and the leukemic stem cell. *Leukemia*, Vol. 18, No. 7, pp. 1169-1175

Rangarajan, A. & Weinberg, R.A. (2003). Opinion: Comparative biology of mouse versus human cells: modelling human cancer in mice. *Nat Rev Cancer*, Vol. 3, No. 12, pp. 952-959

Rego, E.M.; He, L.Z.; Warrell, R.P.; Wang, Z.G. & Pandolfi, P.P. (2000). Retinoic acid (RA) and As2O3 treatment in transgenic models of acute promyelocytic leukemia (APL) unravel the distinct nature of the leukemogenic process induced by the PML-RAR alpha and PLZF-RAR alpha oncoproteins. *Proceedings of the National Academy of Sciences of the United States of America*, Vol. 97, No. 18, pp. 10173-10178

Rhoades, K.L.; Hetherington, C.J.; Harakawa, N.; Yergeau, D.A.; Zhou, L.; Liu, L.Q.; Little, M.T.; Tenen, D.G. & Zhang, D.E. (2000). Analysis of the role of AML1-ETO in leukemogenesis, using an inducible transgenic mouse model. *Blood*, Vol. 96, No. 6, pp. 2108-2115

Rizo, A.; Horton, S.J.; Olthof, S.; Dontje, B.; Ausema, A.; van Os, R.; van den Boom, V.; Vellenga, E.; de Haan, G. & Schuringa, J.J. (2010). BMI1 collaborates with BCR-ABL in leukemic transformation of human CD34+ cells. *Blood*, Vol. 116, No. 22, pp. 4621-4630

Robinson, C.R. & Sauer, R.T. (1998). Optimizing the stability of single-chain proteins by linker length and composition mutagenesis. *Proc Natl Acad Sci U S A*, Vol. 95, No. 11, pp. 5929-5934

Roe, T.Y.; Reynolds, T.C.; Yu, G. & Brown, P.O. (1993). Integration of Murine Leukemia-Virus DNA Depends on Mitosis. *Embo Journal*, Vol. 12, No. 5, pp. 2099-2108

Ryan, M.D.; King, A.M.Q. & Thomas, G.P. (1991). Cleavage of Foot-and-Mouth-Disease Virus Polyprotein Is Mediated by Residues Located within a 19 Amino-Acid-Sequence. *Journal of General Virology*, Vol. 72, No. pp. 2727-2732

Sawyers, C.L. (1999). Chronic myeloid leukemia. *N Engl J Med*, Vol. 340, No. 17, pp. 1330-1340

Sawyers, C.L.; Hochhaus, A.; Feldman, E.; Goldman, J.M.; Miller, C.B.; Ottmann, O.G.; Schiffer, C.A.; Talpaz, M.; Guilhot, F.; Deininger, M.W.; Fischer, T.; O'Brien, S.G.; Stone, R.M.; Gambacorti-Passerini, C.B.; Russell, N.H.; Reiffers, J.J.; Shea, T.C.; Chapuis, B.; Coutre, S.; Tura, S.; Morra, E.; Larson, R.A.; Saven, A.; Peschel, C.; Gratwohl, A.; Mandelli, F.; Ben-Am, M.; Gathmann, I.; Capdeville, R.; Paquette, R.L. & Druker, B.J. (2002). Imatinib induces hematologic and cytogenetic responses in patients with chronic myelogenous leukemia in myeloid blast crisis: results of a phase II study. *Blood*, Vol. 99, No. 10, pp. 3530-3539

Schnittger, S.; Dicker, F.; Kern, W.; Wendland, N.; Sundermann, J.; Alpermann, T.; Haferlach, C. & Haferlach, T. (2011). RUNX1 mutations are frequent in de novo AML with noncomplex karyotype and confer an unfavorable prognosis. *Blood*, Vol. 117, No. 8, pp. 2348-2357

Schuringa, J.J.; van den Boom, V. & Horton, S.J. (2010). *Genetic & Epigenetic Alterations That Drive Leukemic Stem Cell Self-Renewal*, Nova Science Publishers Inc, ISBN 978-1-61728-379-6, New York, USA

Song, J.; Mercer, D.; Hu, X.; Liu, H. & Li, M.M. (2011). Common leukemia- and lymphoma-associated genetic aberrations in healthy individuals. *J Mol Diagn*, Vol. 13, No. 2, pp. 213-219

Szilvassy, S.J.; Bass, M.J.; Van Zant, G. & Grimes, B. (1999). Organ-selective homing defines engraftment kinetics of murine hematopoietic stem cells and is compromised by ex vivo expansion. *Blood*, Vol. 93, No. 5, pp. 1557-1566

Szymczak, A.L.; Workman, C.J.; Wang, Y.; Vignali, K.M.; Dilioglou, S.; Vanin, E.F. & Vignali, D.A. (2004). Correction of multi-gene deficiency in vivo using a single 'self-cleaving' 2A peptide-based retroviral vector. *Nature Biotechnology*, Vol. 22, No. 5, pp. 589-594

Takeda, A.; Goolsby, C. & Yaseen, N.R. (2006). NUP98-HOXA9 induces long-term proliferation and blocks differentiation of primary human CD34+ hematopoietic cells. *Cancer Res*, Vol. 66, No. 13, pp. 6628-6637

Terpe, K. (2003). Overview of tag protein fusions: from molecular and biochemical fundamentals to commercial systems. *Applied Microbiology and Biotechnology*, Vol. 60, No. 5, pp. 523-533

Trumpp, A. & Wiestler, O.D. (2008). Mechanisms of Disease: cancer stem cells--targeting the evil twin. *Nat Clin Pract Oncol*, Vol. 5, No. 6, pp. 337-347

Weber, K. (2007). Homepage of the Lentiviral Gene Ontology Vectors, Available from: http://www.lentigo-vectors.de/vectors.htm

Weber, K.; Bartsch, U.; Stocking, C. & Fehse, B. (2008). A multicolor panel of novel lentiviral " gene ontology" (LeGO) vectors for functional gene analysis. *Molecular Therapy*, Vol. 16, No. 4, pp. 698-706

Weber, K.; Mock, U.; Petrowitz, B.; Bartsch, U. & Fehse, B. (2010). Lentiviral gene ontology (LeGO) vectors equipped with novel drug-selectable fluorescent proteins: new building blocks for cell marking and multi-gene analysis. *Gene Therapy*, Vol. 17, No. 4, pp. 511-520

Wei, J.; Wunderlich, M.; Fox, C.; Alvarez, S.; Cigudosa, J.C.; Wilhelm, J.S.; Zheng, Y.; Cancelas, J.A.; Gu, Y.; Jansen, M.; Dimartino, J.F. & Mulloy, J.C. (2008). Microenvironment determines lineage fate in a human model of MLL-AF9 leukemia. *Cancer Cell*, Vol. 13, No. 6, pp. 483-495

Wichmann, C.; Becker, Y.; Chen-Wichmann, L.; Vogel, V.; Vojtkova, A.; Herglotz, J.; Moore, S.; Koch, J.; Lausen, J.; Mantele, W.; Gohlke, H. & Grez, M. (2010). Dimer-tetramer transition controls RUNX1/ETO leukemogenic activity. *Blood*, Vol. 116, No. 4, pp. 603-613

Wiernik, P.H. (2010). FLT3 inhibitors for the treatment of acute myeloid leukemia. *Clin Adv Hematol Oncol*, Vol. 8, No. 6, pp. 429-436, 444

Wu, X.L.; Li, Y.; Crise, B. & Burgess, S.M. (2003). Transcription start regions in the human genome are favored targets for MLV integration. *Science*, Vol. 300, No. 5626, pp. 1749-1751

Wunderlich, M.; Krejci, O.; Wei, J. & Mulloy, J.C. (2006). Human CD34+ cells expressing the inv(16) fusion protein exhibit a myelomonocytic phenotype with greatly enhanced proliferative ability. *Blood*, Vol. 108, No. 5, pp. 1690-1697

Xu, W.; Yang, H.; Liu, Y.; Yang, Y.; Wang, P.; Kim, S.H.; Ito, S.; Yang, C.; Wang, P.; Xiao, M.T.; Liu, L.X.; Jiang, W.Q.; Liu, J.; Zhang, J.Y.; Wang, B.; Frye, S.; Zhang, Y.; Xu, Y.H.; Lei, Q.Y.; Guan, K.L.; Zhao, S.M. & Xiong, Y. (2011). Oncometabolite 2-hydroxyglutarate is a competitive inhibitor of alpha-ketoglutarate-dependent dioxygenases. *Cancer Cell*, Vol. 19, No. 1, pp. 17-30

Yan, M.; Burel, S.A.; Peterson, L.F.; Kanbe, E.; Iwasaki, H.; Boyapati, A.; Hines, R.; Akashi, K. & Zhang, D.E. (2004). Deletion of an AML1-ETO C-terminal NcoR/SMRT-interacting region strongly induces leukemia development. *Proc Natl Acad Sci U S A*, Vol. 101, No. 49, pp. 17186-17191

Yan, M.; Kanbe, E.; Peterson, L.F.; Boyapati, A.; Miao, Y.; Wang, Y.; Chen, I.M.; Chen, Z.; Rowley, J.D.; Willman, C.L. & Zhang, D.E. (2006). A previously unidentified alternatively spliced isoform of t(8;21) transcript promotes leukemogenesis. *Nat Med*, Vol. 12, No. 8, pp. 945-949

Yang, L.; Bryder, D.; Adolfsson, J.; Nygren, J.; Mansson, R.; Sigvardsson, M. & Jacobsen, S.E. (2005). Identification of Lin(-)Sca1(+)kit(+)CD34(+)Flt3- short-term hematopoietic stem cells capable of rapidly reconstituting and rescuing myeloablated transplant recipients. *Blood*, Vol. 105, No. 7, pp. 2717-2723

Yu, S.F.; Vonruden, T.; Kantoff, P.W.; Garber, C.; Seiberg, M.; Ruther, U.; Anderson, W.F.; Wagner, E.F. & Gilboa, E. (1986). Self-Inactivating Retroviral Vectors Designed for Transfer of Whole Genes into Mammalian-Cells. *Proceedings of the National Academy of Sciences of the United States of America*, Vol. 83, No. 10, pp. 3194-3198

Zhang, X.W.; Yan, X.J.; Zhou, Z.R.; Yang, F.F.; Wu Z.Y.; Sun, H.B.; Liang, W.X.; Song, A.X.; Lallemand-Breitenbach, V.; Jeanne, M.; Zhang, Q.Y.; Yang, H.Y.; Huang, Q.H.; Zhou, G.B.; Tong, J.H.; Zhang, Y.; Wu, J.H.; Hu, H.Y.; de Thé, H.; Chen, S.J. & Chen, Z. (2010). Arsenic trioxide controls the fate of the PML-RAR alpha oncoprotein by directly binding PML (vol 328, pg 240, 2010). *Science*, Vol. 328, No. 5981, pp. 974-974

4

New Molecular Markers in Acute Myeloid Leukemia

Silvia de la Iglesia Iñigo[1], María Teresa Gómez Casares[1],
Carmen Elsa López Jorge[1,2], Jezabel López Brito[1]
and Pedro Martin Cabrera[3]
[1]Servicio de Hematología, Hospital de Gran Canaria Doctor Negrín,
Las Palmas de GranCanaria
[2]Unit Research, Hospital de Gran Canaria Doctor Negrín,
Las Palmas de GranCanaria
[3]Secció de Citologia Hematològica, Servei d'Anatomia Patològica
Hospital Universitari de Bellvitge,
Barcelona,
Spain

1. Introduction

Acute leukemia is characterized by abnormal proliferation, inhibition of differentiation and expansion of leukemic cells blocked at the early stage of hematopoiesis. Acute myeloid leukemia (AML) is a malignant hematological disease of hematopoietic precursor cells of non-lymphoid lineage. Recent insights into the molecular mechanisms of AML are challenging the traditional diagnostic classification, prognostic significance and clinical practice of this hematological disorder.

1.1 Concept and classification

AML is a clinically heterogeneous disorder with distinct clinical and biological features. Until the 1970s, diagnosis was based on morphological examination of bone marrow and peripheral blood samples. In 1976, French, American, and British hematologists (the FAB group) defined six subgroups of AML morphological variants (Bennett et al., French-American-British Cooperative Group [FAB], 1976). This classification allowed us to identify several types of AML: M1-M6. Blastic populations were identified using standard staining techniques and consequently classified depending on reactivity to certain cytochemicals, namely, myeloperoxidase and Sudan black B (markers of myeloid differentiation) and nonspecific esterase reactions such as alpha-naphthyl acetate esterase and alpha-naphthyl butyrate esterase (for monocytic lineage). Later on, this group identified two new types of AML (M0 and M7) according to cytochemical and inmunophenotypical features (Bennett et al., FAB, 1985). Over the past decade, refinement in the diagnosis of subtypes of AML and advances in therapeutic approaches have improved the outlook for patients with AML (Döhner et al., 2010).

FAB classification
M0: AML minimally differentiated
M1: AML without maturation
M2: AML with maturation
M3: Acute promyelocytic leukemia
M4: Acute myelomonocytic leukemia
M5: Acute monoblastic leukemia
M6: Acute erythroleukemia
M7: Acute megakaryoblastic leukemia

Table 1. FAB classification of acute myeloid leukemia (AML).

Since several specific cytogenetic and genetic abnormalities in AML are associated with a characteristic morphology and have distinctive clinical behavior (Harris et al., World Health Organization [WHO], 1999). The World Health Organization (WHO), classification of myeloid neoplasms and acute leukemias integrates genetic, clinical data, and morphological features.

Three prognostic groups have been described classically according to cytogenetic findings. The favorable prognostic group includes the following chromosomal abnormalities: t(15;17), t(8;21) and inv(16). Normal karyotype and cytogenetic abnormalities not classified as favorable or adverse comprise the intermediate group. The adverse prognosis group includes patients with complex karyotype, del (5q), 5 or 7 monosomy, 3q abnormalities and t(6;9) (Dohner et al., 2010).

Recently the WHO published a revised and updated edition of the 1998 WHO classification where the importance of gene mutations as diagnostic and prognostic markers in myeloid neoplasms was acknowledged. This group recommended that fluorescence in situ hybridization (FISH), reverse transcriptase–polymerase chain reaction (RT-PCR) and mutational status studies should be guided through clinical, laboratory, and morphologic information. Mutational studies for mutated *NPM1, CEBPA, FLT3, KIT, WT1,* and *MLL* are recommended in all cytogenetically normal AML. Table 2 lists the major subgroups of AML in the WHO classification (WHO, 2009).

The genes involved in the pathogenesis of leukemia are normal genes (proto-oncogenes) with either structural alterations or deregulated expression patterns, which generates in turn a novel gene (an oncogene) whose protein product acts on the host cell to enhance malignancy-related characteristics. Oncogene activation and the loss of tumor-suppressor genes are consistently associated with some types of leukemia (Cline, 1994). Some of the molecular alterations involved in the pathogenesis of AML are: translocations, mutations and overexpression of normal genes, which often characterizes a particular subtype of AML. Therefore, there are also activating mutations which lead to increased proliferation or survival, or both, of haematopoietic progenitor cells through the stimulation of tyrosine kinases such as FLT3 or RAS family members. These are considered class I mutations (Haferlach et al., 2007; Schlenk et al., 2008). Class II mutations interfere with transcription and lead to a maturation arrest either through a direct alteration of transcription factors due to gene fusions (CBF-leukemias or PML-RARA positive leukemia) or by indirect interference with transcription (MLL-rearrangements). Cytogenetic and molecular analysis of leukemic blasts, provide critical diagnostic, therapeutic and prognostic information.

Acute myeloid leukemia with recurrent genetic abnormalities
AML with t(8;21)(q22;q22); *RUNX1-RUNX1T1*
AML with inv(16)(p13.1q22) or t(16;16)(p13.1;q22); *CBFB-MYH11*
APL with t(15;17)(q22;q12); *PML-RARA*
AML with t(9;11)(p22;q23); *MLLT3-MLL*
AML with t(6;9)(p23;q34); *DEK-NUP214*
AML with inv(3)(q21q26.2) or t(3;3)(q21;q26.2); *RPN1-EVI1*
AML (megakaryoblastic) with t(1;22)(p13;q13); *RBM15-MKL1*
Provisional entity: AML with mutated NPM1
Provisional entity: AML with mutated CEBPA
Acute myeloid leukemia with myelodysplasia-related changes
Therapy-related myeloid neoplasms
Acute myeloid leukemia, not otherwise specified
AML with minimal differentiation
AML without maturation
AML with maturation
Acute myelomonocytic leukemia
Acute monoblastic/monocytic leukemia
Acute erythroid leukemia
Pure erythroid leukemia
Erythroleukemia, erythroid/myeloid
Acute megakaryoblastic leukemia
Acute basophilic leukemia
Acute panmyelosis with myelofibrosis
Myeloid sarcoma
Myeloid proliferations related to Down syndrome
Transient abnormal myelopoiesis
Myeloid leukemia associated with Down syndrome
Blastic plasmacytoid dendritic cell neoplasm

Table 2. WHO classification of acute myeloid leukemia and related neoplasms.

1.2 Molecular markers
1.2.1 Useful at diagnosis and to evaluate Minimal Residual Disease (MRD)

Molecular techniques allow us to diagnose and classify AML, establishing groups of patients with different disease behaviour and prognosis. In the same way, the development of more specific therapies and the application of risk-adjusted therapeutic approaches have been made possible. Disease relapse can be favored by persistent low numbers of leukemic cells undetectable by conventional techniques. Monitoring of AML patients has given rise to a higher insight into the effectiveness of treatment. At diagnosis, some types of myeloid leukemias display a molecular change that might be useful as a marker of neoplastic disease and MRD (Hilden et al., 1995; Nakao et al., 1996; Foroni et al., 1999; Lo Coco et al., 1999a). Specific molecular alterations of certain hematologic malignancies are useful in the detection of MRD. Translocations are the most widely involved chromosomal abnormalities in AML. These can give rise to an altered function or activity of oncogenes located at or near the translocated breakpoint. The first molecular cytogenetic marker described in AML was t(15;17), which originates a single morphologic phenotype (hyper- or micro-granular French-American-British [FAB] AML-M3 acute myeloid leukemia) (Bernstein et al., 1980). This rearrangement disappears with complete remission and is able to predict a relapse very accurately. The presence of this translocation or its fusion gene (PML/ RARα) is thus a detectable tumor marker in leukemic cells, which allows assessment of the molecular response to therapy in AML-M3 patients (Lo Coco et al., 1999b). *RUNX1-RUNX1T1* and CBFβ-MYH11 are other genetic alterations less likely to predict relapse, since they may persist even when complete remission (CR) has been achieved. However, the applicability of this strategy has been limited to those leukemia subsets characterized by genetic markers. Recent interest has focused on identifying new molecular markers that might prove significant in the diagnosis and follow-up of MRD in AML patients. In recent years, a variety ot potential molecular markers have been identified (see table 2 and table 3) (Radich & Thomson, 1997; Inoue et al., 1994; Kreuzer et al., 2001; Alberta et al., 2003; Lin et al., 2005; Gilliland & Griffin, 2002; Morishita et al., 1992).

Involvement of transcription				
	Prevalence	Prognostic value	Associated mutations	Utility in MRD
CBF-leukemias: Inv 16/t(16;16) CBFB/MYH11 t(8;21);*RUNX1-RUNX1T1*	15%	Favorable (Poor with KIT in normal karyotype leukemia)	FLT3 NRAS KIT	Possible
PML-RARA	10-15%	Favorable	FLT3 (40%)	Yes
MLL mutation	10-30%	Poor	-	Yes
CEBPA mutation	15-20%	Favorable if biallelic	-	Yes
AML1 mutation	1-20%	Poor	FLT3 (in 20% M0)	Yes
Activating mutations				
FLT3-ITD mutation	28-34%	Poor		Possible
FLT3-TKD mutation	20-30%	Controversial	CBF, NPM1	
c-KIT mutation	6-48%	Poor	CBF-leukemias	Yes
RAS mutation	NRAS 11% KRAS 5%	Not influence	FLT3-ITD (24-26%)	-
Other genes alterations				
NPM1 mutation	35%	Favorable (without FLT3)	FLT3	Yes
BAALC overexpression	65%	Poor	-	Possible
EVI-1 overexpression	10-22%	Poor	-	Possible
WT1 overexpression	10-15%	Poor	-	Yes
DNMT3A mutation	20%	Poor	FLT3-ITD	-
IDH1/2 mutation	15%	Controversial	NPM1, FLT3-ITD	-

Table 3. Molecular markers in AML: prevalence, prognostic, associated mutations, genetic alterations and utility in MDR.

1.2.2 Genetic alterations with prognosis value

In recent years, the availability of new genetic and molecular prognostic markers in AML has grown considerably. This is particularly important in the case of patients with normal cytogenetics who comprise the largest subgroup of AML patients (approximately 45%) where many new prognostic factors have been identified. These include gene mutations in FLT3 (Fms-like tyrosine kinase 3; generally FLT3-ITD has been associated with significantly worse survival (Sheikhha et al, 2003)), NPM1 (nucleophosmin 1) and CEBPA (CCAAT enhancer-binding protein-α; generally favorable in cases of biallelic mutations) and gene overexpression as BAALC, WT1, EVI1 and MN1 (Foran, 2010).

Identifying alterations in these genes might provide independent prognostic value in predicting the outcome of acute leukemia, as in the case of the NPM1 mutation gene, which is a relatively frequent abnormality in AML patients and is useful in detecting MRD (Falini et al., 2007).

2. Detailed description of molecular markers

Next, we will describe the most common molecular markers in AML.

2.1 Core Binding Factor (CBF)

Leukemias affecting CBF are characterized by rearrangements of genes that code for components of the heterodimeric transcription factor CBF, which plays an essential role in haematopoiesis (Gabert et al., 2006). CBF complex is a heterodimer composed of RUNX1 (also called AML1) and CBFβ and is the target of at least three common transloctions in AML: t(8;21)/RUNX1-RUNX1T1, t(3;21)/RUNX1-EVI1 and inv(16) or t(16;16) resulting in CBFβ-MYH11. Rearrangements of *AML1* and *CBFB* with other genes lead to chimeric proteins that disrupt the CBF complex, suppressing the activation of transcription.

2.1.1 AML1 (RUNX1) rearrangements

AML1, also called, RUNX1, is normally expressed in all hematopoietic lineages and regulates the expression of several genes specifically linked to hematopoiesis, including the granulocyte colony-stimulating factor receptor, interleukin 3, T-cell receptor, and myeloperoxidase (MPO) genes. The *AML1* gene (on 21q22) is one of the genes most frequently deregulated in leukemias, generally through translocations that produce chimeric messenger RNA. Chimeric protein AML1-ETO (*RUNX1-RUNX1T1*) results from the t(8;21)(q22;q22) involving the AMLI gene on chromosome 21 and the ETO gene on chromosome 8. This rearrangement is detected in approximately 8% of AML cases in children and young adults. *RUNX1-RUNX1T1* is a marker for favourable outcome and an important PCR target for MRD detection. Most patients achieve a CR after induction therapy and those patients benefit most from a postremission therapy with high-dose cytarabin (Bloomfield et al., 1998; Perea et al., 2006). Hence, this marker permits to single out a relatively small subgroup of patients who are more likely to relapse (Gabert et al., 2003). *RUNX1-RUNX1T1* is also frequently associated with c-kit mutations which determine an adverse outcome within this group of patients with favorable prognosis. In addition, the loss of Y chromosome in male patients with t(8;21) leukemia is a negative prognostic factor for the overall survival (Schlenk et al., 2004). While the molecular diagnosis is performed by qualitative and quantitative Real Time RT-PCR (QRT-PCR), MRD monitoring is performed by quantitative QRT-PCR. The rare balanced t(3;21)(q26;q22) was described in AML, mainly after treatment with topoisomerase II inhibitors. This translocation fuses the AML1 gene on 21q22 and the EVI-1 gene on 3q26 resulting in t(3;21)(q26;q22). This translocation is associated with higher WBC and platelets counts but is not, however, predictive for relapse-free or overall survival (Preudhomme et al., 2000; Meyers et al., 1993; Lutghart et al., 2010).

2.1.2 AML1 mutations

AML1 mutations can be found in *de novo* leukemia, particularly subtypes FAB M0 and M7, as well as in patients with trisomy 21 and myelodysplastic syndromes. Testing for mutations can be performed By real time PCR or PCR-single stranded conformational polymorphism (SSCP). A multivariate analysis carried out by Schnittger et al., showed an independent unfavourable prognostic significance of AML1 (or RUNX1) mutations for overall survival (Schnittger et al., 2011).

2.1.3 CBFb-MYH11

Inv(16)(p13;q22) or t(16;16)(p13;q22) are among the most frequent recurring chromosomal rearrangements detected in AML, generally observed in cases showing myelomonocytic differentiation and having abnormal bone marrow eosinophils (M4 Eo AML in the French American British (FAB) classification). Inv(16)(p13;q22) is found in approximately 10-12% of cases of AML. It can occur in all age groups but is predominantly seen in younger patients. This rearrangement results in the disruption of the myosin heavy chain (MYH) gene at 16p13 and the core binding factor β(CBFβ) gene at 16q22 (FAB, 1976). Ten different CBFβ-MYH11 transcripts have been reported, but the frequency of each transcript is variable. CBFB-MYH11 positive patients are considered to have a favourable prognosis. This rearrangement is frequently associated with c-kit and FLT3 mutations which worsen the prognosis. Quantitative QRT-PCR allows monitoring of CR (Gabert et al., 2003; Perea et al., 2005).

2.1.4 CEBPA

The CCAAT/enhancer binding alpha protein (C/EBPα) is the founding member of a family of related leucine zipper transcription factors. Mutations in CEBPA are found in 5-14% of AML and have been associated with a relatively favourable outcome only in biallelic mutations of this gene. There are two main classes of mutation situated at the N- terminal or

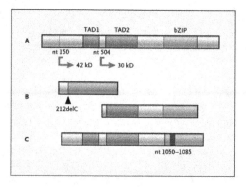

Fig. 1. Schematic representation of CEBPA (by Smith, 2004).

C-terminal basic leucine zipper (bZIP) regions (Figure 1). The latter affect both DNA binding and homo and heterodimerization with other CEBP-proteins. The former introduce a premature stoppage of the translation of the p42 CEBPA protein, preserving a p30 isoform, which was shown to inhibit DNA binding and transactivation by C/EBPα p42. CEBPA mutations are exclusively related to the intermediate risk group karyotype AML. CEBPA insertion, deletions and point mutations are detected usually by DNA sequencing (Wouters et al., 2009; Pabst et al., 2001; Fuchs et al., 2008).

2.2 PML-RARα

Acute promyelocytic leukemia is a distinct subtype of AML (AML-M3) according to the FAB classification. AML-M3 is characterized by t(15;17) that involves the retinoic acid receptor a (RARα) gene on chromosome 17 and the promyelocytic leukemia gene (PML) on chromosome 15. At the molecular level, t(15;17) results in a hybrid PML/ RARα gene, which is easily identified by reverse transcriptase-polymerase chain reaction (RT-PCR). This test provides a rapid and refined diagnosis. The usefulness of minimal residual disease monitoring during follow up (Lo Coco et al., 1992; Lo Coco et al., 1999a) has been well established. The different breakpoints within the PML gene cluster can be located in three regions: bcr1, 2 and 3.

The assessment of remission status at the molecular level by RT-PCR of PML-RARα represents a significant clinical advance with respect to other poorly sensitive methods (morphology, karyotype). The treatment of this disease (arsenicals, liposomal ATRA, other retinoid derivatives, etc) needs to be assessed taking into account the response at the RT-PCR level. The detection of residual PML-RARα transcripts during clinical remission predicts subsequent hematologic relapse. This determines the need for additional treatment given the benefits of anticipating salvage therapy in AML-M3. Figure 3 shows the statistically significant difference between patients treated for molecular relapse and the historical series treated for hematologic relapse (Lo Coco et al., 1999b).

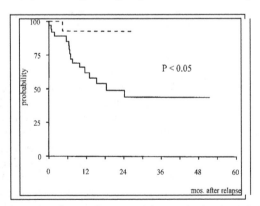

Fig. 2. Kaplan-Meier estimates of overall survival from relapse in patients treated at the time of molecular relapse (dotted line) and in the historical series of patients treated for hematologic relapse (continuous line).

Around 40% of all cases of PML-RARα-positive AML show FLT3 mutations. FLT3-ITD mutations, but not *FLT3-D835*, are associated with characteristic diagnostic hematological features of acute promyelocytic leukemia, in particular with high WBC counts. Also, FLT3 mutations, especially ITD, can adversely affect overall survival and disease-free survival in PML-RARα-positive AML (Beitinjaneh et al., 2010). However, in a large series of 739 patients with acute promyelocytic leukemia treated with ATRA and anthracycline-based chemotherapy, we were unable to demonstrate an independent prognostic value of *FLT3* mutations (Barragan et al., 2011).

2.3 DEK-CAN

AML defined by t(6;9) is a relatively rare disease, associated with specific clinical and morphological features (Garcon et al., 2005). Especially in young adults, the leukemic phase can be preceded by dysplastic features, conferring a bad prognosis. Morphological findings usually correlate with FAB M2 (60%), M4 (30%), or Ml (von Lindern et al., 1990). A chimeric protein is generated, resulting from the fusion between DEK and the 30- terminus of the CAN gene, also known as NUP214 (von Lindern et al., 1990). DEK is a component of metazoan chromatin capable of modifying the structure of DNA by introducing supercoils. CAN is a nuclear pore complex protein implicated in nucleocytoplasmic trafficking. The CAN gene is also involved in several fusion transcripts described in acute leukemia other than DEK in t(6;9)(p23;q34) AML, such as the SET gene and recently with ABL in T-cell acute lymphoblastic leukaemia (ALL). The DEK-CAN transcript can be used as a marker of t(6;9) AML which can be sensitively monitored by the polymerase chain reaction. This offers a great advantage in the diagnosis, monitoring of response to chemotherapy, and detection of minimal residual disease after bone marrow transplantation (von Lindern et al., 1992). DEK-CAN is related with an adverse prognosis (Dohner et al., 2010).

2.4 NPM1

NPM1 gene is located in 5q35 and encodes a phosphoprotein, nucleophosmin, which moves between the nucleus and the cytoplasm. The gene product is thought to be involved in several processes including regulation of the ARF/p53 pathway. Mutations in exon 12 in this gene are associated with AML with normal karyotype (50%) and especially correlate with monocytic leukemias. Patients with *NPM1* mutations have a significantly higher rate of complete remissions (CRs) after standard induction chemotherapy except for cases associated with internal tandem duplications mutations of FLT3 (Falini et al., 2007; Gale et al., 2008). Gale et al. (2008) identified 3 prognostic groups among the NPM1+ AML patients: good in those with only a NPM1 mutation and absence of a FLT3-ITD; intermediate in those with either absence of FLT3-ITD or NPM1 mutations or mutations in both genes; and poor in those with only FLT3-ITD. Monitoring can be performed by quantitative PCR (Schnittger et al., 2009). In our group, the incidence of NPM1 mutation was 30% (17 of 55 patients with AML), being this prevalence similar to that found for FLT3-ITD in the same population (29 %). The 17 NPM1+ AML patients were distributed as follows: eight M1-M2 (47.1 %), four M4-M5 (23.5%), and five not labelled (29.4 %) because cytogenetic studies were not informative due to several reasons. 64.7% of the NPM1+ patients had a normal karyotype, while 5.8% of them had cytogenetic anomalies. FLT3-ITD mutations were found in 41.2 % of the NPM1+ AML cases. In contrast to what has been described in the literature our group did not find a higher incidence of M4 or M5 subtypes (Thiede et al., 2002). In our case, a higher incidence of M1 and M2 subtypes was detected (Table 4). However the differences are most likely attributable to the small sample size of our cohort as compared to the Thiede cohort. The global mortality was analyzed disregarding risk factors, with a mortality of 67 % in the NPM1+/FLT3-ITD- group standing in clear contrast to a 100% death rate in the NPM1+/FLT3-ITD+ group (Lopez Jorge et al., 2006). This was confirmed in another study where we analysed the incidence and prognostic relevance of CD34/CD7/DR surface markers in a group of forty two NPM1positive patients and related it to FLT3-ITD mutations. We found that 84% of the NPM1 positive patients had normal karyotypes. Mutations in FLT3-ITD were detected in 23.8% of the NPM1+ patients. The screening for this mutation could be very useful in the future as patients with normal karyotype and expression of this molecular marker is included in a better prognostic subgroup (Gomez Casares et al., 2009; Dohner et al., 2010).

	N° patients	NPM1+	NPM1-
Patients (%)	55	17 (30.9)	38(69)
Median (range age) (years)	60 (18-95)	58 (18-82)	60 (19-95)
Age, rFAB subtype			
M0	5	0	5
M1/M2	8/10	4/4	4/6
M4/M5	12/4	3/1	9/3
M6	1	0	1
Not labeled	15	5	10
Cytogenetic:			
Normal karyotype	24	11	13
del(5)	2	0	2
del(7)	5	0	5
trisomy 8	1	1	0
t(4;11)	1	0	1
t(8;21)	2	0	2
t(10;11)	1	0	1
t(9;11)	1	0	1
t(12;13)	1	0	1
t(3;10)	1	0	1
+11	2	0	2
-Y	2	0	2
Complex: >3 abnormalities	2	0	2
Non determinated	14	5	9
FLT3-ITD+ (%)	16 (29)	7(41.2)	9(23.6)

Table 4. Cytogenetics and demographic characteristics in a group of 55 AML patients (Lopez Jorge et al., 2006).

2.5 c-KIT

KIT is a proto-oncogene located on chromosome band 4q11-12 and encodes a 145-kDa transmembrane glycoprotein member of the type III receptor tyrosine kinase family. Ligand independent activation of KIT results from mutations in the extracellular portion of the receptor (exon 8), transmembrane and juxtamembrane domains (exons 10 and 11, respectively), and activation loop of the tyrosine kinase domain (exon 17). *c-KIT* mutations have been found in a variable but relatively high frequency (up to 50%) in patients with CBF

AML, including both t(8;21) and the other major type of CBF AML inv(16)(p13q22) or t(16;16)(p13;q22). This appears to confer a quite unfavourable prognosis with higher relapse risk (associated to inv(16) or t(8;21)). An adverse effect on OS in AML with inv(16) has been described, particularly those that occur in exon 17 (Paschka et al., 2006). Such patients may warrant more aggressive or alternative therapy. The presence of the c-KIT mutation would be also important because it provides a target for novel tyrosine kinase inhibitor (TKI) therapy (Pollard et al., 2010).

2.6 FLT3

Flt3 is a member of the class III tyrosine kinase receptor family that includes the c-kit, c-fms, and PDGF receptors. The Flt3 receptor is preferentially expressed on hematopoietic stem cells and mediates stem cell differentiation and proliferation. Interaction of the Flt3 receptor with Flt3 ligand causes receptor dimerization, leading to the activation of the receptor tyrosine kinase and receptor autophosphorylation. The phosphorylated Flt3 transduces activation signals through associations with various cytoplasmic proteins, including ras GTPase-activating protein, phospholipase C, and Src family tyrosine kinases. Activation of the Flt3 receptor by ligand-dependent phosphorylation induces cellular proliferation via activation of cytoplasmic mediators. Thus, constitutive activation of the Flt3 pathway may lead to disease proliferation and may block cellular apoptotic response to conventional chemotherapy. An internal tandem duplication of the juxtamembrane (JM) domain-coding sequence of the FLT3 (FLT3-IT) gene on chromosome 13 has been identified in a group of patients with AML. Constitutive activation of the Flt3 receptor tyrosine kinase, either by internal tandem duplication (ITD) mutations of the juxtamembrane domain or point mutations clustering in the second tyrosine kinase domain (TKD mutations as D835), has been found in 20% to 30% of patients with AML and in 30% to 45% of patients with normal karyotype (reviewed by Stirewalt and Radich (2003)). ITD mutations have been associated with an increased risk of treatment failure after conventional chemotherapy (overall survival and disease-free survival were worse for ITD positive patients versus FLT3 wildtype patients), whereas the prognostic relevance of FLT3 point mutations is less evident (D835 mutants did not appear to have a worse median overal suvival or disease-free survival compared with the wildtype group) (Sheikhha et al., 2003). Recently, Spassov et al analyzed for WT1 and FLT3-internal tandem duplication (FLT3-ITD) expression in 30 samples of AML patients and determined that high WT1 expression correlated with the presence of FLT3-ITD (P = 0.014) and with a lower rate of complete remissions (P = 0.023) (Spassov et al., 2011). The detection of both molecular markers (WT1 and FLT3-ITD) may be helpful in defining high risk AML patients that need special therapeutic strategies.

Several studies described that a higher mutational load as determined by calculation of FLT3-ITD/FLT3 wildtype ratio indicates a worse prognosis in mutation carriers. Therefore, it was suggested that not the FLT3-ITD per se, but more likely loss of heterozygosity is associated with the unfavorable outcome in FLT3-ITD mutated AML (Meshinchi et al., 2001; Yanada et al., 2005; Thiede et al., 2002; Schnittger et al., 2011).

2.7 EVI1 overexpression

The ectopic viral integration site 1 (EVI1), located in chromosome 3q26, has been recognized in the last years as one of the most aggressive oncogenes associated to human leukemia (Gröschel et al., 2010). The inappropriate expression of EVI1 in hematopoietic cells has been implicated in the development or progress of myeloid disorders (Lugthart et al., 2008). Previous studies, applying microarray technology, indicate that high levels of EVI1 expression are detected in 10% -22% of patients with AML (Barjesteh et al., 2003). Although the higher expression of EVI1 gene was clearly associated with myeloid malignancies, is not restricted to this group. It is noteworthy that overexpression of EVI1 was also observed in 13.8% of patients with acute lymphoid leukemia. The correlation between overexpression of EVI1 in bone marrow and poor outcome in AML is a frequent issue of discussion in the literature (Lugthart et al., 2008; Luzardo et al., 2007).

We analyzed the incidence of EVI1 overexpression in haematological malignancies and its value as a prognostic factor. EVI1 overexpression (EVI1+) was examined by RT-PCR in bone marrow and/or peripheral blood samples of 113 AML patients at diagnosis and during follow-up. We found that 23.8% of AML overexpressed EVI1, as established by our previously determined cut-off point. Correlation with FAB subtypes stands as follows: 2M0, 1 M1,3 M2, 6 M4, 7 M5, 1 M6, 4 secondary AML and 3 not labeled. Survival curves in the AML group didn´t show any significant differences in overall survival and disease free survival when comparing EVI1+ to EVI1- populations. In AML samples a greater than expected incidence of EVI1 expression was observed (22.8% vs 11% previously described). When survival curves were analyzed in the AML group with ages ranging from 14 to 60 years, all of them treated with similar chemotherapy schemes, no significant difference was observed. However, a recent collaboration with other groups, showed that EVI1 overexpression is a poor prognostic marker in patients <65 years in an independent large cohort, and showed that the total absence of EVI1 expression has a prognostic impact in the outcome of acute myeloid leukemia patients (Vazquez et al.,2011).

2.8 BAALC AND MN1

The Brain and Acute Leukemia Cytoplasmic (BAALC), human gene located on chromosome 8q22.3, has also been found to be an important adverse prognostic factor if overexpressed in normal karyotype AML, suggesting a role for BAALC overexpression in acute leukemia. This gene is highly conserved in mammals. Normally, BAALC is almost exclusively expressed in neuroectoderm-derived tissues. Though little is known about the biological function of BAALC, it is highly expressed in hematopoietic precursor cells as well as leukemic blasts and is down-regulated during differentiation. BAALC has been postulated to play its role in the cytoskeleton network due to its cellular location. BAALC expression is an independent adverse prognostic factor and is associated with a specific gene-expression profile. Recent studies revealed the prognostic impact of BAALC expression in AML and also as a marker in minimal residual disease. Currently, determination of BAALC expression is performed by qualitative and quantitative real-time PCR, although the lack of validation or standardization studies limits its utility (Tanner et al., 2001; Gregory et al., 2009; Baldus et al., 2003; Najima et al., 2010).

The meningioma 1 (MN1) gene is localized on human chromosome 22. MN1 overexpression is a prognostic marker in patients with AML with normal karyotype characterized by an intermediate prognosis. Patients with high MN1 expression had a significantly worse prognosis (the overall survival was shorter and relapse rate was higher in this group compared to low MN1 expression group). High MN1 expression has as well been associated with other AML characteristics like inv(16) or overexpression of EVI-1 (Heuser et al, 2007). In addition, MN1 is able to induce myeloid leukemias in a murine model (Heuser et al, 2011). This suggested that MN1 may play a functional role in the pathogenesis of AML.

We performed a retrospective analysis of MN1 expression in a group of 49 AML patients with a mean age of 52 years (43 de novo AML and 6 secondary AML). In order to analyze response to chemotherapy, overall survival and correlation to other molecular markers (NPM1, FLT3-ITD, EVI1 and BAALC), patients were further classified into three groups depending on prognosis (favourable with 11 patients, intermediate with 25 and poor with 12). We analysed by real-time PCR the expression of MN1 in patients samples. We used as positive control of expression RNA of KG1 cell line that overexpress MN1. The incidence of MN1 overespression was 65.3%. The study showed that MN1 overexpression correlated to BAALC expression. We did not find relation with other markers, such as EVI-1, NPM-1 and FLT3. MN1 and BAALC overexpression have been associated to induction treatment refractoriness. However, due to the limited sample size in our series, determining whether MN1 or BAALC were actually involved with refractoriness was not possible. The 2-year overall survival was 52% and 53% for MN1 overexpressed and MN1 not overexpressed patients respectively. The 5-year overall survival was 52% and 42% respectively, showing no significant differences. Survival analysis for the intermediate risk AML group did not show significant differences either. MN1 overexpression was not associated with a worse prognosis in any of the studied patients, probably due to a small sample size (Rodriguez et al., 2010).

2.9 WT1

The Wilms' tumor locus was identified as a tumor suppressor gene, which is inactivated in Wilms' tumor, a pediatric kidney cancer. This protein, displaying characteristic features of a transcription factor, and with an expression restricted to kidney and haematopoetic cells, was called Wilms' tumor gene 1 (*WT1*). This gene is located on chromosome 11p13 and encodes a zinc-finger transcription factor influencing the expression of several growth factors and their corresponding receptors. It is also known to be involved in the early stage of hematological cell differentiation. Aberrant expression may be one mechanism by which the normal function of *WT1* is disrupted. However, the exact role of *WT1* in hematopoiesis and leukemogenesis still remains unclear. The abundant overexpression of *WT1* in leukemia creates a very attractive target for quantitative MRD studies in AML, especially in those samples with no specific fusion gene available. The method used to determine the expression of *WT1* gene is the RT-PCR, which will reveal its value as a marker to detect minimal residual disease (Keilholz et al., 2005; Weisser et al., 2005; Inoue et al., 1994; Garg et al., 2003).

Mutations of the coding region (most frequently in 7 and 9 exons) of the *WT1* gene have also been described and occur in 10–15% of AML (figure 3). Gaidzik et al. concluded that *WT1* mutation as a single molecular marker did not have an impact on outcome. On the other hand, Hou et al. demonstrated that *WT1* mutations disappeared in *WT1*-mutated studied patients who achieved complete remission, suggesting its potential use as MRD marker (Gaidzik et al., 2009; Hou et al., 2010).

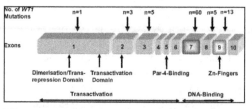

Fig. 3. Structure of the *WT1* gene and localization of the 87 mutations identified by Gaidzik et al.

2.10 MLL rearrangement and MLL-PTD

The *MLL* (mixed lineage leukemia) gene located at 11q23, is fused to a variety of partner genes through chromosomal translocations in acute leukemias. Up to now, more than 40 different *MLL* partner genes have been identified. *MLL* gene contains 100 kb of DNA, but nearly all breakpoints are clustered within a 8.3 kb region. Molecular analysis shows that fusion of the amino terminus of *MLL* to the carboxy terminus of partner genes generates the critical leukemogenic fusion proteins. Abnormalities of the mixed-lineage leukemia (*MLL*) gene can be detected in *de novo* acute myeloid leukemia (AML) and acute lymphoblastic leukemia (ALL) as well as in therapy-related AML, particularly after treatment with DNA topoisomerase II inhibitors (generally less than 5–10% of patients carried this rearrangements).The most common translocation involving 11q23 in acute myeloid leukemia (AML) is t(9;11)(p22;q23), which results in the generation of a fusion transcript of *MLL-AF*. The other common translocations involving 11q23 in AML are t(6;11)(q27;q23), t(10;11)(p12;q23), t(11;19)(q23;p13.1) and t(11;19)(q23;p13.3); these translocations result in the generation of fusion transcripts *MLL-AF6*, *MLL-AF10*, *MLL-ELL* or *MLL-ENL*, respectively. In AML, *MLL-AF9* has generally been associated with a more favourable outcome although this finding is controversial. This rearrangement is related to a superior event-free and overall survival as compared to patients with other chromosomal abnormalities or with no detectable rearrangements (Dimartino et al., 1999; Balgobind et al., 2005). In contrast, the other traslocation involving Cr 11q23 are asociated with poor prognostic in more cases (Dimartino et al., 1999; Balgobind et al., 2005). t(9;11)(p22;q23) is classified as intermediate and t(v;11)(v;q23) as adverse prognostic group (Döhner et al., 2010). Therefore, detection and identification of the different types of *MLL* rearrangements is of clinical importance. A recent study indicated that quantification by RQ-PCR of the fusion gene transcript levels at diagnosis may be of prognostic relevance (Shih et al., 2006; Jansen et al., 2005). One type of *MLL* rearrangement not detectable by classic cytogenetic is the partial tandem duplication of *MLL* (*MLL*-PTD). This rearrangement results most commonly from a duplication of a genomic region encompassing either *MLL* exons 5 through 11 or *MLL* exons 5 through 12 that is inserted into intron 4 of a full-length *MLL* gene, thus fusing introns 11 or 12 with intron 4. At a transcriptional level, this results in a unique in-frame fusion of exons 11 or 12 upstream of exon 5. In adult de novo AML with a normal karyotype, the presence of the *MLL*-PTD has been associated with a worse prognosis (ie, shorter duration of remission) when compared with normal karyotype AML without the *MLL*-PTD (Whitman et al., 2005).

2.11 Other molecular markers in research: Renin expression

There have been reports of experimental findings that relate the renin-angiotensin system (RAS) with hematopoiesis. Some studies have identified RAS components located in the bone marrow (Haznedaroglu & Buyukasik, 1997) that might functionally affect cellular proliferation and differentiation in physiological or pathological states (Huckle & Earp, 1994; Comte et al., 1997). It has been demonstrated that the RAS component renin is expressed in the bone marrow microenvironment as well as in hematopoietic cells (Abali et al., 2002). Bone marrow blast cells of some types of AML (M4 and M5 FAB types) express renin (Wulf et al., 1998), however no expression has been detected in normal bone marrow from healthy donors (Gómez Casares et al., 2002). Our group also detected renin expression in AML patients, but it did not relate to monocytic differentiation or to the existence of other cytogenetic risk markers (Gómez Casares et al., 2002). Moreover, renin expression has been found to be related to disease activity, disappearing with AML remission and returning with relapse (De la Iglesia et al., 2006).

We did not found statistically significant differences in the outcome between renin-positive and renin-negative patients (De la Iglesia et al., 2006).

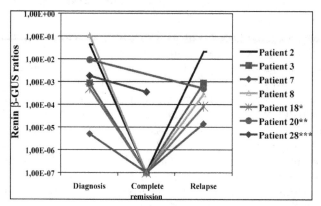

Fig. 4. Renin:βglucuronidase ratios vs clinical state of the quantified patients. *This data belong to third relapse, CR and fourth relapse, respectively. **This patient did not reach CR, continuing the positivity of the renin gene expression. ***Patient 28 in morphological CR was presented with 1% blasts in BM that later disappeared (De la Iglesia et al., 2006).

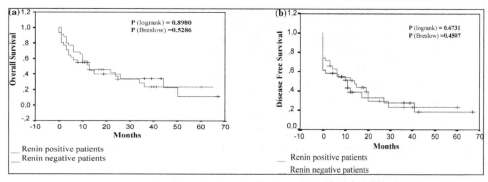

Fig. 5. (a) Overall survival of renin-positive and renin-negative patients with AML. Kaplan-Meier plot showing the correlation between overall survival and renin expression in AML patients. (b)Disease-free survival of renin-positive and renin-negative patients with AML. Kaplan-Meier plot showing the correlation between disease-free survival and renin expression in AML patients. (De la Iglesia et al., 2006).

Renin expression is related to undifferentiated phenotypic cell lines (K562, KU812), since no expression of the renin gene was found in cellular lines that showed a highly differentiated phenotype like HL60 and U937 (Gómez Casares et al., 2002). ACE inhibitors (captopril and trandolapril) and AT1 receptor blocker (losartan) produce a stop in proliferation in K562 cells with captopril (C) 10 mM and trandolapril (T) 2 mM (figure 6a) as well as an increase in the apoptotic rate in renin positive leukemia cell lines (K562) after the treatment with captopril (data not shown) and trandolapril (figure 6b) (De la Iglesia et al., 2009).

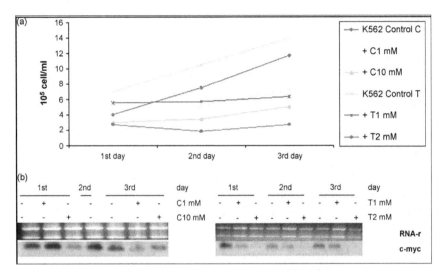

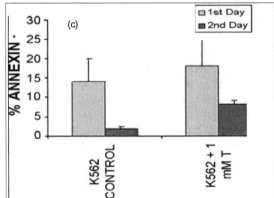

Fig. 6. **(a)** Proliferation in K562 after the treatment with captopril (C) and trandolapril (T). **(b)** C-myc gene expression in K562 after the treatment with the same drugs. **(c)** Apoptosis determined by annexin V binding in K562 and K562 transfected with bcl-2 and bcl-x (Kbcl2 and Kbclx) cells treated with 1mM trandolapril (T) (De la Iglesia et al., 2009). All experiments were performed in triplicate.

The leukaemogenic role of renin gene expression and the implicated molecular pathways have not yet been elucidated but it may offer novel therapeutic approaches in pathological or neoplastic conditions (Haznedaroglu & Öztürk, 2003).

3. Conclusion

The AML embraces very heterogeneous entities with different clinical behaviours. Some of these leukemias have certain chromosomal alterations that are related to specific morphological and clinical subtypes. Their identification has had great impact on different management aspects of these diseases, either from the standpoint of diagnosis, prognosis or development of a treatment plan tailored to the risk of relapse. This has been largely possible thanks to the application of molecular biology studies, which have provided a better and deeper understanding of the pathogenesis of leukemia.

The genetic alterations that occur at different stages fall into two broad groups: those that activate signal transduction as c-KIT and FLT3 (type I) and those which alter transcription factors such as CBF, RAR-α, CEBPA and NPM1 (type II). These two groups work together in leukemogenesis, being very frequent the coexistence of alterations of the two groups in the same patient.

The knowledge of these molecular markers helps us to classify patients within certain prognostic groups. In this way, in patients with normal cytogenetics, it is very important to know if there is a mutation of the FLT3 gene as well as its kind (ITD or TKD), because this information is of great relevance in order to select the appropriate treatment scheme. Moreover, the overexpression of the genes BAALC (under OS, DFS), MN1 (induction failure in patients with normal karyotype) or EVI1 (adverse impact) has been shown to have prognostic significance in AML.

In a laboratory setting there are different ways to classify leukemias. One of them is the rationale showed in the figure 5. According to the cytogenetic or molecular biology at diagnosis, it is possible to perform different determinations which will allow us to classify the patients within a favourable or unfavourable prognostic group. AML patients are classified at the time of diagnosis into three different prognostic groups based on their cytogenetic profiles.

There are plenty of algorithms which allow us to classify patients into different prognostic groups. They are undergoing continuous changes with the enrichment of new data. If we are in the presence of a CBF leukemia (by showing RUNX1-RUNXT1 or inv (16)), mutational analysis of c-kit should be performed, as this mutation translates into a higher risk of relapse. In patients with AML with normal karyotype, we recommend to analyze for FLT3-ITD first, as FLT-ITD3 is a well-known adverse prognostic factor. We then recommend screening for NPM1 mutations as a next step, because it is another mutation with clinical relevance of this subgroup of patients in the absence of FLT3-ITD. Then, given the favourable prognosis of NK-AML with biallelic CEBPA mutation, we recommend a CEBPA mutational analysis in those patients non-carriers of FLT3-ITD or NPM1. Also, FLT3-TKD an others mutations can be analyze in a context of clinical trials, even though there is no prognostic relevance.

There after, it is possible to perform other studies such as the detection of mutations in MLL/AF9 or BAALC, MN1 and EVI1 gene overexpression in order to make a better stratification of the prognosis. Besides working with prognostic and follow up markers with a recognized utility, we are also carrying out experimental work with new, not yet validated markers which will probably help us in the follow up, prognosis, classification and monitoring of AML patients. Renin, EVI1 and WT1 would be markers applicable to AML patients, especially in those with normal karyotype where they will facilitate the monitoring of minimal residual disease.

GENETIC GROUP	SUBSET
Favorable	t(8;21)(q22;q22); *RUNX1-RUNX1T1* inv(16)(p13.1q22) or t(16;16)(p13.1;q22); *CBFB-MYH11* Mutated *NPM1* without *FLT3*-ITD (normal karyotype) Mutated *CEBPA* (normal karyotype)
Intermediate-1	Mutated *NPM1* and *FLT3*-ITD (normal karyotype) Wild-type *NPM1* and *FLT3*-ITD (normal karyotype) Wild-type *NPM1* without *FLT3*-ITD (normal karyotype)
Intermediate-2	t(9;11)(p22;q23); *MLLT3-MLL* Cytogenetic abnormalities not classified as favorable or adverse
Adverse	inv(3)(q21q26.2) or t(3;3)(q21;q26.2); *RPN1-EVI1* t(6;9)(p23;q34); *DEK-NUP214* t(v;11)(v;q23); *MLL* rearranged -5 or del(5q); -7; abnl(17p); complex karyotype

Table 5. Standardized reporting for correlation of cytogenetic and molecular genetic data in AML with clinical data (Döhner. European LeukemiaNet , 2010)

In recent past, treatments had an empirical basis, lack of specificity and, therefore, limited effectiveness combined with high toxicity. The treatment of AML pioneered the search for specific therapies with the use of ATRA in APL. Currently, the ultimate goal of the understanding and classification of molecular aberrations in every AML subtype is to design a targeted therapy, which will reduce the risk of relapse and treatment side effects. That is because the future of AML therapy should be in the search and development of drugs that are directed against specific molecular or fusion proteins aberrations. On the other hand, due to the interaction between different molecular aberrations that arise in AML, the design of these new drugs has to be focused on the combined inhibition of several signalling pathways to achieve maximum clinical benefit.

4. References

Abali H, Haznedaroglu IC, Goker H, Celik I, Ozatli D, Koray Z & Caglar M. (2002). Circulating and Local Bone Marrow Renin-angiotensin System in Leukemic Hematopoiesis: Preliminary Evidences. Hematology, Vol. 7, No.75-82.

Alberta, J. A., Springett, G. M., Rayburn, H., Natoli, T. A., Loring, J., Kreidberg, J. A., & Housman, D. (2003). Role of the WT1 tumor suppressor in murine hematopoiesis. Blood, Vol. 101, No.7, 2570-2574.

Baldus, C. D., Tanner, S. M., Kusewitt, D. F., Liyanarachchi, S., Choi, C., Caligiuri, M. A., Bloomfield, C. D., & Chapelle, A. d. l. (2003). BAALC, a novel marker of human hematopoietic progenitor cells. Experimental Hematology, Vol. 31, No.11, 1051-1056, 0301-472X.

Balgobind, B.V., Raimondi, S.C., Harbott, J., Zimmermann, M., Alonzo, T.A., Auvrignon, A., Beverloo, H.B., Chang, M., Creutzig, U., Dworzak, M.N., Forestier, E., Gibson, B., Hasle, H., Harrison, C.J., Heerema, N.A., Kaspers, G.J., Leszl, A., Litvinko, N., Nigro, L.L., Morimoto, A., Perot, C., Pieters, R., Reinhardt, D., Rubnitz, J.E., Smith, F.O., Stary, J., Stasevich, I., Strehl, S., Taga, T., Tomizawa, D., Webb, D., Zemanova, Z., Zwaan, C.M. & van den Heuvel-Eibrink, M.M. (2009). Novel prognostic subgroups in childhood 11q23/MLL-rearranged acute myeloid leukemia: results of an international retrospective study. Blood, Vol. 114, No. 12, 2489-96.

Barjesteh van Waalwijk van Doorn-Khosrovani, S., Erpelinck, C., van Putten, W. L. J., Valk, P. J. M., van der Poel-van de Luytgaarde, S., Hack, R., Slater, R., Smit, E. M. E., Beverloo, H. B., Verhoef, G., Verdonck, L. F., Ossenkoppele, G. J., Sonneveld, P., de Greef, G. E., Löwenberg, B., & Delwel, R. (2003). High EVI1 expression predicts poor survival in acute myeloid leukemia: a study of 319 de novo AML patients. Blood, Vol. 101, No.3, 837-845.

Barragan, E., Montesinos, P., Camos, M., Gonzalez, M., Calasanz, M. J., Roman-Gomez, J., Gomez-Casares, M. T., Ayala, R., Lopez, J., Fuster, O., Colomer, D., Chillon, C., Larrayoz, M. J., Sanchez-Godoy, P., Gonzalez-Campos, J., Manso, F., Amador, M. L., Vellenga, E., Lowenberg, B., & Sanz, M. A. (2011). Prognostic value of FLT3 mutations in patients with acute promyelocytic leukemia treated with all-trans retinoic acid and anthracycline Haematologica, Vol. 96, No. 10, 1470-1477.

Beitinjaneh, A., Jang, S., Roukoz, H. & Majhail, N.S (2010). Prognostic significance of FLT3 internal tandem duplication and tyrosine kinase domain mutations in acute promyelocytic leukemia: a systematic review. Leuk Res. Vol. 34, No.7:831-6.

Bennett, J. M., Catovsky, D., Daniel, M. T., Flandrin, G., Galton, D. A. G., Gralnick, H. R., & Sultan, C. (1976). Proposals for the Classification of the Acute Leukaemias French-American-British (FAB) Cooperative Group. British Journal of Haematology, Vol. 33, No.4, 451-458, 1365-2141.

Bennett J.M.; Catovsky D.A.N.I.; Daniel,Marie T.; Flandrin G.E.O.R.; Galton D.; Gralnick R.& Sultan C.L.A.U. (1985). Proposed Revised Criteria for the Classification of Acute Myeloid Leukemia. Annals of Internal Medicine, Vol. 103, No.4, 620-625.

Bernstein, R., Mendelow, B., Pinto, M. R., Morcom, G., & Bezwoda, W. (1980). Complex translocations involving chromosomes 15 and 17 in acute promyelocityc leukaemia. British Journal of Haematology, Vol. 46, No.2, 311-314, 1365-2141.

Bloomfield, C.D., Lawrence, D., Byrd, J.C., Carroll, A., Pettenati, M.J., Tantravahi, R., Patil, S.R., Davey, F.R., Berg, D.T., Schiffer, C.A., Arthur, D.C. & Mayer, R.J. (1998). Frequency of prolonged remission duration after high-dose cytarabine intensification in acute myeloid leukemia varies by cytogenetic subtype. Cancer Res, Vol. 58, No.18, 4173-9.

Chellappan, S. P., Hiebert, S., Mudryj, M., Horowitz, J. M., & Nevins, J. R. (1991). The E2F transcription factor is a cellular target for the RB protein. Cell, Vol. 65, No.6, 1053-1061, 0092-8674.

Cline M.J. (1994). The Molecular Basis of Leukemia. New England Journal of Medicine, Vol. 330, No.5, 328-336, 0028-4793.

Comte, L., Lorgeot, V., Volkov, L., Roullet, B., Tubiana, N., & Praloran, V. (1997). AcSDKP plasma concentrations in patients with solid tumors: comparison of two chemotherapeutic regimens. Cancer Letters, Vol. 112, No.1, 1-4, 0304-3835.

De la Iglesia Iñigo, S., Lopez-Jorge, C. E., Gomez-Casares, M. T., Lemes Castellano, A., Martin Cabrera, P., Lopez Brito, J., Suarez Cabrera, A., & Molero Labarta, T. (2009). Induction of apoptosis in leukemic cell lines treated with captopril, trandolapril and losartan: A new role in the treatment of leukaemia for these agents. Leukemia Research, Vol. 33, No.6, 810-816, 0145-2126.

De la Iglesia, S., Gomez-Casares, M.T., Lopez-Jorge, C. E., Gonzalez-Leiza, S.M., Santana, G., Jimenez, S., Gonzalez-San Miguel, J.D., Caballero, A., Perera, M., Lemes, A., Luzardo, H., & Molero,T. (2006). Relevance of renin expression by real-time PCR in acute myeloid leukemia. Leukemia & Lymphoma, Vol. 47, No.3, 409-416, 1042-8194.

Dimartino, J.F., & Cleary, M.L. (1999). Mll rearrangements in haematological malignancies: lessons from clinical and biological studies. Br J Haematol, Vol. 106, No.3, 614-26.

Döhner, H., Estey, E.H., Amadori, S., Appelbaum, F.R., Büchner, T., Burnett, A.K., Dombret, H., Fenaux, P., Grimwade, D., Larson, R.A., Lo-Coco, F., Naoe, T., Niederwieser, D., Ossenkoppele, G.J., Sanz, M.A., Sierra, J., Tallman, M.S., Löwenberg, B. & Bloomfield, C.D.European LeukemiaNet (2010). Diagnosis and management of acute myeloid leukemia in adults: recommendations from an international expert panel, on behalf of the European LeukemiaNet. Blood, Vol 115, No 3, 453-74.

Falini, B., Nicoletti, I., Martelli, M. F., & Mecucci, C. (2007). Acute myeloid leukemia carrying cytoplasmic/mutated nucleophosmin (NPMc+ AML): biologic and clinical features. Blood, Vol. 109, No.3, 874-885.

Foran, J. M. (2010). New Prognostic Markers in Acute Myeloid Leukemia: Perspective from the Clinic. Hematology, Vol. 2010, No.1, 47-55.

Foroni, L., Harrison, C. J., Hoffbrand, A. V., & Potter, M. N. (1999). Investigation of minimal residual disease in childhood and adult acute lymphoblastic leukaemia by molecular analysis. British Journal of Haematology, Vol. 105, No.1, 7-24, 1365-2141.

Fuchs, O., Provaznikova, D., Kocova, M., Kostecka, A., Cvekova, P., Neuwirtova, R., Kobylka, P., Cermak, J., Brezinova, J., Schwarz, J., Markova, J., Salaj, P., Klamova, H., Maaloufova, J., Lemez, P., Novakova, L., & Benesova, K. (2008). CEBPA polymorphisms and mutations in patients with acute myeloid leukemia, myelodysplastic syndrome, multiple myeloma and non-Hodgkin's lymphoma. Blood Cells, Molecules, and Diseases, Vol. 40, No.3, 401-405, 1079-9796.

Gabert, J., Beillard, E., van der Velden, V. H. J., Bi, W., Grimwade, D., Pallisgaard, N., Barbany, G., Cazzaniga, G., Cayuela, J. M., Cave, H., Pane, F., Aerts, J. L. E., De Micheli, D., Thirion, X., Pradel, V., Gonzalez, M., Viehmann, S., Malec, M., Saglio, G., & van Dongen, J. J. M. (2003). Standardization and quality control studies of /`real-time/' quantitative reverse transcriptase polymerase chain reaction of fusion gene transcripts for residual disease detection in leukemia - A Europe Against

Cancer Program. Leukemia : official journal of the Leukemia Society of America, Leukemia Research Fund, U.K, Vol. 17, No.12, 2318-2357, 0887-6924.

Gaidzik, V. I., Schlenk, R. F., Moschny, S., Becker, A., Bullinger, L., Corbacioglu, A., Krauter, J., chlegelberger, B., anser, A., öhner, H., & öhner, K. (2009). Prognostic impact of WT1 mutations in cytogenetically normal acute myeloid leukemia: a study of the German-Austrian AML Study Group. Blood, Vol. 113, No.19, 4505-4511.

Gale, R. E., Green, C., Allen, C., Mead, A. J., Burnett, A. K., Hills, R. K., & Linch, D. C. (2008). The impact of FLT3 internal tandem duplication mutant level, number, size, and interaction with NPM1 mutations in a large cohort of young adult patients with acute myeloid leukemia. Blood, Vol. 111, No.5, 2776-2784.

Garcon, L., Libura, M., Delabesse, E., Valensi, F., Asnafi, V., Berger, C., Schmitt, C., Leblanc, T., Buzyn, A., & Macintyre, E. (2005). DEK-CAN molecular monitoring of myeloid malignancies could aid therapeutic stratification. Leukemia : official journal of the Leukemia Society of America, Leukemia Research Fund, U.K, Vol. 19, No.8, 1338-1344, 0887-6924.

Garg, M., Moore, H., Tobal, K., & Liu Yin, J. A. (2003). Prognostic significance of quantitative analysis of WT1 gene transcripts by competitive reverse transcription polymerase chain reaction in acute leukaemia. British Journal of Haematology, Vol. 123, No.1, 49-59, 1365-2141.

Gomez Casares, M.T., Lemes, A.,Navarro, N., González-San Miguel, J.D., Fumero, S., Bosch, J.M., Martín, P., Fiuza, M.D., López-Jorge, C.E., Luzardo, H., De la Iglesia, S. & Molero T. (2009). Prognostic value of inmunophenotype in AML patients with NPM1 mutation. Poster 0296.14th Congress of EHA.

Gomez Casares, M. T., de la Iglesia, S., Perera, M., Lemes, A., Campo, C., Gonzalez San Miguel, J. D., Bosch, J. M., Suarez, A., Guerra, L., Rodriguez-Perez, J. C., & Molero, T. (2002). Renin Expression in Hematological Malignancies and its Role in the Regulation of Hematopoiesis. Leukemia & Lymphoma, Vol. 43, No.12, 2377-2381, 1042-8194.

Gregory, T., Wald, D., Chen, Y., Vermaat, J., Xiong, Y., & Tse, W. (2009). Molecular prognostic markers for adult acute myeloid leukemia with normal cytogenetics. Journal of Hematology & Oncology, Vol. 2, No.1, 1756-8722.

Gröschel, S., Lugthart, S., Schlenk, R. F., Valk, P. J. M., Eiwen, K., Goudswaard, C., van Putten, W. J. L., Kayser, S., Verdonck, L. F., Lübbert, M., Ossenkoppele, G. J., Germing, U., Schmidt-Wolf, I., Schlegelberger, B., Krauter, J., Ganser, A., Döhner, H., Löwenberg, B., Döhner, K., & Delwel, R. (2010). High EVI1 Expression Predicts Outcome in Younger Adult Patients With Acute Myeloid Leukemia and Is Associated With Distinct Cytogenetic Abnormalities. Journal of Clinical Oncology, Vol. 28, No.12, 2101-2107.

Haferlach, T., Bacher, U., Haferlach, C., Kern, W., & Schnittger, S. (2007). Insight into the molecular pathogenesis of myeloid malignancies. Current Opinion in Hematology, Vol. 14, No.2, 1065-6251.

Harris, N. L., Jaffe, E. S., Diebold, J., Flandrin, G., Muller-Hermelink, H. K., Vardiman, J., Lister, T. A., & Bloomfield, C. D. (1999). World Health Organization Classification of Neoplastic Diseases of the Hematopoietic and Lymphoid Tissues: Report of the Clinical Advisory Committee Meeting-ùAirlie House, Virginia, November 1997. Journal of Clinical Oncology, Vol. 17, No.12, 3835-3849.

Haznedaroglu IC, B. Y. (1997). Current evidence for the existence of a local renin-angiotensin system affecting physiological and pathological haemopoiesis in the bone marrow. British Journal of Haematology, Vol. 99, No.2, 471-471, 1365-2141.

Haznedaroglu, I. C. , Oztürk M.A. (2003). Towards the understanding of the local hematopoietic bone marrow renin-angiotensin system. The International Journal of Biochemistry & Cell Biology, Vol. 35, No.6, 867-880, 1357-2725.

Heuser, M., Argiropoulos, B., Kuchenbauer, F., Yung, E., Piper, J., Fung, S., Schlenk, R. F., Dohner, K., Hinrichsen, T., Rudolph, C., Schambach, A., Baum, C., Schlegelberger, B., Dohner, H., Ganser, A., & Humphries, R. K. (2007). MN1 overexpression induces acute myeloid leukemia in mice and predicts ATRA resistance in patients with AML. Blood, Vol. 110, No.5, 1639-1647.

Heuser, M., Yun, H., Berg, T., Yung, E., Argiropoulos, B., Kuchenbauer, F., Park, G., Hamwi, I., Palmqvist, L., Lai, C.K., Leung, M., Lin, G., Chaturvedi, A., Thakur, B.K., Iwasaki, M., Bilenky, M., Thiessen, N., Robertson, G., Hirst, M., Kent, D., Wilson, N.K., Göttgens, B., Eaves, C., Cleary, M.L., Marra, M., Ganser ,A. & Humphries, R.K.(2011). Cell of origin in AML: susceptibility to MN1-induced transformation is regulated by the MEIS1/AbdB-like HOX protein complex. Cancer Cell. Vol. 20, No.1, 39-52.

Hilden, J. M., Frestedt, J. L., Moore, R. O., Heerema, N. A., Arthur, D. C., Reaman, G. H., & Kersey, J. H. (1995). Molecular analysis of infant acute lymphoblastic leukemia: MLL gene rearrangement and reverse transcriptase-polymerase chain reaction for t(4; 11)(q21; q23). Blood, Vol. 86, No.10, 3876-3882.

Hou, H. A., Huang, T. C., Lin, L. I., Liu, C. Y., Chen, C. Y., Chou, W. C., Tang, J. L., Tseng, M. H., Huang, C. F., Chiang, Y. C., Lee, F. Y., Liu, M. C., Yao, M., Huang, S. Y., Ko, B. S., Hsu, S. C., Wu, S. J., Tsay, W., Chen, Y. C., & Tien, H. F. (2010). WT1 mutation in 470 adult patients with acute myeloid leukemia: stability during disease evolution and implication of its incorporation into a survival scoring system. Blood, Vol. 115, No.25, 5222-5231.

Huckle, W. R. , Earp, H. S. (1994). Regulation of cell proliferation and growth by angiotensin II. Progress in Growth Factor Research, Vol. 5, No.2, 177-194, 0955-2235.

Inoue, K., Sugiyama, H., Ogawa, H., Nakagawa, M., Yamagami, T., Miwa, H., Kita, K., Hiraoka, A., Masaoka, T., & Nasu, K. (1994). WT1 as a new prognostic factor and a new marker for the detection of minimal residual disease in acute leukemia. Blood, Vol. 84, No.9, 3071-3079.

Jansen, M. W. J. C., van der Velden, V. H. J., & van Dongen, J. J. M. (2005). Efficient and easy detection of MLL-AF4, MLL-AF9 and MLL-ENL fusion gene transcripts by multiplex real-time quantitative RT-PCR in TaqMan and LightCycler. Leukemia : official journal of the Leukemia Society of America, Leukemia Research Fund, U.K, Vol. 19, No.11, 2016-2018, 0887-6924.

Keilholz, U., Menssen, H. D., Gaiger, A., Menke, A., Oji, Y., Oka, Y., Scheibenbogen, C., Stauss, H., Thiel, E., & Sugiyama, H. (2005). Wilms' tumor gene 1 (WT1) in human neoplasia. Leukemia : official journal of the Leukemia Society of America, Leukemia Research Fund, U.K, Vol. 19, No.8, 1318-1323, 0887-6924.

Kreuzer, K. A., Saborowski, A., Lupberger, J., Appelt, C., Na, I. K., Le Coutre, P., & Schmidt, C. A. (2001). Fluorescent 5'-exonuclease assay for the absolute quantification of

Wilms' tumor gene (WT1) mRNA: implications for monitoring human leukaemias. British Journal of Haematology, Vol. 114, No.2, 313-318, 1365-2141.

Lin, L. I., Chen, C. Y., Lin, D. T., Tsay, W., Tang, J. L., Yeh, Y. C., Shen, H. L., Su, F. H., Yao, M., Huang, S. Y., & Tien, H. F. (2005). Characterization of CEBPA Mutations in Acute Myeloid Leukemia: Most Patients with CEBPA Mutations Have Biallelic Mutations and Show a Distinct Immunophenotype of the Leukemic Cells. Clinical Cancer Research, Vol. 11, No.4, 1372-1379.

Lo Coco , F., Diverio, D., Falini, B., Biondi, A., Nervi, C., & Pelicci, P. G. (1999). Genetic Diagnosis and Molecular Monitoring in the Management of Acute Promyelocytic Leukemia. Blood, Vol. 94, No.1, 12-22.

Lo Coco, F., Diverio, D., Avvisati, G., Arcese, W., Petti, M. C., Meloni, G., Mandelli, F., Pandolfi, P. P., Grignani, F., Pelicci, P. G., Biondi, A., Rossi, V., Masera, G., Barbui, T., & Rambaldi, A. (1992). Molecular evaluation of residual disease as a predictor of relapse in acute promyelocytic leukaemia. The Lancet, Vol. 340, No.8833, 1437-1438, 0140-6736.

Lo Coco, F., Diverio, D., Avvisati, G., Petti, M. C., Meloni, G., Pogliani, E. M., Biondi, A., Rossi, G., Carlo-Stella, C., Selleri, C., Martino, B., Specchia, G., & Mandelli, F. (1999). Therapy of Molecular Relapse in Acute Promyelocytic Leukemia. Blood, Vol. 94, No.7, 2225-2229.

Lopez-Jorge, C.E., Martin, P.,Lopez Brito, J., Gomez Casares, M.T., Gonzalez San Miguel, J.D., Lemes, A., Ramirez, T., Santana, G., Mataix, R., De La Iglesia, S., Luzardo, H.& Molero, T. (2006). Prevalence of NPM1 mutation in AML and MDR. Póster 0695.11th Congress of the EHA.

Lugthart, S., van Drunen, E., van Norden, Y., van Hoven, A., Erpelinck, C. A. J., Valk, P. J. M., Beverloo, H. B., Löwenberg, B., & Delwel, R. (2008). High EVI1 levels predict adverse outcome in acute myeloid leukemia: prevalence of EVI1 overexpression and chromosome 3q26 abnormalities underestimated. Blood, Vol. 111, No.8, 4329-4337.

Lugthart, S., Groschel, S., Beverloo, H.B., Kayser, S., Valk, P.J., van Zelderen-Bhola, S.L., Jan Ossenkoppele, G., Vellenga, E., van den Berg-de Ruiter, E., Schanz, U., Verhoef, G., Vandenberghe, P., Ferrant, A., Kohne, C.H., Pfreundschuh, M., Horst, H.A., Koller, E., von Lilienfeld-Toal, M., Bentz, M., Ganser, A., Schlegelberger, B., Jotterand, M., Krauter, J., Pabst, T., Theobald, M., Schlenk, RF., Delwel, R., Döhner, K., Löwenberg, B. & Döhner, H. (2010). Clinical, molecular, and prognostic significance of WHO type inv(3)(q21q26.2)/t(3;3)(q21;q26.2) and various other 3q abnormalities in acute myeloid leukemia. J Clin Oncol, Vol.28, No.24, 3890-8.

Luzardo, H., Gómez-Casares, M.T., Gonzalez-San Miguel, J.D., Lopez-Brito, J., Calvo-Villas, J.M., Molines, A., De la Iglesia, S, Caballero, A., López-Jorge, C.E., Santana, G., Suarez, A.& Molero, T. (2007). EVI1 overexpression in a serie of 212 hematological malignancies. Poster 0171.12th Congress of EHA.

Meshinchi, S., Woods, W. G., Stirewalt, D. L., Sweetser, D. A., Buckley, J. D., Tjoa, T. K., Bernstein, I. D., & Radich, J. P. (2001). Prevalence and prognostic significance of Flt3 internal tandem duplication in pediatric acute myeloid leukemia. Blood, Vol. 97, No.1, 89-94.

Meyers, S., Downing, J. R., & Hiebert, S. W. (1993). Identification of AML-1 and the (8;21) translocation protein (AML-1/ETO) as sequence-specific DNA-binding proteins:

the runt homology domain is required for DNA binding and protein-protein interactions. Molecular and Cellular Biology, Vol. 13, No.10, 6336-6345.

Morishita, K., Parganas, E., William, C. L., Whittaker, M. H., Drabkin, H., Oval, J., Taetle, R., Valentine, M. B., & Ihle, J. N. (1992). Activation of EVI1 gene expression in human acute myelogenous leukemias by translocations spanning 300-400 kilobases on chromosome band 3q26. Proceedings of the National Academy of Sciences, Vol. 89, No.9, 3937-3941.

Najima, Y., Ohashi, K., Kawamura, M., Onozuka, Y., Yamaguchi, T., Akiyama, H., & Sakamaki, H. (2010). Molecular monitoring of BAALC expression in patients with CD34-positive acute leukemia. International Journal of Hematology, Vol. 91, No.4, 636-645, 0925-5710.

Nakao, M., Yokota, S., Horiike, S., Taniwaki, M., Kashima, K., Sonoda, Y., Koizumi, S., Takaue, Y., Matsushita, T., Fujimoto, T., & Misawa, S. (1996). Detection and quantification of TEL/AML1 fusion transcripts by polymerase chain reaction in childhood acute lymphoblastic leukemia. Leukemia : official journal of the Leukemia Society of America, Leukemia Research Fund, U.K, Vol. 10, No.9, 1463-1470.

Pabst, T., Mueller, B. U., Zhang, P., Radomska, H. S., Narravula, S., Schnittger, S., Behre, G., Hiddemann, W., & Tenen, D. G. (2001). Dominant-negative mutations of CEBPA, encoding CCAAT/enhancer binding protein-[alpha] (C/EBP[alpha]), in acute myeloid leukemia. Nat Genet, Vol. 27, No.3, 263-270, 1061-4036.

Paschka, P., Marcucci, G., Ruppert, A.S., Mrozek, K., Chen, H., Kittles, R.A., Vukosavljevic, T., Perrotti, D., Vardiman, J.W., Carroll, A.J., Kolitz, J.E., Larson, R.A. & Bloomfield, C.D.; Cancer and Leukemia Group B. (2006). Adverse prognostic significance of KIT mutations in adult acute myeloid leukemia with inv(16) and t(8;21): a Cancer and Leukemia Group B Study. J Clin Oncol, Vol.24, No.24, 3904-11.

Perea, G., Lasa, A., Aventin, A., Domingo, A., Villamor, N., Paz Queipo de Llano, M., Llorente, A., Junca, J., Palacios, C., Fernandez, C., Gallart, M., Font, L., Tormo, M., Florensa, L., Bargay, J., Marti, J. M., Vivancos, P., Torres, P., Berlanga, J. J., Badell, I., Brunet, S., Sierra, J., & Nomdedeu, J. F. (2005). Prognostic value of minimal residual disease (MRD) in acute myeloid leukemia (AML) with favorable cytogenetics t(8;21) and inv(16). Leukemia : official journal of the Leukemia Society of America, Leukemia Research Fund, U.K, Vol. 20, No.1, 87-94, 0887-6924.

Pollard, J. A., Alonzo, T. A., Gerbing, R. B., Ho, P. A., Zeng, R., Ravindranath, Y., Dahl, G., Lacayo, N. J., Becton, D., Chang, M., Weinstein, H. J., Hirsch, B., Raimondi, S. C., Heerema, N. A., Woods, W. G., Lange, B. J., Hurwitz, C., Arceci, R. J., Radich, J. P., Bernstein, I. D., Heinrich, M. C., & Meshinchi, S. (2010). Prevalence and prognostic significance of KIT mutations in pediatric patients with core binding factor AML enrolled on serial pediatric cooperative trials for de novo AML. Blood, Vol. 115, No.12, 2372-2379.

Preudhomme, C., Warot-Loze, D., Roumier, C., Grardel-Duflos, N., Garand, R., Lai, J. L., Dastugue, N., Macintyre, E., Denis, C., Bauters, F., Kerckaert, J. P., Cosson, A., & Fenaux, P. (2000). High incidence of biallelic point mutations in the Runt domain of the AML1/PEBP2αB gene in Mo acute myeloid leukemia and in myeloid malignancies with acquired trisomy 21. Blood, Vol. 96, No.8, 2862-2869.

Radich, J. & Thomson, B. (1997). Advances in the detection of minimal residual disease. Current Opinion in Hematology, Vol. 4, No.4, 1065-6251.

Rodríguez ,C., Gómez Casares, MT., Santana, G., Guedes, S.,Calvo-Villas, JM, López Jorge, CE.,García Bello, MA.,González San Miguel JD., Jiménez, S.,Quiroz, K., Fumero, S., Ramos, Y., Navarro, N. & Molero, T. (2010). Sobreexpresión de MN1 en leucemias agudas de estirpe mieloide. Correlación con otros marcadores moleculares y relación con respuesta al tratamiento y supervivencia global. Poster 0154.LII Reunión Nacional de la SEHH y XXVI Congreso Nacional de la SETH.

Stirewalt, D.L. & Radich, J.P. (2003). The role of FLT3 in haematopoietic malignancies. Nat Rev Cancer. Vol. 3, No.9,:650-65.

Sasaki, O., Meguro, K., Tohmiya, Y., Funato, T., Shibahara, S., & Sasaki, T. (2002). Altered expression of retinoblastoma protein-interacting zinc finger gene, RIZ, in human leukaemia. British Journal of Haematology, Vol. 119, No.4, 940-948, 1365-2141.

Schlenk, RF., Benner, A., Krauter, J., Büchner, T., Sauerland, C., Ehninger, G., Schaich, M., Mohr, B., Niederwieser, D., Krahl, R., Pasold, R., Döhner, K., Ganser, A., Döhner, H. & Heil, G. (2004). Individual Patient Data–Based Meta-Analysis of Patients Aged 16 to 60 Years With Core Binding Factor Acute Myeloid Leukemia: A Survey of the German Acute Myeloid Leukemia Intergroup. J Clin Oncol, Vol. 22, No.18, 3741-50.

Schlenk, RF., Döhner, K., Krauter, J., Fröhling, S., Corbacioglu, A., Bullinger, L., Habdank, M., Späth, D., Morgan, M., Benner, A., Schlegelberger, B., Heil, G., Ganser, A.& Döhner, H.; German-Austrian Acute Myeloid Leukemia Study Group. (2008). Mutations and treatment outcome in cytogenetically normal acute myeloid leukemia. N Engl J Med; Vol. 358, No.18, 1909-18.

Schnittger, S., Kern, W., Tschulik, C., Weiss, T., Dicker, F., Falini, B., Haferlach, C. & Haferlach, T. (2009). Minimal residual disease levels assessed by NPM1 mutation-specific RQ-PCR provide important prognostic information in AML. Blood, Vol. 114, No.11, 2220-31.

Schnittger, S., Bacher, U., Kern, W., Alpermann, T., Haferlach, C., & Haferlach, T. (2011). Prognostic impact of FLT3-ITD load in NPM1 mutated acute myeloid leukemia. Leukemia : official journal of the Leukemia Society of America, Leukemia Research Fund, U.K, 1476-5551.

Schnittger, S., Dicker, F., Kern, W., Wendland, N., Sundermann, J., Alpermann, T., Haferlach, C., & Haferlach, T. (2011). RUNX1 mutations are frequent in de novo AML with noncomplex karyotype and confer an unfavorable prognosis. Blood, Vol. 117, No.8, 2348-2357.

Sheikhha, M.H., Awan, A., Tobal, K. & Liu Yin, J.A. (2003). Prognostic significance of FLT3 ITD and D835 mutations in AML patients. Hematol J, Vol. 4, No.1,41-6.

Shih, L., Liang, D., Fu, J., Wu, J., Wang, P., Lin, T., Dunn, P., Kuo, M., Tang, T., Lin, T., & Lai, C. (2006). Characterization of fusion partner genes in 114 patients with de novo acute myeloid leukemia and MLL rearrangement. Leukemia : official journal of the Leukemia Society of America, Leukemia Research Fund, U.K, Vol. 20, No.2, 218-223, 0887-6924.

Spassov, BV., Stoimenov, AS., Balatzenko, GN., Genova, ML., Peichev, DB. & Konstantinov, SM. (2011). Wilms' tumor protein and FLT3-internal tandem duplication expression in patients with de novo acute myeloid leukemia. Hematology. Vol.16, No.1, 37-42.

Tanner, S. M., Austin, J. L., Leone, G., Rush, L. J., Plass, C., Heinonen, K., Mrózek, K., Sill, H., Knuutila, S., Kolitz, J. E., Archer, K. J., Caligiuri, M. A., Bloomfield, C. D., & de la Chapelle, A. (2001). BAALC, the human member of a novel mammalian neuroectoderm gene lineage, is implicated in hematopoiesis and acute leukemia. Proceedings of the National Academy of Sciences, Vol. 98, No.24, 13901-13906.

Thiede, C., Steudel, C., Mohr, B., Schaich, M., Schäkel, U., Platzbecker, U., Wermke, M., Bornhäuser, M., Ritter, M., Neubauer, A., Ehninger, G., & Illmer, T. (2002). Analysis of FLT3-activating mutations in 979 patients with acute myelogenous leukemia: association with FAB subtypes and identification of subgroups with poor prognosis. Blood, Vol. 99, No.12, 4326-4335.

Vardiman, J. W., Thiele, J., Arber, D.A., Brunning, R.D., Borowitz, M. J., Porwit, A., Harris, N. L., Le Beau, M. M., Hellström-Lindberg, E., Tefferi, A., & Bloomfield, C. D. (2009). The 2008 revision of the World Health Organization (WHO) classification of myeloid neoplasms and acute leukemia: rationale and important changes. Blood, Vol. 114, No.5, 937-951.

Vazquez, I., Maicas, M., Cervera, J., Agirre, X., Marin-Bejar, O., Marcotegui, N., Vicente, C., Lahortiga, I., Gomez-Benito, M., Carranza, C., Valencia, A., Brunet, S., Lumbreras, E., Prosper, F., Gomez-Casares, M.T., Hernandez-Rivas, J.M., Calasanz, M.J., Sanz, M.A., Sierra, J. & Odero, M.D. (2011). Downregulation of EVI1 is associated with epigenetic alterations and good prognosis in patients with acute myeloid leukemia. Haematologica; Vol. 96, No.10, 448-56.

von Lindern, M., Poustka, A., Lerach, H., & Grosveld, G. (1990). The (6;9) chromosome translocation, associated with a specific subtype of acute nonlymphocytic leukemia, leads to aberrant transcription of a target gene on 9q34. Molecular and Cellular Biology, Vol. 10, No.8, 4016-4026.

von Lindern, M., Fornerod, M., van Baal, S., Jaegle, M., de Wit, T., Buijs, A., & Grosveld, G. (1992). The translocation (6;9), associated with a specific subtype of acute myeloid leukemia, results in the fusion of two genes, dek and can, and the expression of a chimeric, leukemia-specific dek-can mRNA. Molecular and Cellular Biology, Vol. 12, No.4, 1687-1697.

Weisser, M., Kern, W., Rauhut, S., Schoch, C., Hiddemann, W., Haferlach, T., & Schnittger, S. (2005). Prognostic impact of RT-PCR-based quantification of WT1 gene expression during MRD monitoring of acute myeloid leukemia. Leukemia : official journal of the Leukemia Society of America, Leukemia Research Fund, U.K, Vol. 19, No.8, 1416-1423, 0887-6924.

Whitman, S. P., Liu, S., Vukosavljevic, T., Rush, L. J., Yu, L., Liu, C., Klisovic, M. I., Maharry, K., Guimond, M., Strout, M. P., Becknell, B., Dorrance, A., Klisovic, R. B., Plass, C., Bloomfield, C. D., Marcucci, G., & Caligiuri, M. A. (2005). The MLL partial tandem duplication: evidence for recessive gain-of-function in acute myeloid leukemia identifies a novel patient subgroup for molecular-targeted therapy. Blood, Vol. 106, No.1, 345-352.

Wouters, B. J., Löwenberg, B., Erpelinck-Verschueren, C. A. J., van Putten, W. L. J., Valk, P. J. M., & Delwel, R. (2009). Double CEBPA mutations, but not single CEBPA mutations, define a subgroup of acute myeloid leukemia with a distinctive gene expression profile that is uniquely associated with a favorable outcome. Blood, Vol. 113, No.13, 3088-3091.

Wulf, G. G., Jahns-Streubel, G., Nobiling, R., Strutz, F., Hemmerlein, B., Hiddemann, W., & Wörmann, B. (1998). Renin in acute myeloid leukaemia blasts. British Journal of Haematology, Vol. 100, No.2, 335-337, 1365-2141.

Yanada, M., Matsuo, K., Suzuki, T., Kiyoi, H., & Naoe, T. (2005). Prognostic significance of FLT3 internal tandem duplication and tyrosine kinase domain mutations for acute myeloid leukemia: a meta-analysis. Leukemia: official journal of the Leukemia Society of America, Leukemia Research Fund, U.K, Vol. 19, No.8, 1345-1349, 0887-6924.

5

The Association of the DNA Repair Genes with Acute Myeloid Leukemia: The Susceptibility and the Outcome After Therapy

Claudia Bănescu, Carmen Duicu and Minodora Dobreanu
Univ Med & Pharm Tg-Mures
România

1. Introduction

Acute myeloid leukemia (AML), the most common acute leukemia in adults, is a clonal hemopoietic disorder that is frequently associated with genetic instability characterized by a diversity of chromosomal and molecular abnormalities. There are a lot of reports that show that human cancer can be initiated by DNA damage caused by ultraviolet (UV), ionizing radiation, and environmental chemical agents. Many genes encode proteins that function to protect cells against genetic instability through numerous mechanisms, including deoxyribonucleic acid (DNA) repair pathways and protection against oxidative stress.

DNA repair pathways play an important role in maintaining the integrity of the genome, and it is obvious that defects in repair pathways are involved in many different types of diseases, including leukemia and cancer (Seedhouse, 2002).

DNA damage repair and cell-cycle checkpoints are the most important defense mechanisms against mutagenic exposures. The most important DNA-repair pathways in human cells are: direct repair, base excision repair (BER), nucleotide excision repair (NER), mismatch repair (MMR), Double Strand Break Repair (DSB repair) and translesion DNA synthesis (TLS). Each pathway repairs a different type of lession (D'Andrea, 2010). The NER pathway mainly removes bulky distortions in the shape of the DNA double helix. The BER pathway is responsible for removal of oxidized DNA bases that may arise endogenously or from exogenous agents. The DSB pathway is responsible for repairing double-strand breaks caused by a variety of exposures, including ionizing radiation. There are two distinct and complementary pathways for DSB repair-namely, homologous recombination (HR) and nonhomologous end joining (NHEJ).

Recent studies have suggested that DNA damage was related to the pathogenesis of some diseases such as AML. Therefore, some DNA repair genes may be involved in AML susceptibility (Allan, 2004; Kuptsova, 2007; Seedhouse, 2002, 2004; Voso, 2007).

Exposure to carcinogenic and genotoxic compounds causes DNA damage, and the cells have developed multiple DNA repair pathways to protect themselves from different types of DNA damage.

Polymorphisms in DNA repair genes, including those involved in base excision repair (BER), nucleotide excision repair, mismatch repair and double strand break repair have been implicated in carcinogenesis. Common polymorphisms in DNA repair genes may alter protein function and an individual's capacity to repair damaged DNA. Deficits in repair capacity may lead to genetic instability and tumorigenesis.

Studies have noted associations between risk of de novo AML and DNA repair gene polymorphisms (Matullo et al., 2006; Seedhouse et al., 2004). Increased risk of therapy-related AML was also linked to several gene polymorphisms in base excision repair (BER; XRCC1 Arg399Gln), nucleotide excision repair (NER; XPD Lys751Gln), and DSB repair (RAD51 G135C and XRCC3 Thr241Met) pathways (Allan et al. 2004; Seedhouse et al., 2002, 2004) and may be linked to secondary AML etiology through failure to recognize or excise accumulated DNA lesions.

2. Mechanism of DNA repair

DNA damage response pathways, some of the genes known to participate in each of these pathways, their modes of action are summarized in Table 1. These categories are not exclusive; there may be functional overlap between repair systems. For example, certain types of base damage can be repaired by base excision repair, nucleotide excision repair or homologous recombinational repair.

DNA repair genes may also have great implications in the therapeutic outcome of certain cancer treatments. Most antileukemic drugs interact with target cell DNA and exert their cytotoxic effects preferentially in replicating cells. In addition to the primary DNA lesions, secondary DNA alterations induced in the course of repair processes also contribute to the cytotoxic effects of DNA-reactive agents (Rajewsky &Müller, 2005).

Although there are several reports on associations between polymorphisms in DNA repair genes and cancer risk (Goode et al., 2002), fewer studies have been conducted to evaluate relationships between DNA repair gene polymorphisms and response to treatment.

2.1 Direct repair mechanism

This is the simplest repair mechanism compared to other repair system regarding number of molecules involved. It is an enzyme-catalyzed process used to correct the most frequent cause of point mutations in humans.

In direct repair mechanisms, the lesion is removed or reversed by a single step reaction restoring the local sequence to its original state. There are several direct repair enzymes, each having a different substrate. For example, O^6- methyl guanine DNA methyltransferase (O^6-MT, the product of the MGMT gene) repairs the alkylation damage. MGMT is important in the repair of alkylation damage. The alkyl group from the lesion is transferred to a cysteine residue in the active site of MGMT (Hazra et al., 1997). In 20% of human tumor cell lines the MGMT activity is decreased and the sensivity to alkylating agent is increased (Sancar, 1995), but there are few data which suggest that mutations in the MGMT gene contribute to cancer (Wang L et al, 1997; Yu Z et al, 1999).

The functional status of the O^6-MT pathway may be important in patients treated with alkylating agents, for O^6-methylation of guanine appears to be an important effect of some members of that class of drugs (Kaina & Christmann, 2002). High levels of O^6-MT are often found in AML blasts, which are thereby rendered resistant to certain alkylators (Gerson & Trey, 1988).

Pathway	Function	Genes Involved	References
Direct Repair Mechanism	Reverses damage to restore DNA integrity.	DNA photolyase, O^6-MGMT	Kaina et al., 2007; Mitra, 2007
Base Excision Repair (BER)	Repair of damaged bases or single-strand DNA breaks	OGG1, XRCC1, APE1, PARP,	Chaudhry, 2007; Yu et al., 1999; Hazra et al., 2007
Nucleotide Excision Repair (NER)	Excision of a variety of helix-distorting DNA lesions	XPA, XPB, XPC, XPD, XPE, XPF, XPG, RAD23, TFIIH, RPA1, RPA2, RPA3, PCNA	Kang et al., 2011; Reardon & Sancar, 2005; Yu et al., 1999
Mismatch Repair (MMR)	Repair of mispaired nucleotides	MSH2, MSH6, MSH4, PMS1, MLH1, PMS2, MLH3, PMS2L3, PCNA, RPA	Jiricny, 2006; Martin et al., 2010; Papouli et al., 2004; Surtees et al., 2004
Homologous recombination (HR)	Repair of double strand DNA break	RAD51, RAD51B, RAD51C, RAD51D, XRCC2, XRCC3, RAD52, RAD54, BRCA1, BRCA2, RAD50, NBS1, MRE11	Li & Heyer, 2008; Sung & Klein, 2006;
Nonhomologous End Joining (NHEJ)	Repair of double strand DNA breaks	XRCC4, XRCC5, XRCC6, XRCC7, LIG4, XLF,	Burma et al., 2006; Shrivastav et al., 2008
Translesion Synthesis (TLS)	Bypass of DNA adducts during DNA replication	POLK, POLI, POLZ, REV7, REV1, POLH,	Lehmann, 2006

Table 1. DNA Damage Response Pathways

2.2 Base Excision Repair

Base excision repair (BER) is the predominant DNA damage repair pathway for the processing of small base lesions, derived from ionizing radiation (Chen et al., 2010), oxidation, hydrolysis, or deamination and alkylation damages. The repair system involves three steps: removal of damaged bases from DNA by DNA glycosylases, then formed abasic site is removed and finally gap is filled by DNA polymerase.

In BER, the removal of a single modified base from one DNA strand is performed by DNA glycosylases, specialized enzymes. Some of these glycosylases show pronounced lesion specificity, others recognize multiple, and structurally different damaged bases. The apurinic/apyrimidinic (AP) site left behind after cleavage of the N-glycosylic bond is hydrolyzed by an AP endonuclease, and the 5'-deoxyribose phosphate is excised by a phosphodiesterase. The resulting single-nucleotide gap is then filled by polymerase β and ligated. Alternatives to this common BER pathway include the excision of a short oligonucleotide patch containing the AP site and filling of the gap by polymerase δ or ε. Base alterations caused by a large variety of agents and processes (e.g. spontaneous deamination, ionizing radiation, alkylating agents, DNA replication errors) are processed by BER. A common feature of the DNA lesions recognized by BER glycosylases is that they do not significantly distort the DNA helix (Yu, 2009).

Common single-nucleotide polymorphisms (SNPs) in the 8-oxoguanine glycosylase 1 (OGG1), X-ray repair cross-complementing group1 (XRCC1), and the apyrimidinic endonuclease-endonuclease 1 (APE1) genes in the BER pathway have been studied for their influences in induction of DNA damage (Chen et al., 2010).

XRCC1

X-ray repair cross-complementing group 1 (XRCC1) is required for repairing single-strand breaks and damaged bases in DNA. The XRCC1 protein interacts with DNA polymerase β, DNA ligase III and polyadenosine diphosphate-ribose polymerases (PARP) involved in excision and recombinational repair pathways (Cardecott, 2003). The XRCC1 has no known enzymatic activity (Thompson et al., 1990) and participates as a scaffold protein in both single-strand break repair and base excision repair activities. The human XRCC1 gene is located on chromosome 19q13.2 which contains 17 exons and encodes a protein of consisting 633 amino acids (Lindahl & Wood, 1999). More than 60 validated single-nucleotide XRCC1 polymorphisms are known. The most studied single nucleotide polymorphisms are Arg194Trp on exon 6, Arg280His on exon 9, and Arg399Gln on exon 10. All these polymorphisms were studied with association to different types of cancer.

The presences of the variant (399Gln and 194Trp) alleles have been shown to be associated with measurable reduced DNA repair capacity and increased risk of several types of cancers (Dufloth et al., 2005; Goode et al., 2002; Hu et al., 2005; Hung et al., 2005). In our study involving 43 patients with acute leukemia and 40 controls, for XRCC1 Arg194Trp and Arg399Gln polymorphism, we observed the relationship of XRCC1 polymorphisms with acute myeloid leukemia (our own unpublished data). Our cases with a codon 194 Trp/Trp homozygous variant as well as the heterozygous Arg/Trp variant had an increased risk of AML with a greater risk in the case of the homozygous codon 194 Trp/Trp allele (OR=2.28, 95% for Trp/Trp). There was a significantly high risk of AML among patients who were carriers of the variant allele 399Gln (OR=2.45, 95% for Gln/Gln and OR=1.90, 95% for Arg/Gln).

A study by Seedhouse et al. (2002) reported that the presence of at least one XRCC1 399Gln allele indicated a protective effect for the allele in controls compared with patients with AML, particularly therapy-related AML (t-AML) (odds ratio OR=0.44; 95% confidence interval CI=0.20~0.93). According to the same study patients who develop AML as a result of therapy for a primary malignancy are more likely to have the wild-type XRCC1 399 arginine allele. El-Din et al. (2010) reported that XRCC1 gene polymorphism is important in the pathogenesis of de novo AML. El-Din et al. (2010) observed that AML patients expressing XRCC1 Arg194Trp polymorphism are at high risk of developing AML; in addition, a significant risk in the development of AML was observed when XRCC1 Arg399Gln polymorphism was present. In a study of 372 patients with acute myeloid leukemia, Kuptsova et al. (2007) reported no significant associations between XRCC1 polymorphisms and treatment outcomes.

hOGG1

The human 8-oxoguanine DNA glycosylase 1 (hOGG1) encoded by the hOGG1 gene can remove 8-hydroxy-2-deoxyguanine (8-OHdG) from damaged DNA as a part of the base excision repair pathway (Kohno et al., 1998). The hOGG1 gene is located on chromosome 3p26.2 (Kohno et al., 1998). Although, several polymorphisms in the hOGG1 gene have been described, the most commonly studied polymorphism is an amino acid change from serine to cysteine at codon 326 (Ser326Cys). Several studies have reported that Ser326Cys polymorphism in OGG1 gene may increase susceptibility to for bladder (Arizono et al., 2008), lung (Park et al., 2004), oesophageal (Xing et al., 2001), gallbladder and gastric (Tsukino et al., 2004) cancer development.

Liddiard et al (2010) provided a study about the importance of 8-oxoguanine in AML including the genotyping of 174 AML patients for the hOGG1 Ser326Cys polymorphism. Using Affymetrix microarrays they showed that the prevalence rate of hOGG1 expression was 33% and correlated strongly with adverse cytogenetics. hOGG1-expressing patients had a worse relapse-free survival and overall survival and an increased risk of relapse at 5-years of follow-up. According to Liddiard et al. (2010) hOGG1 is an important prognostic marker that could be used to sub-stratify AML patients to predict those likely to fail conventional chemotherapies and those likely to benefit from novel therapeutic approaches that modulate DNA repair activity. In a recent study Stanczyk et al. (2011) have demonstrated that Cys/Cys variant of the OGG1 Ser326Cys polymorphism may increase the risk of ALL (OR=5.36, P<0.001).

APE1

The human apurinic/apyrimidinic endonuclease (APE1) plays a central role in the base excision repair pathway, which is the primary mechanism for the repair of DNA damage caused by oxidation and alkylation. The APE1 gene is located on chromosome 14q11.2–q12 and contains five exons. A total of 18 polymorphisms in APE1 have been reported, but the most extensively studied polymorphism is Asp148Glu (Gu et al., 2009). The damaged bases of purine and pyrimidine are recognized and excised by specific DNA glycosylases, leaving abasic sites. Apurinic/apyrimidinic endonuclease then incise the DNA 5' to the abasic sites; further repair proceeds to short-patch (when the gap is only one nucleotide) or long-patch (when the gap is two or more nucleotides) subpathways of base excision repair (Lo et al., 2009). In a hospital-based matched case-control study with 730 lung cancer cases and 730 cancer-free controls Lo et al. (2009) found that the -656T>G variant in the APE1 promoter was associated with a significantly decreased risk for lung cancer. In a study of 320 pediatric patients with acute leukemia, Krajinovic et al. (2002) reported no significant associations between polymorphic APE1 148Glu and XRCC1 194Trp variants and event-free survival. Ji et al. (2020) performed a meta-analysis to explore the association between the APE1 Asn148Glu gene polymorphisms and lung cancer risk. They suggested that the APE1 T1349G (Asp148Glu) polymorphism was not associated with lung cancer risk among Asians or Caucasians. But, the APE1 G allele was an increased risk factor for developing lung cancer among smokers. Pre-clinical and clinical data indicate a role for APE1 in the pathogenesis of cancer and in resistance to DNA-interactive drugs, particularly monofunctional alkylators and antimetabolites (Wilson & Simeonov, 2010).

2.3 Nucleotide Excision Repair

Nucleotide excision repair is the most studied DNA repair system in humans (de Laat et al., 1999). The NER pathway is responsible for repair of bulky distortions in the shape of the DNA double helix such as chemical adducts, pyrimidine dimers, and cross-links caused by endogenous and environmental lesions (Riedl et al., 2003; van der Wees et al., 2007; Wood, 1989). This pathway may also be important in conferring resistance to chemotherapeutic agents such as platinum-based chemotherapy (Kennedy & D'Andrea, 2006).

NER has five stages: recognition of the bulky damage which distorts the DNA helix; hydrolyzing a phosphodiester bond in the deoxyribose backbone on the 5' side of the lesion; excising the damage; filling in the resultant gap using the information from the complementary strand; closing the nicked DNA to generate intact strand (Yasbin, 2002).

NER can be divided into two subpathways (Transcription coupled NER and Global genomic NER) that differ only in their recognition of helix-distorting DNA damage (Hanawalt, 2002). Global genome repair is a slow process of inspecting the entire genome for damage (Kennedy & D'Andrea AD, 2006). Transcription-coupled repair is more rapid, highly specific and efficient and repairs DNA damage that blocks the progression of RNA polymerase II.

The actual repair mechanism appears to be identical in transcription-coupled and in global-genome repair. However, the damage recognition in global-genome repair does not involve the RNA polymerase, but is performed by the XPC and HHR23 proteins. Following lesion recognition, however, both repair systems use TFIIH components such as XPB and XPD, as well as the single-strand binding protein RPA and the XPA protein to fully unwind and mark the lesion. The damaged segment of DNA is excised through 5'-incision by the XPF endonuclease and 3'-incision by the XPG endonuclease. The DNA gap is filled by DNA polymerases δ or ε supported by PCNA and sealed by a DNA ligase, presumably DNA ligase I (Kennedy & D'Andrea, 2006; Yu et al., 1999).

XPD

The XPD gene (xeroderma pigmentosum group D, also known as ERCC2) encodes a DNA helicase involved in nucleotide excision repair pathway. The XPD gene maps to chromosome 19q13.3 and consists of 23 exons (Wang et al., 2008). Its protein is 761 amino acids in length. The XPD protein repairs a wide range of structurally unrelated lesions, such as bulky adducts and thymidine dimers (Braithwaite et al., 1999). The DNA repair process and gene transcription are coupled via activity of the TFIIH complex, a protein complex with functions including transcription, NER, transcription-coupled repair, apoptosis, and cell cycle regulation. XPD protein is involved in maintaining the stability of the TFIIH complex. The XPD gene product has an ATP-dependent DNA helicase activity (Laine et al, 2007).

Because of the biological significance of XPD, the XPD Lys751Gln (2251A>C) polymorphism has been a common subject of studies in different malignant diseases in the last years. Although the XPD 751Gln variant was associated with an increased risk of esophageal cancer and acute lymphoid leukemia (Wang et al., 2008) Allan et al. (2004) investigated XPD Lys751Gln polymorphism in 341 adult British AML patients and observed that the XPD codon 751 polymorphism is an independent prognostic marker for disease-free survival and overall survival in elderly AML patients treated with chemotherapy, and specifically that the glutamine variant was associated with a poorer prognosis relative to the lysine variant. In a pediatric study, Mehta et al. (2006) found no influence of XPD751 genotype on susceptibility to de novo AML in children. In another study, Kuptsova-Clarkson et al. (2010)

evaluated the role of XPD and XRCC1 gene polymorphic variation in response to induction
chemotherapy, toxicities and survival in a population of 293 predominantly Caucasian adult
patients treated for AML. Kuptsova-Clarkson et al. (2010) had reported that in AML,
variation in the XPD gene may be associated with suboptimal DNA repair activity and may
thus predispose to therapy-related AML development. In a UK study by Seedhouse et al.
(2002), therapy-related AML was not associated with XPD genotypes.

There have been studies of XPD, involved in NER, and survival of patients with AML (Allan
et al., 2004). In a study of elderly patients with AML conducted by researchers in the United
Kingdom, modestly increased hazard ratio (HR) of 1.30 and 1.19 were found for disease-free
and overall survival, respectively, by XPD variant genotypes. However, in a study of
pediatric patients with acute myeloid leukemia conducted by the the Children's Oncology
Group (Mehta et al., 2006) survival and treatment-related mortality were not associated with
XPD codon 751 genotypes.

2.4 Mismatch repair

DNA mismatch repair (MMR) plays a critical role in maintaining genomic integrity. MMR is
responsible for correction of mismatched basepairs which occurs through processes
including misincorporations during DNA replication, formation of heteroduplexes, and
secondary structure such as imperfect palindromes (Bishop et al., 1985).

In addition, MMR can also process some types of DNA damage. MMR deficient tumors
display widespread alterations in simple repetitive DNA sequences, a phenomenon also
called microsatellite instability; MSI (Li, 2008). The repair mechanism is similar to that of
excision repair; a patch of nucleotides is removed from one strand, and followed by
resynthesis and ligation processes.

There are two types of mismatch repair, long-patch and short-patch which have been found
in human cells. In short-patch repair system there are three enzymes possessing nicking
activities specific for mismatch repair; T/G specific (Wiebauer & Jiricny, 1989), A/G specific,
and all type mismatch nicking enzymes (Yeh et al., 1991). That enzymes have different mode
of action, but in either an A/G mismatch or a T/G mismatch, it is usually the guanine that
remains untouched by mismatch specific glycosylases (Wiebauer & Jiricny, 1989).

Long patch can repair all types of mismatches. Long-patch MMR removes a patch of one of
the DNA strands from an incision on the to-be-removed strand to 90~170 nucleotides
beyond the mismatch (Fang & Modrich, 1993; Yu et al., 1999).

Defects in the MMR pathway significantly increase the mutation frequency and promote
oncogenesis. It has been documented that defects in MMR genes, are the genetic basis for
certain types of hereditary and sporadic cancers, including hereditary nonpolyposis
colorectal cancer (Mao et al., 2008). There are some studies looking at the incidence of MMR
deficiency (microsatellite instability; MSI) in AML (Mao et al., 2008). Genomic instability in
AML has led to a search for MSI in AML patients, but the results are quite controversial.
While several studies have reported MSI in AML (Das-Gupta et al., 2001; Sheikhha et al.,
2002), a study of 132 cases failed to confirm the previous results (Rimsza et al., 2000).
According to Rimsza et al. (2000) MMR deficiency was associated with all stages of AML,
but the rate of the deficiency was much higher in patients with refractory and relapsed AML
than in de novo AML patients, suggesting that the loss of MMR function could contribute to
the refractory and relapsed disease.

2.5 Double Strand Break repair

Double strand break repair (DSB) is responsible for the repair of double strand DNA breaks. DNA double strand breaks represent the most important class of DNA damage because, if unrepaired, they can result in a loss of genetic material, chromosome abnormalities and possibly cell death. Moreover, the breaks are prone to nuclease attack with subsequent destruction (Rufer & Morgan, 1992). Double strand breaks (DSBs) can be produced by exogenous agents such as ionizing radiation, some chemotherapeutic drugs, endogenous formed reactive oxygen species. When DNA replication forks encounter DNA single strand breaks or other types of lesion, it might result in formation of DSBs. In addition, DSBs are generated to initiate recombination between homologues chromosomes during meiosis, and also during the immunoglobulin class-switch recombination. Repair of DSBs is more difficult than other type of DNA damage because there is no undamaged template available (Khanna & Jackson, 2001).

Direct DSBs are mainly repaired by non-homologous end joining (Sargent et al., 1997), whereas replication-associated DSBs are repaired by homologous recombination (HR) and related replication repair pathways (Iliakis et al., 2004).

2.5.1 Non-homologous End Joining

Non homologous end joining (NHEJ) is active in all phases of the cell cycle and is considered to be the most important DSB repair pathway in mammalian cells. The NHEJ pathway is simpler than HR and requires no complementary template. The protein components of NHEJ include the catalytic subunit of DNA protein kinase (DNA-PKCS), the two regulatory subunits of the DNA-PK complex Ku70 and Ku80, DNA ligase IV with its cofactor XRCC4 (the X-ray cross complementing group 4 protein) and the nuclease artemis (Drouet et al., 2005; Khanna & Jackson, 2001). The Ku70/Ku80 (Ku) heterodimer is the first protein to bind to the damaged DNA ends. When bound to the DSB, Ku recruits and activates DNA-PKcs. These proteins play an important role in DNA DSB repair and will act as tumor suppressors. However, either the DNA protein kinase complex, or its three subunits individually, can also act as oncogenes, depending on the compartment of the cell in which they are expressed and on the cell cycle phase (Gullo et al., 2006).

XRCC4

The X-ray cross-complementing group 4 (XRCC4) gene is one of the specific members of the NHEJ system. Some of the SNPs of XRCC4 have been found to be associated with the susceptibility to different types of cancer. Two single nucleotide polymorphisms (SNPs) of XRCC4, one splicing-site polymorphism (SNP14 rs1805377:A4G) and one intronic polymorphism (SNP1 rs2075685:G4T), have been studied, and the results are conflicting (Allen-Brady et al., 2006; Fu et al., 2003). The protein encoded by XRCC4 consists of 336 amino acid residues distributed among 8 exons, and has a long helical stem domain responsible for multimerization and interaction with DNA ligase IV (Junop et al., 2000). By forming a complex with DNA ligase IV and DNA-dependent protein kinase, XRCC4 functions in the repair of DNA double-strand breaks by non-homologous end joining (NHEJ) and the completion of V(D)J recombination events (Hayden et al, 2007). The NHEJ pathway is required not only for normal development but also for suppression of tumors. Since it is one of the ubiquitous NHEJ components, XRCC4 might be considered as a potential tumor suppressor gene in cancer and leukemia.

There have been several studies showing that variations of the XRCC4 gene are associated with prostate (Chang et al., 2008), gastric (Chiu et al., 2008), and breast cancer (Fu et al., 2003). Therefore, XRCC4 and the DNA double-strand break repair pathway may serve as a common mechanism of early carcinogenesis. In a recent study, Wu et al. (2008) investigated the association between XRCC4 gene polymorphisms and oral cancer. Their findings suggest that the presence of the A allele of XRCC4 codon 247 was associated with a higher susceptibility to oral cancer, and the A allele of XRCC4 codon 247 may be a useful novel marker in oral oncology for primary prevention and intervention.

XRCC5, XRCC6, XRCC7

A key component of the NHEJ pathway is the DNA-dependent Protein Kinase (DNA-PK), which consists of a heterodimeric DNA targeting subunit (i.e., Ku70/Ku80, encoded by XRCC6/XRCC5 genes) and a catalytic subunit DNA-PKcs, encoded by XRCC7 gene (Smith & Jackson, 1999).

XRCC5 (X-ray repair cross-complementing 5) is a gene involved in repair of DNA double-strand breaks. Abnormal expression of the XRCC5 protein is associated with genomic instability and an increased incidence of cancers. The XRCC5 gene mapped to chromosome 2q35, encodes the 80-kDa subunit of the Ku heterodimer protein, the DNA-binding component of the DNA-dependent protein kinase. The Ku80 is essential for maintaining genomic integrity through its ability to bind DNA double-strand breaks and to facilitate repair by the nonhomologous end-joining pathway in mammalian cells (Taccioli et al., 1994).

XRCC6 (X-ray repair complementing defective repair in Chinese hamster cells 6) is a helicase involved in DNA repair and chromatin remodeling. The XRCC6 gene (also called Ku70) maps to chromosome 22q13.2-q1. Ku70 plays an important role in the DNA double-strand breaks repair and maintenance of genomic integrity. Genetic variations within human Ku70 have been demonstrated to be associated with increased risk of several types of cancers (Wenshan et al., 2011).

XRCC7 (X-ray repair cross complementing group 7) is located on chromosome 8q12, span about 110-180 kb and contains 100 exons. The human XRCC7 gene encodes DNA-PKcs, which is recruited to the site of DSBs by the Ku70/Ku80 heterodimer to form an active DNA-PK complex (Sipley et al., 1995). The expression of Ku70 and XRCC7 is elevated in bladder tumor tissue and head and neck cancer cell lines, respectively (Stronati et al., 2001; Sturgis et al., 1999) and Ku70 may function as a caretaker gene for the development of T-cell lymphomas (Li et al., 1998). XRCC7 encodes DNA-PKcs, which also may have a caretaker role in colon carcinogenesis. Therefore, the variants of the Ku70 and XRCC7 genes could be expected to have an effect on DSB repair, and thus, on carcinogenesis. The Ku70 polymorphism is associated with risk of breast cancer (Fu et al., 2003), and the XRCC7 polymorphism is associated with risk of glioma (Wang et al., 2004). According to Wang et al. (2008) the XRCC7 polymorphism appears to be involved in the etiology of human bladder cancer. This data support the notion that the XRCC7 polymorphism is implicated in cancer risk.

Given the crucial roles of the NHEJ pathway in DNA repair (Gullo et al., 2006), it is possible that the XRCC5, XRCC6 and XRCC7 variants may modulate the risk of cancer, including leukemia. It has been shown that increased NHEJ activity is due to the presence of XRCC5 and XRCC6 protein, which results in genomic instability in myeloid leukemia cells (Gaymes et al., 2002). XRCC5 and XRCC6 may function as a caretaker gene for the development of T-cell lymphomas, while XRCC7 may have a caretaker role in colon carcinogenesis (Wang et al., 2009). In a recent study, Wang et al. (2009) have investigated the association between the X-ray repair cross complementing group XRCC5, XRCC6 and XRCC7 polymorphisms and risk of AML in Chinese population. In this case-control study in a southern Chinese population three polymorphisms, XRCC5 2R/1R/0R, XRCC6 -61C>G and XRCC7 6721G>T were investigated. For the XRCC7 6721G>T polymorphism among AML cases and controls no significant association was observed (P=0.68). Significant association was observed (P=0.04) for the XRCC6 -61C > G polymorphism. Their analysis revealed that compared with the XRCC6 -61CC wild type homozygote, the -61CG heterozygotes had a significant 43% decreased risk of AML (adjusted OR=0.57; 95% CI=0.35~0.92) and subjects carrying -61CG/GG variant genotypes had 45% decrease in risk of AML (adjusted OR=0.55; 95% CI=0.34~0.89). For the XRCC5 2R/1R/0R polymorphism, Wang et al. (2009) found that XRRC5 1R/0R genotype was associated with a 2.60-fold increase in risk of AML (95% CI=1.42~5.92) compared with the 2R/2R genotype. They found a significant association with the polymorphisms of XRCC5 2R/1R/0R, XRCC6 -61C>G and the risk of AML, but there was no evidence for an association between the XRCC7 6721G>T variants and AML.

2.5.2 Homologous recombination

Homologous recombination (HR) is one of the main pathways for the repair of DNA double strand breaks (DSBs). HR is thought to be particularly important in DNA repair occurring during cellular replication (Rollinson et al., 2007). Although HR is indispensable for maintaining genome integrity, it must be tightly regulated to avoid harmful outcomes. The repair process is complex and involves many proteins working coordinately. Key players include MRE11, RAD50, NBS1 (MRN), RAD51, RAD51B, RAD51C, RAD51D, XRCC2, XRCC3, RAD52, RAD54 and BRCA2 (Lieberman, 2008). A number of polymorphic genes involved in this pathway have been studied in AML.

Homologous recombination mechanism starts with degradation of the DNA next to the double-strand break, leaving single-strand ends. Next the single-strand end of the damaged strand invades and binds to its complementary DNA sequence on the homologous duplex. This is associated with the displacement of the cross-complementary strand toward the gap site, where it serves as a template for gap-filling DNA synthesis. The repair sequence is terminated by religation of the repair patches. This mechanism requires the presence of undamaged homologous DNA, and increased activity of this repair pathway has been observed.

RAD51 protein catalyzes homologous recombination through its homologous pairing and strand exchange activities. RAD52 may modulate these activities through its RAD51-interacting region. The ability of RAD52 to induce homologous recombination requires its binding to the p34 subunit of RPA. This RPA binding domain is at amino acids 221–280. Recall that RPA is also involved in NER—this may provide a linkage between these two repair systems (Yu Z et al., 1999).

XRRC3

The X-ray repair cross-complementing group 3 (XRCC3), codes for a protein participating in homologous recombination repair of DNA double-strand breaks. XRCC3 is a member of the RAD-51-related protein family. RAD-51-like proteins are known to participate in homologous recombination to maintain chromosome stability and repair DNA damage (Brenneman et al., 2000). XRCC3-deficient cells demonstrated genetic instability and increased sensitivity to DNA damaging agents (Griffin, 2002). The human XRCC3 gene is located on chromosome 14q32.3 and consists of 17870 bases. The protein product of XRCC3 gene contains 346 amino acids. According to NCBI SNP database, XRCC3 gene has 111 SNPs. The main polymorphism in this gene involves the change of threonine (Thr) to methionine (Met) at codon 241 in exon 7 (Shen et al., 1998). Little is known about the functional consequences of this variation, although some studies observed a positive relation between the Thr241Met polymorphism and an increased risk for skin (Winsey et al., 2000), bladder (Matullo et al., 2001), breast (Garcia-Closas et al., 2006) and lung (Jacobsen et al., 2004) cancers.

A meta-analysis of 48 case–control studies, including 24975 cancer patients and 34209 controls, investigated the associations of the three DNA repair gene XRCC3 polymorphisms (Thr241Met; 4541A4G; 17893A4G) with cancer risk (Han et al., 2006). According to this meta-analysis individuals carrying the XRCC3 Met/Met genotype have a smaller cancer risk compared with the individuals with the Thr/Thr or Thr/Met genotype (OR=1.07; P=0.008; 95% CI=1.02~1.13) (Han et al., 2006). For A4541G, a significantly increased risk was associated with the variant genotypes (G/G+A/G), compared with the wild homozygote A/A genotype (OR=1.09; P=0.004; 95% CI, 1.03~1.15). For A17893G, individuals with the variant genotypes (G/G+A/G) had a significantly decreased cancer risk, compared with individuals with the A/A genotype under a dominant genetic model (OR=0.92; P=0.0004; 95% CI=0.87~0.96). Han et al. (2006) consider that the XRCC3 could not be a major increased risk factor for cancer but it might represent a low-penetrance susceptible gene especially for cancer of breast, bladder, head and neck, and non-melanoma skin cancer

In their study Seedhouse et al. (2004) have observed that the presence of variant XRCC3 241Met was associated with an increase in the risk of developing therapy-related AML of more than 8 fold, whereas the increase in risk for the development of de novo AML was nearly 4 fold.

RAD 51

The RAD51 gene plays an important role in homologous recombination and in maintaining the genetic stability of the cell. In HR, RAD51 interacts with and is stabilized by XRCC3, during strand invasion and cross-strand resolution. RAD51 is a central protein in the HR repair pathway binding to DNA and promoting ATP-dependent homologous pairing and strand transfer reactions.

The RAD51 gene is located on chromosome 15q15.1 and consists of 36998 bases. The protein product of RAD51 has 6 domains, one for DNA binding, one for ATPase activity, and the other domains are specific to action of RAD51. According to NCBI SNP database, RAD51 gene has 296 SNPs. The most important polymorphism identified for RAD51 is G135C SNP in 5′ untranslated region. The RAD51 G135C polymorphism is associated with RAD51 protein over-expression (Richardson et al., 2004). Regarding the role of RAD51 in the homologous DNA repair mechanism, several studies have examined the relationship between RAD51 G135C polymorphism and risk of certain cancers. However the results from these studies are conflicting. Further studies are needed to establish the role of RAD51 G135C polymorphism in human carcinogenesis.

Voso et al. (2007) found an increased frequency of the RAD51 135C allele in AML, mainly in de novo AML, when compared with controls, but not between therapy-related AML (t-AML) and controls. Other reports found increased frequency of the RAD51 135C allele in t-AML patients compared with controls (Seedhouse et al., 2004), suggesting an effect of RAD51 over-expression during leukemogenesis induced by chemotherapy or radiotherapy. According to Bhatla et al. (2008) RAD51 gene polymorphism did not influence the outcome of AML therapy in the study of de novo AML patients. On the contrary, Liu et al. (2008) concluded that RAD51 gene polymorphism was significantly related to response to therapy, adverse effects, and prognosis of AML and reported that detection of the RAD51 gene polymorphism genotypes may be useful in selecting individual chemotherapy regimens for patients with AML. Also, Bolufer et al. (2007) reported that the RAD51 gene polymorphism showed significant unfavorable outcome among AML patients.

In their study, Bathla et al. (2008) observed a doubling of risk of AML in children with a RAD51 G135C variant allele and a wild-type XRCC3 Thre241Met genotype. In addition risk of AML was significantly increased in children with at least one variant XRCC3 Thr241Met allele. In antithesis, risk was not significantly elevated in children with variant alleles at both wild-type XRCC3 Thre241Met and RAD51 G135C. Liu et al. (2008) found that XRCC3 gene polymorphism was significantly related to response to therapy and prognosis of AML and reported that detection of the XRCC3 gene polymorphism genotypes may be useful in selecting individual chemotherapy regimens for AML patients.

2.6 Translesion synthesis

Translesion synthesis is an important mechanism by which cells replicate past DNA damage. The sliding clamp DNA polymerase processivity factors play a central role in this process. The clamps are dimeric in bacteria and trimeric in eukaryotes and archaea, raising the question of whether more than one polymerase can interact with the clamp simultaneously (Lehmann, 2006).

3. Inherited human disease with leukemia susceptibility

Several studies have demonstrated that the genes involved in DNA repair and maintenance of genome integrity are critically in protecting against mutations that lead to cancer and/or inherited human disease (Table 2).

Syndrome	Gene(s) involved	Chromosome	References
Fanconi anaemia (FA)	FANC-A to FANC-N	16q24.3	Levitus et al., 2004; Steensma, 2007;
Ataxia-telangiectasia (AT)	Ataxia-telangiectasia (AT)	11q22.3	Savitsky et al., 1995; Thompson & Schild, 2002
Nijmegen breakage syndrome (NBS)	NBS1 (Nibrin)	8p21	Digweed et al., 1999; Varon et al. 2003
Bloom syndrome (BLM)	BLM (RECQL3)	15q26.1	Ellis & German, 1996; Thompson & Schild, 2002
Seckel Syndrome	ATR	3q22-24	Casper et al., 2002;

Table 2. DNA repair defective syndromes

Several of these diseases include an inherent predisposition to hematologic malignancies, including AML. The clinical features and molecular characteristics of several of the inherited disorders with leukemia risk are described below.

Fanconi anemia (FA) is a rare disorder with a birth incidence around 3 per million. FA is an autosomal recessive and rarely X-linked syndrome which is characterised by congenital abnormalities, defective haemopoiesis (bone marrow failure) and a high risk of developing AML and certain solid tumours.

Affected individuals can have mild growth retardation, hypo- or hyperpigmented areas of the skin, skeletal defects including radial limb defects (absent thumb with or without radial aplasia), abnormalities of ribs and hips and scoliosis, cardiac and renal malformations, genital abnormalities (especially undescended testes, testicular agenesis, hypospadias). Other associated anomalies include micropthalmia and developmental delay (Grompe & D'Andrea, 2001). The phenotypic abnormalities are variable and there is marked variability between affected individuals in the same family (Alter, 1993).

The Fanconi anemia defect results from biallelic mutation of any one of thirteen known Fanconi anemia genes (A, B, C, D1, D2, E, F, G, I, J, L, M, N). The proteins encoded by these Fanconi anemia genes cooperate in a common DNA repair pathway, referred to as the Fanconi anemia /BRCA pathway. In this pathway, eight of the Fanconi anemia proteins (A, B, C, E, F, G, L, M) are assembled into a core complex that functions as an E3 ubiquitin ligase. This ligase activates in response to DNA damage from a crosslinking drug, adding a 76-amino acid moiety onto two other Fanconi proteins, D2 and I. This monoubiquinated D2/I complex is translocated into chromatin, where it interacts with the downstream Fanconi proteins BRCA2, N, and J. This combination of proteins mediates the DNA repair process. After the repair has occurred, there is another enzyme complex, called USP1, which removes the ubiquitin and inactivates the pathway. Knocking out any of the proteins in this pathway causes FA (D'Andrea, 2010).

FANCA, located on chromosome 16q24.3, is the most commonly mutated gene and is altered in 60-65% of FA patients (Steensma, 2007). FANCC and G mutations account for almost 25%, and FANCE and FANCF for a further 8%.

Approximately one third of patients homozygous for a Fanconi anemia gene mutation will develop a hematologic or solid tumors by the age of 40 years (Kennedy & D'Andrea, 2006). Fanconi anemia patients develop predominately myeloid malignancies (the most common hematologic maliganancy is AML), although numerous other cancers arise, including squamous cell carcinomas of the head and neck or gynecologic system, skin cancers, esophageal cancers and liver tumors (Alter, 2003; Rosenberg et al, 2008).

Fanconi anemia patients have a systemic DNA repair defect that results in a low tolerance for DNA damaging chemotherapeutic agents.

Ataxia–telangiectasia (AT) is a rare autosomal recessive disorder. This human disease is characterized by cerebellar degeneration, immunodeficiency, hypogonadism, growth retardation, genome instability, extreme sensitivity to radiation and predisposition to cancer (Taylor & Byrd, 2005). The disease is caused by homozygous mutations in the gene encoding the ATM protein kinase that plays a critical role in DNA damage detection and regulates DNA double-strand break repair (Mavrou et al, 2008). The ATM gene is located on chromosome 11q23. When ATM is dysfunctional or absent, cells are able to progress from G1 to S phase and initiate DNA replication in the presence of DNA damage.

Approximately one third of AT patients develop cancer, mainly leukemias and lymphomas which develop in childhood and are a common cause of death (Ball & Xiao, 2005; Gumy-Pause et al, 2004). Solid tumors in AT patients are usually adenocarcinoma of the stomach, dysgerminoma, gonadoblastoma and medulloblastoma (Mavrou et al, 2008).

Bloom's syndrome (BS) is a rare autosomal recessive syndrome of growth retardation, telangiectasia manifest by facial erythema, immunodeficiency, and skull abnormalities. BS patients also are predisposed to cancer, as they develop mostly leukemias and lymphomas in about half of the patients. This disorder is most commonly found in the Ashkenazi Jewish population resulting from a founder mutation (Ellis et al, 1998). It is characterised by low birth weight, growth deficiency, characteristic facies (long thin face, prominent nose) sun-sensitivity, immunodeficiency and infertility in males.

Bloom's syndrome arise through mutations in both copies of the BLM gene, which is located on chromosome 15 at 15q26.1. This gene encodes a member of the RecQ family of DNA helicases (BLM) that is important in maintaining appropriate DNA conformation during chromosomal recombination and repair. Together with topoisomerase III, BLM resolves Holliday junctions during homologous recombination (HR) by a mechanism called double-junction dissolution that is distinct from classical Holliday junction resolution and that prevents erroneous exchange of flanking sequences (Steensma, 2007).

Nijmegen breakage syndrome (NBS) is an autosomal recessive disorder that is most commonly found in Eastern Europe. NBS is caused by abnormalities in the NBN gene at 8p21 (Varon et al, 2003), which encodes the protein NBN (NBS1). Complete loss of this polypeptide is lethal. The NBS gene encodes a 95-kDa protein that binds with MRE11 and RAD50 to form a nuclease-containing protein complex that appears to be involved in homologous and nonhomologous recombination. Clinical features include growth retardation, microcephaly, skin findings such as vitiligo and café au lait spots, skeletal defects, immunodeficiency and propensity to infection. Radiation hypersensitivity is a hallmark of the disease, along with a predisposition to cancer, most notably lymphomas (Digweed et al, 1999). The most common cause of death for NBS patients is neoplasia (Steensma, 2007). Although the predominant neoplasm is lymphoma, both lymphoid and myeloid leukemia have been reported (Resnick et al, 2002).

Seckel syndrome (SCKL) is a rare autosomal recessive disorder associated with short stature, prenatal and postnatal growth retardation, characteristic craniofacial dysmorphism (bird-headed face including prominent beaked nose, micrognathia and malformed ears), mental deficiency, microcephaly, and skeletal defects (Faivre et al, 2002). Hematological abnormalities, including pancytopenia, myelodysplasia and acute myeloid leukemia, have been reported in some patients with Seckel syndrome (Chanan-Khan et al, 2003; Hayani et al,1994). A gene for Seckel syndrome was mapped on chromosome 3q22.1-q24. The ataxia-telancgiectasia and RAD3-related (ATR) gene is mutated in Seckel syndrome, and encodes an phosphotidylinositol-3-kinase-like kinase which has distinct, but overlapping functions with ATM in co-ordinating the response to DNA damage. ATR is activated by single stranded DNA whilst ATM responds to DNA double strand breaks (Casper et al, 2002; Steensma, 2007).

4. Conclusion

Genetic variations in genes involved in DNA repair may influence both cancer susceptibility and treatment response. However, in AML, the relevance of these genetic variations remains to be fully established. There is evidence that some polymorphisms in DNA repair genes play a role in carcinogenesis, notably hOGG1 Ser326Cys, XRCC1 Arg194Trp, XRCC3 Thr241Met, RAD51 G135C and XPD Lys751Gln. Additional studies of these and other DNA repair polymorphisms will provide essential information about the relationships between the DNA repair mechanisms and risk of AML.

5. Acknowledgement

This paper is partly supported by the Sectorial operational programme human resources development (SOP HRD), financed from the European social Fund and by the Romanian Government under the contract number POSDRU 60782.

6. References

Allan JM, Smith AG, Wheatley K, Hills RK, Travis LB, Hill DA, Swirsky DM, Morgan GJ, Wild CP. (2004). Genetic variation in XPD predicts treatment outcome and risk of acute myeloid leukemia following chemotherapy. *Blood*, Vol.104 (December 2004), pp. 3872–3877, ISSN: 1528-0020

Allen-Brady K, Cannon-Albright LA, Neuhausen SL, Camp NJ. (2006). A role for XRCC4 in age at diagnosis and breast cancer risk. *Cancer Epidemiol Biomarkers Prev*, Vol.15, No.7 (July 2006), pp. 1306–1310, ISSN: 1538-7755

Alter BP. (1993). Fanconi's anaemia and its variability. *Br J Haematol*, Vol.85, No.1 (1993 Sep), pp.9-14, ISSN: 1365-2141.

Alter BP. (2003). Cancer in Fanconi anemia, 1927-2001. *Cancer*, Vol. 97, No. 2 (January 2003), pp.425-440, ISSN: 1097-0142.

Arizono K, Osada Y, Kuroda Y. (2008). DNA repair gene hOGG1codon 326 and XRCC1 codon 399 polymorphisms and bladder cancer risk in a Japanese population. *Jpn J Clin Oncol*, Vol.38, No.3 (February 2008) pp.186–191, ISSN: 1465-3621

Ball LG, Xiao W. (2005). Molecular basis of ataxia telangiectasia and related diseases. *Acta Parmacologica Sinica*, Vol. 26, No.8 (August 2005), pp.897-907, ISSN: 1745-7254.

Bhatla D, Gerbing R, Alonzo T. (2008). DNA repair polymorphisms and outcome of chemotherapy for acute myelogenous leukemia: a report from the Children's Oncology Group. *Leukemia*, Vol.22, No.2 (February 2008), pp. 265–272, ISSN: 0887-6924

Bishop JO, Selman GG, Hickman J, Black L, Saunders RD, Clark AJ. (1985) The 45-kb unit of major urinary protein gene organization is a gigantic imperfect palindrome. *Mol Cell Biol*, Vol.5, No.7 (July 1985), pp.1591–1600, ISSN: 1098-5549

Bolufer P, Collado M, Barragán E, Cervera J, Calasanz MJ, Colomer D, Roman-Gómez J, Sanz MA. (2007). The potential effect of gender in combination with common genetic polymorphisms of drug-metabolizing enzymes on the risk of developing acute leukemia. *Haematologica*, Vol.92, No.3 (March 2007), pp. 308–314, ISSN: 1592-8721

Braithwaite E, Wu X, Wang Z.(1999). Repair of DNA lesions: mechanisms and relative repair efficiencies. *Mutat Res*, Vol. 424, No.1-2 (1999 Mar 8), pp.207–219, ISSN: 0027-5107

Brenneman MA, Weiss AE, Nickoloff JA, Chenet DJ. (2000). XRCC3 is required for efficient repair of chromosome breaks by homologous recombination. *Mutat Res*, Vol.459, No.2 (March 2000), pp. 89–97, ISSN: 1568-7864

Burma S, Chen BP, Chen DJ. (2006). Role of non-homologous end joining (NHEJ) in maintaining genomic integrity. *DNA Repair*, Vol.5, No.9-10 (September 2006), pp. 1042-1048, ISSN: 1568-7864

Cardecott KW.(2003). XRCC1 and DNA stand break repair. *DNA Repair*, Vol.2, No.9 (September 2003), pp. 955-969, ISSN: 1568-7864

Casper AM, Nghiem P, Arlt MF, Glover TW. (2002). ATR regulates fragile site stability. *Cell*, Vol.111, No.6 (December 2002), pp.779-789.

Chanan-Khan A, Holkova B, Perle MA, Reich E, Wu CD, Inghirami G, Takeshita K. (2003). T-cell clonality and myelodysplasia without chromosomal fragility in a patient with features of Seckel syndrome. *Haematologica*, Vol.88, No. 5 (May 2003), ECR14, ISSN: 1592-8721.

Chang CH, Chiu CF, Wu HC, Tseng HC, Wang CH, Lin CC, Tsai CW, Liang SY, Wang CL, Bau DT. (2008). Significant association of XRCC4 single nucleotide polymorphisms with prostate cancer susceptibility in Taiwanese males. *Mol Med Report*, Vol.1, No.4 (July 2008), pp.525-30, ISSN: 1791-3004

Chen PL, Yeh KT, Tsai YY, Koeh H, Liu YL, Lee H, Cheng YW. (2010). XRCC1, but not APE1 and hOGG1 gene polymorphisms is a risk factor for pterygium. *Mol Vis*, Vol.16 (June 2010), pp.991-996.

Chiu CF, Wang CH, Wang CL, Lin CC, Hsu NY, Weng JR, Bau DT. (2008). A novel single nucleotide polymorphism in XRCC4 gene is associated with gastric cancer susceptibility in Taiwan. *Ann Surg Oncol*, Vol.15, No.2 (February 2008), pp.514-518, ISSN: 1534-4681

D'Andrea AD. Targeting DNA repair pathways in AML. (2010). *Best Pract Res Clin Haematol*, Vol.23, No.4 (December 2010), pp.469-73, ISSN: 1521-6926

Das-Gupta EP, Seedhouse CH, Russell NH. (2001). Microsatellite instability occurs in defined subsets of patients with acute myeloblastic leukaemia. *Br J Haematol*, Vol.114, No.2 (August 2001), pp.307-312.

de Laat W L, Jaspers N G, Hoeijmakers J H.(1999). Molecular mechanism of nucleotide excision repair. *Genes & Dev*, Vol.13, pp.768-785, ISSN: 1549-5477

Digweed M, Reis A, Sperling K. (1999). Nijmegen breakage syndrome: consequences of defective DNA double strand break repair. *BioEssays*, Vol.21, No.8 (August 1999), pp.649-656, ISSN: 1521-1878

Drouet J, Delteil C, Lefrançois J, Concannon P, Salles B, Calsou P. (2005). DNA-dependent protein kinase and XRCC4-DNA ligase IV mobilization in the cell in response to DNA double strand breaks. *J Biol Chem*, Vol.280, No.8 (February 2005), pp.7060-7069, ISSN: 1521-1878

Dufloth RM, Costa S, Schmitt F, Zeferino LC. (2005). DNA repair gene polymorphisms and susceptibility to familial breast cancer in a group of patients from Campinas, Brazil. *Genet Mol Res*, Vol.4, No.4 (Decembrie 2005), pp.771-782.

El-Din M, Raslan H, Abdel-Hamid S, Makhlouf M. (2010). Detection of XRCC1 gene polymorphisms in Egyptian patients with acute myeloid leukemia. *Comparative Clinical Pathology* (November 2010), 1-9

Ellis NA, Ciocci S, Proytcheva M, Lennon D, Groden J, German I. (1998). The Ashkenazic Jewish Bloom syndrome mutation blmAsh is present in non-Jewish Americans of Spanish ancestry. *Am J Hum Genet*, Vol. 63, No. 6 (December 1998), pp.1685-1693, ISSN: 0002-9297.

Ellis NA, German J. (1996). Molecular genetics of Bloom's syndrome. *Hum Mol Genet*, Vol.5
    Spec, pp.1457–1463, ISSN: 1460-208
Faivre L, Le Merrer M, Lyonnet S, Plauchu H, Dagoneau N, Campos-Xavier AB, Attia-Sobol
    J, Verloes A, Munnich A, Cormier-Daire V. (2002). Clinical and genetic
    heterogeneity of Seckel syndrome. *Am J Med Genet*, Vol.112, No.4 (November 2002),
    pp.379-83, ISSN: 1552-4833.
Fang WH, Modrich P. (1993). Human strand-specific mismatch repair occurs by a
    bidirectional mechanism similar to that of the bacterial reaction. J Biol Chem,
    Vol.268, (June 1993), pp.11838 –11844, ISSN: 1083-351X
Fu YP, Yu JC, Cheng TC, Lou MA, Hsu GC, Wu CY, Chen ST, Wu HS, Wu PE, Shen CY.
    (2003). Breast cancer risk associated with genotypic polymorphism of the
    nonhomologous end-joining genes: a multigenic study on cancer susceptibility.
    Cancer Res, Vol.63 (May 2003), pp.2440–2446, ISSN: 1538-7445
Garcia-Closas M, Egan KM, Newcomb PA, Brinton LA, Titus-Ernstoff L, Chanock S, Welch
    R, Lissowska J, Peplonska B, Szeszenia-Dabrowska N, Zatonski W, Bardin-
    Mikolajczak A, Struewing JP. (2006). Polymorphisms in DNA double-strand break
    repair genes and risk of breast cancer: two population-based studies in USA and
    Poland, and meta-analyses. *Hum Genet*, Vol.119, No.4 (May2006), pp.376–88, ISSN:
    0014-4266
Gaymes TJ, Mufti GJ, Rassool FV. (2002). Myeloid leukemias have increased activity of the
    nonhomologous end-joining pathway and concomitant DNA misrepair that is
    dependent on the Ku70/86 heterodimer. *Cancer Res*, Vol.62, No.10 (May 2002),
    pp.2791–2797, ISSN: 1538-7445
Gerson SL, Trey JE. 1988. Modulation of nitrosourea resistance in myeloid leukemias. *Blood*,
    Vol.71, No.5 (May 1988), pp.1487–1494, ISSN: 1528-0020
Goode EL, Ulrich CM, Potter JD. (2002). Polymorphisms in DNA repair genes and
    associations with cancer risk. *Cancer Epidemiol Biomarkers Prev*, Vol.11 (December
    2002), pp.1513–1530, ISSN: 1538-7755
Griffin CS. (2002). Aneuploidy, centrosome activity and chromosome instability in cells
    deficient in homologous recombination repair. *Mutat Res*, Vol.504, No.1-2 (July
    2002,), pp.149– 155, ISSN: 0027-5107
Grompe M, D'Andrea A. (2001). Fanconi anemia and DNA repair. *Hum Mol Genet*, Vol. 10,
    No. 20 (October 2001), pp.2253-2259, ISSN 1460-2083.
Gu D, Wang M, Wang M, Zhang Z, Chen J. (2009). The DNA repair gene APE1 T1349G
    polymorphism and cancer risk: a meta-analysis of 27 case-control studies.
    Mutagenesis, Vol. 24, No. 6 (November 2009), pp.507-512, ISSN 1464-3804
Gullo C, Au M, Feng G, Teoh G. (2006). The biology of Ku and its potential oncogenic role in
    cancer. *Biochim Biophys Acta*, Vol.1765, No.2 (April 2006), pp.223–234, ISSN: 0304-
    419X
Gumy-Pause F, Wacker P, Sappino AP. (2004). ATM gene and lymphoid malignancies.
    Leukemia, Vol.18, (November 2003), pp.238-242, ISSN: 1476-555.
Han S, Zhang HT, Wang Z, Xie Y, Tang R, Mao Y, Li Y. (2006). DNA repair gene XRCC3
    polymorphisms and cancer risk: a meta-analysis of 48 case-control studies. *Eur J
    Hum Genet*, Vol.14, No.10 (June 2006), pp.1136–1144, ISSN: 1018-4813
Hanawalt PC. (2002). Subpathways of nucleotide excision repair and their regulation.
    Oncogene, Vol.21, No.58 (December 2002), pp.8949–8956, ISSN: 0950-9232

Hayani A, Suarez CR, Molnar Z, LeBeau M, Godwin. (1994). Acute myeloid leukaemia in a patient with Seckel syndrome. *J Med Genet*, Vol.31, No.2 (February 1994), pp.148–149, ISSN: 0022-2593

Hayden PJ, Tewari P, Morris DW, Staines A, Crowley D, Nieters A, Becker N, de Sanjosé S, Foretova L, Maynadié M, Cocco PL, Boffetta P, Brennan P, Chanock SJ, Browne PV, Lawler M. (2007). Variation in DNA repair genes XRCC3, XRCC4, XRCC5 and susceptibility to myeloma. *Hum Mol Genet*, Vol.16, No.24 (December 2007), pp.3117–3127, ISSN: 0964-6906

Hazra TK, Das A, Das S, Choudhury S, Kow YW, Roy R. (2007). Oxidative DNA damage repair in mammalian cells: a new perspective. *DNA Repair*, Vol.6, No.4 (April 2007), pp.470–80, ISSN: 1568-7864

Hazra TK, Roy R, Biswas T, Grabowski DT, Pegg AE, Mitra S. (1997). Specific recognition of O6-methylguanine in DNA by active site mutants of human O6-methylguanine-DNA methyltransferase. *Biochemistry*, Vol.36, No.19 (May 1997), pp.5769 –5776, ISSN: 0006-2960

He W, Luo S, Huang T, Ren J, Wu X, Shao J, Zhu Q. (2011). The Ku70 -1310C/G promoter polymorphism is associated with breast cancer susceptibility in Chinese Han population. *Mol Biol Rep*. May 10. [Epub ahead of print], ISSN: 1573-4978.

Hu Z, Ma H, Chen F, Wei Q, Shen H. (2005). XRCC1 polymorphisms and cancer risk: a meta-analysis of 38 case-control studies. *Cancer Epidemiol Biomarkers Prev*, Vol.14, No.7 (July 2005), pp.1810–1818, ISSN: 1538-7755

Hung RJ, Hall J, Brennan P, Boffetta P. (2005). Genetic polymorphisms in the base excision repair pathway and cancer risk: a HuGE review. *Am J Epidemiol*, Vol.162, No.10 (November 2005), pp.925–942, ISSN: 1476-6256

Iliakis G, Wang H, Perrault AR, Boecker W, Rosidi B, Windhofer F, Wu W, Guan J, Terzoudi G, Pantelias G. (2004). Mechanisms of DNA double strand break repair and chromosome aberration formation. *Cytogenet Genome Res*, Vol.104, No.1-4, pp.14–20.

Jacobsen NR, Raaschou-Nielsen O, Nexo B, Wallin H, Overvad K, Tjonneland A, Vogel U. (2004). XRCC3 polymorphisms and risk of lung cancer. Cancer Lett, Vol.213, No.1 (September 2004) pp.67–72, ISSN: 0304-3835

Ji YN, Zhan P, Wang J, Qiu LX, Yu LK. (2010). APE1 Asp148Glu gene polymorphism and lung cancer risk: a meta-analysis. *Mol Biol Rep*, Epub December 2010 Dec,

Jiricny J. (2006). The multifaceted mismatch-repair system. *Nat Rev Mol Cell Biol*, Vol.7, No.5 (May2006), pp.335–346, ISSN: 1471-0072

Junop MS, Modesti M, Guarne A, Ghirlando R, Gellert M, Yang W. (2000). Crystal structure of the Xrcc4 DNA repair protein and implications for end joining. *EMBO J*, Vol.19, No.22 (November 2000), pp.5962–5970.

Kaina B, Christmann M, Naumann S, Roos WP. MGMT: key node in the battle against genotoxicity, carcinogenicity and apoptosis induced by alkylating agents. *DNA Repair*, Vol.6, No.8 (August 2007), pp.1079–1099, ISSN: 1568-7864

Kaina B, Christmann M. (2002). DNA repair in resistance to alkylating anticancer drugs. *Int J Clin Pharmacol Ther*, Vol.40, No.8 (August 2002), pp.354–367, ISSN: 0946-1965

Kang TH, Reardon JT, Sancar A. (2011). Regulation of nucleotide excision repair activity by transcriptional and post-transcriptional control of the XPA protein. *Nucleic Acids Res*, Vol.39, No.8 (December 2010), pp.3176–87, ISSN: 0305-1048

Kennedy RD, D'Andrea AD.(2006). DNA repair pathways in clinical practice: lessons from pediatric cancer susceptibility syndromes. *J Clin Oncol*, Vol.24, No.23 (August 2006), pp.3799–3808, ISSN: 0732-183X

Khanna KK, Jackson SP. (2001). DNA double-strand breaks: signaling, repair and the cancer connection. *Nat Genet*, Vol.27, No.3 (March 2001), pp.247–254, ISSN: 1061-4036

Kohno T, Shinmura K, Tosaka M, Tani M, Kim SR, Sugimura H, Nohmi T, Kasai H, Yokota J. (1998). Genetic polymorphisms and alternative splicing of the hOGG1 gene, that is involved in the repair of 8-hydroxyguanine in damaged DNA. *Oncogene*, Vol.16, No.25 (June 1998), pp.3219–3225, ISSN: 0950-9232

Krajinovic M, Labuda D, Mathonnet G, Labuda M, Moghrabi A, Champagne J, Sinnett D. (2002). Polymorphisms in genes encoding drugs and xenobiotic metabolizing enzymes, DNA repair enzymes, and response to treatment of childhood acute lymphoblastic leukemia. *Clin Cancer Res*, Vol. 8, No.2 (March 2002), pp.802-810, ISSN: 1557-3265.

Kuptsova N, Kopecky KJ, Godwin J, Anderson J, Hoque A, Willman CL, Slovak ML, Ambrosone CB. (2007). Polymorphisms in DNA repair genes and therapeutic outcomes of AML patients from SWOG clinical trials. *Blood*, Vol.109, No.9 (May2007), pp.3936–3944, ISSN: 1528-0020

Kuptsova-Clarkson N, Ambrosone CB, Weiss J, Baer MR, Sucheston LE, Zirpoli G, Kopecky KJ, Ford L, Blanco J, Wetzler M, Moysich KB. (2010). XPD DNA nucleotide excision repair gene polymorphisms associated with DNA repair deficiency predict better treatment outcomes in secondary acute myeloid leukemia. *Int J Mol Epidemiol Genet*, Vol.1, No.4 (August2010), pp.278–294, ISSN: 1948-1756

Laine JP, Mocquet V, Bonfanti M, Braun C, Egly JM, Brousset P. (2007). Common XPD (ERCC2) polymorphisms have no measurable effect on nucleotide excision repair and basal transcription. *DNA Repair*, Vol.6, No.9 (September 2007),pp.1264 –1270, ISSN: 1568-7864

Lehmann AR. (2006). Clubbing together on clamps: The key to translesion synthesis. *DNA Repair*, Vol.5, No.3 (March 2006), pp.404–407, ISSN: 1568-7864

Levitus M, Rooimans MA, Steltenpool J, Cool NF, Oostra AB, Mathew CG, Hoatlin ME, Waisfisz Q, Arwert F, de Winter JP, Joenje H. (2004). Heterogeneity in Fanconi anemia: evidence for 2 new genetic subtypes. *Blood*, Nol.103, No.7 (April 2004), pp.2498–2503, ISSN: 1528-0020

Li GC, Ouyang H, Li X, Nagasawa H, Little JB, Chen DJ, Ling CC, Fuks Z, Cordon-Cardo C. (1998). Ku70: a candidate tumor suppressor gene for murine T cell lymphoma. *Mol Cell*, Vol.2, No.1(July 1998), pp.1–8.

Li GM. (2008). Mechanisms and functions of DNA mismatch repair. *Cell Res*, Vol.18, No.1 (January 2008), pp.85–98, ISSN: 1001-0602

Li X, Heyer WD. (2008). Homologous recombination in DNA repair and DNA damage tolerance. *Cell Res*, Vol.18, No.1 (January 2008), pp.99–113, ISSN: 1001-0602

Liddiard K, Hills R, Burnett AK, Darley RL, Tonks A. (2010). OGG1 is a novel prognostic indicator in acute myeloid leukaemia. *Oncogene*, Vol.29, No.13 (April 2010), pp.2005-2012 ISSN: 0950-9232

Lieberman HB.(2008). DNA damage repair and response proteins as targets for cancer therapy. *Curr Med Chem*, Vol.15, No.4 (February 2008), pp.360-367, ISSN 0929-8673

Lindahl T, Wood RD. (1999). Quality control by DNA repair. *Science*, Vol.286, No.5446 (December 1999), pp.1897–905, ISSN: 0036-8075

Liu L, Yang L, Zhang Y, Wei J, Zou Z, Qian X, Nakamura T, Ding Y, Feng J, Yu L. (2008). Polymorphisms of RAD51 (G135C) and XRCC3 (C241T) genes and correlations there of with prognosis and clinical outcomes of acute myeloid leukemia. *Mol. Cell*, Vol.88, No.6 (February 2008), pp.378–382

Lo YL, Jou YS, Hsiao CF, Chang GC, Tsai YH, Su WC, Chen KY, Chen YM, Huang MS, Hu CY, Chen CJ, Hsiung CA. (2009). A polymorphism in the APE1 gene promoter is associated with lung cancer risk. *Cancer Epidemiol Biomarkers Prev*, Vol. 18, No. 1 (Jabuary 2009), pp.223–229, ISSN: 1538-7755

Mao G, Yuan F, Absher K, Jennings CD, Howard DS, Jordan CT, Gu L. (2008). Preferential loss of mismatch repair function in refractory and relapsed acute myeloid leukemia: potential contribution to AML progression. *Cell Res*, Vol.18, No.2 (February 2008), pp.281–289, ISSN: 1001-0602

Martin SA, Lord CJ, Ashworth A. (2010). Therapeutic targeting of the DNA mismatch repair pathway. *Clin Cancer Res*, Vol.16, No.21(November 2010), pp.5107–5113, ISSN: 1557-3265

Matullo G, Dunning AM, Guarrera S, Baynes C, Polidoro S, Garte S, Autrup H, Malaveille C, Peluso M, Airoldi L, Veglia F, Gormally E, Hoek G, Krzyzanowski M, Overvad K, Raaschou-Nielsen O, Clavel-Chapelon F, Linseisen J, Boeing H, Trichopoulou A, Palli D, Krogh V, Tumino R, Panico S, Bueno-De-Mesquita HB, Peeters PH, Lund E, Pera G, Martinez C, Dorronsoro M, Barricarte A, Tormo MJ, Quiros JR, Day NE, Key TJ, Saracci R, Kaaks R, Riboli E, Vineis P. (2006). DNA repair polymorphisms and cancer risk in non-smokers in a cohort study. *Carcinogenesis*, Vol.27, No.5 (May 2006), pp.997–1007, ISSN: 1460-2180

Matullo G, Guarrera S, Carturan S, Peluso M, Malaveille C, Davico L, Piazza A, Vineis P. (2001). DNA repair gene polymorphisms, bulky DNA adducts in white blood cells and bladder cancer in a case-control study. *Int J Cancer*, Vol.92, No.4 (May 2001), pp.562–567, ISSN: 1097-0215

Mavrou A, Tsangaris GT, Roma E, Kolialexi A. (2008). The ATM gene and ataxia telangiectasia. *Anticancer Res*, Vol. 28, No. 1B (February 2008), pp.401-405, ISSN: 1791-7530.

Mehta PA, Alonzo TA, Gerbing RB, Elliott JS, Wilke TA, Kennedy RJ, Ross JA, Perentesis JP, Lange BJ, Davies SM. (2006). XPD Lys751Gln polymorphism in the etiology and outcome of childhood acute myeloid leukemia: a Children's Oncology Group report. *Blood*, Vol.107, No.1 (January 2007), pp.39–45, ISSN: 1528-0020

Mitra S. (2007). MGMT: a personal perspective. *DNA Repair*, Vol.6, No.8 (August 2007), pp.1064–1670, ISSN: 0036-8075

NCBI, http://www.ncbi.nlm.nih.gov, last accessed on 20/05/2011

Papouli E, Cejka P, Jiricny J. (2004). Dependence of the cytotoxicity of DNA-damaging agents on the mismatch repair status of human cells. *Cancer Res*, Vol.64, No. 10 (May 2004), pp.3391–3394, ISSN: 1538-7445

Park J, Chen L, Tockman MS, Elahi A, Lazarus P. (2004). The human 8-oxoguanine DNA N-glycosylase 1 (hOGG1) DNA repair enzyme and its association with lung cancer risk. *Pharmacogenetics*. Vol.14, No.2 (February 2004), pp. 103-109, ISSN: 1744-6880

Rajewsky MF, Müller R. (2005). DNA Repair and the Cell Cycle as Targets in Cancer
    Therapy in *The Cancer Handbook* 1st Ed, Malcolm R. Alison, John Wiley & Sons, Ltd,
    Available from:< http://hasdl.kau.edu.sa/encyclopedia/2/h6 20archive/24.pdf>

Reardon JT, Sancar A. (2005). Nucleotide excision repair. *Prog Nucleic Acid Res Mol Biol*,
    Vol.79 (August 2005), pp.183–235, ISBN: 10: 0-12-540066-7

Resnick IB, Kondratenko I, Togoev O, Vasserman N, Shagina I, Evgrafov O, Tverskaya S,
    Cerosaletti KM, Gatti RA, Concannon P. (2002). Nijmegen breakage syndrome:
    clinical characteristics and mutation analysis in eight unrelated Russian families. *J
    Pediatr*, Vol. 140, No. 3 (March 2002), pp. 355-361.

Richardson C, Stark JM, Ommundsen M, Jasin M. (2004). Rad51 overexpression promotes
    alternative double-strand break repair pathways and genome instability. *Oncogene*,
    Vol. 23, No.2 (January 2004), pp.546–553, ISSN: 0950-9232

Riedl T, Hanaoka F, Egly JM. (2003). The comings and goings of nucleotide excision repair
    factors on damaged DNA. *EMBO J*, Vol.22, No.19 (October 2003), pp.5293–5303.

Rimsza LM, Kopecky KJ, Ruschulte J, Chen IM, Slovak ML, Karanes C, Godwin J, List A,
    Willman CL. (2000). Microsatellite instability is not a defining genetic feature of
    acute myeloid leukemogenesis in adults: results of a retrospective study of 132
    patients and review of the literature. *Leukemia*, Vol.14, No.6 (June 2000), pp.1044–
    1051, ISSN: 0887-6924

Rollinson S, Smith AG, Allan JM, Adamson PJ, Scott K, Skibola CF, Smith MT, Morgan GJ.
    (2007). RAD51 homologous recombination repair gene haplotypes and risk of acute
    myeloid leukaemia. *Leuk Res*, Vol.31, No.2 (February 2007), pp.169–74, ISSN: 0145-
    2126

Rosenberg PS, Alter BP, Ebell W. (2008). Cancer risks in Fanconi anemia: findings from the
    German Fanconi Anemia Registry. *Haematologica*, Vol. 93, No. 4 (Aprilie 2008), pp.
    511-517, ISSN: 1592-8721.

Rufer JT, Morgan WF. (1992). Potentiation of DNA damage by inhibition of poly (ADP-
    ribosyl)ation: A test of the hypothesis for random nuclease action. *Exp Cell Res*,
    Vol.200, No.2 (June 1992), pp.506–512, ISSN: 0014-4827

Sargent RG, Brenneman MA, Wilson JH. (1997). Repair of site-specific double-strand breaks
    in a mammalian chromosome by homologous and illegitimate recombination. Mol
    Cell Biol, Vol.17, No.1 (January 1997), pp.267–277, ISSN: 1098-5549

Savitsky K, Bar-Shira A, Gilad S, Rotman G, Ziv Y, Vanagaite L, Tagle DA, Smith S, Uziel T,
    Sfez S, Ashkenazi M, Pecker I, Frydman M, Harnik R, Patanjali SR, Simmons A,
    Clines GA, Sartiel A, Gatti RA, Chessa L, Sanal O, Lavin MF, Jaspers NG, Taylor
    AM, Arlett CF, Miki T, Weissman SM, Lovett M, Collins FS, Shiloh Y. (1995). A
    single ataxia telangiectasia gene with a product similar to PI-3 kinase. *Science*,
    Vol.268, No.5218 (June 1995), pp.1749–1753, ISSN: 1095-9203

Seedhouse C, Bainton R, Lewis M, Harding A, Russell N, Das-Gupta E. (2002). The genotype
    distribution of the XRCC1 gene indicates a role for base excision repair in the
    development of therapy-related acute myeloblastic leukemia. *Blood*, Vol.100, No.10
    (November 2002), pp.3761–66, ISSN: 1528-0020

Seedhouse C, Faulkner R, Ashraf N, Das-Gupta E, Russell N. (2004). Polymorphisms in
    genes involved in homologous recombination repair interact to increase the risk of
    developing acute myeloid leukemia. *Clin Cancer Res*; Vol.10, No.8 (April 2004),
    pp.2675–2680, ISSN: 1557-3265

Sheikhha MH, Tobal K, Liu Yin JA. (2002). High level of microsatellite instability but not hypermethylation of mismatch repair genes in therapy-related and secondary acute myeloid leukaemia and myelodysplastic syndrome. *Br J Haematol*, Vol.117, No.2 (May 2002), pp.359–365, ISSN: 1365-2141

Shen MR, Jones IM, Mohrenweiser H. (1998). Nonconservative amino acid substitution variants exist at polymorphic frequency in DNA repair genes in healthy humans. *Cancer Res*, Vol.58, No.4 (february 1998), pp.604–608, ISSN: 1538-7445

Shrivastav M, De Haro LP, Nickoloff JA. (2008). Regulation of DNA double-strand break repair pathway choice. *Cell Res*, Vol.18, No.1 (December 2007), pp.134–47, ISSN: 1001-0602

Sipley JD, Menninger JC, Hartley KO, Ward DC, Jackson SP, Anderson CW. (1995). Gene for the catalytic subunit of the human DNA-activated protein kinase maps to the site of the XRCC7 gene on chromosome 8. *Proc Natl Acad Sc. USA*, Vol.92, pp.7515–19.

Smith GC, Jackson SP. (1999). The DNA-dependent protein kinase. *Genes Dev*, Vol.13, No.8 (April 1999), pp.916–934, ISSN: 1549-5477

Stanczyk M, Sliwinski T, Cuchra M, Zubowska M, Bielecka-Kowalska A, Kowalski M, Szemraj J, Mlynarski W, Majsterek I. (2011). The association of polymorphisms in DNA base excision repair genes XRCC1, OGG1 and MUTYH with the risk of childhood acute lymphoblastic leukemia. *Mol Biol Rep*,Vol.38, No.1 (January, 2011), pp.445-451, n.d.

Steensma DP. (2007). The DNA Damage Response, DNA Repair, and AML. In: *Acute Myelogenous Leukemia*. Karp JE. pp.97-132, Humana Press, ISBN-13: 978-1-58829-621-4, Totowa, New Jersey

Stronati L, Gensabella G, Lamberti C, Barattini P, Frasca D, Tanzarella C, Giacobini S, Toscano M, Santacroce C, Danesi DT. (2001). Expression and DNA binding activity of the Ku heterodimer in bladder carcinoma. *Cancer*, Vol.92, No.9 (November 2001), pp.2484–2492, ISSN: 1097-0142

Sturgis EM, Clayman GL, Guan Y, Guo Z, Wei Q. (1999). DNA repair in lymphoblastoid cell lines from patients with head and neck cancer. *Arch Otolaryngol Head Neck Surg*, Vol.125, No.2 (February 1999), pp.185–90.

Sung P, Klein H. (2006). Mechanism of homologous recombination: mediators and helicases take on regulatory functions. *Nat Rev Mol Cell Biol*, Vol.7, No.10 (October 2006), pp.739–50, ISSN: 1471-0072

Surtees JA, Argueso JL, Alani E. (2004). Mismatch repair proteins: key regulators of genetic recombination. *Cytogenet Genome Res*, Vol.107, No.3-4, pp.146–59.

Taccioli GE, Gottlieb TM, Blunt T, Priestley A, Demengeot J, Mizuta R, Lehmann AR, Alt FW, Jackson SP, Jeggo PA. (1994). Ku80: product of the XRCC5 gene and its role in DNA repair and V(D)J recombination. *Science*, Vol.265, No.5177 (September 1994):1442-1445, ISSN: 0036-8075

Taylor AM, Byrd PJ. (2005). Molecular pathology of ataxia telangiectasia. *J Clin Pathol*, Vol.58, no. 10 (October 2005), pp.1009-1015, ISSN: 1472-4146.

Thompson LH, Brookman KW, Jones NJ, Allen SA, Carrano AV. (1990). Molecular cloning of the human XRCC1 gene, which corrects defective DNA strand break repair and sister chromatid exchange. *Mol Cell Biol*, Vol.10, No.12 (December 1990), pp.6160–6171 ISSN: 1098-5549

Thompson LH, Schild D. (2002). Recombinational DNA repair and human disease. *Mutat Res*; Vol.509, No.1-2 (November 2002), pp.49–78, ISSN: 0027-5107

Tsukino H, Hanaoka T, Otani T, Iwasaki M, Kobayashi M, Hara M, Natsukawa S, Shaura K, Koizumi Y, Kasuga Y, Tsugane S. (2004). hOGG1 Ser326Cys polymorphism, interaction with environmental exposures, and gastric cancer risk in Japanese populations. *Cancer Sci*, Vol.95, No.12 (December 2004), pp.977–83, ISSN: 1349-7006

van der Wees C, Jansen J, Vrieling H, van der LaarseA, Van Zeeland A, Mullenders L. (2007). Nucleotide excision repair in differentiated cells. *Mutat Res*, Vol.614, No.1-2 (January 2007), pp.16–23, ISSN: 0027-5107

Varon R, Schoch C, Reis A, Hiddemann WC, Sperling K, Schnittger S. (2003). Mutation analysis of the Nijmegen breakage syndrome gene (NBSl) in nineteen patients with acute myeloid leukemia with complex karyotypes. *Leuk Lymphoma*, Vol.44, No.11 (January 2003), pp.1931–1934, ISSN: 1042-8194

Voso MT, Fabiani E, D'Alo' F, Guidi F, Di Ruscio A, Sica S, Pagano L, Greco M, Hohaus S, Leone G. (2007). Increased risk of acute myeloid leukemia due to polymorphisms in detoxification and DNA repair enzymes. *Ann Oncol*, Vol.18, No.9 (September 2007), pp.1523–1528, ISSN: 1569-8041

Wang F, Chang D, Hu FL, Sui H, Han B, Li DD, Zhao YS. (2008). DNA repair gene XPD polymorphisms and cancer risk: a metaanalysis based on 56 case-control studies. Cancer Epidemiol Biomarkers Prev, Vol.17, No.3 (March 2008), pp.507–517, ISSN: 1538-7755

Wang G, Wang S, Shen Q, Yina S, Li C, Lia A, Li J, Zhoua J, Liu Q. (2009). Polymorphisms in XRCC5, XRCC6, XRCC7 genes are involved in DNA double-strand breaks (DSBs) repair associated with the risk of acute myeloid leukemia (AML) in Chinese population. *Journal of Nanjing Medical University*, Vol.23, No.2 (March 2009), pp.93–99, ISSN: 1007-4376

Wang L, Zhu D, Zhang C, Mao X, Wang G, Mitra S, Li BF, Wang X, WuM. (1997). Mutations of O6-methylguanine-DNA methyltransferasegene in esophageal cancer tissues from Northern China. *Int J Cancer*, Vol.7, No. 5 (May 1997), pp.719 –723, ISSN: 1097-0215.

Wang LE, Bondy ML, Shen H, El-Zein R, Aldape K, Cao Y, Pudavalli V, Levin VA, Yung WK, Wei Q. (2004). Polymorphisms of DNA repair genes and risk of glioma. *Cancer Res*, Vol.64, No.16 (August 2004), pp.5560–5563, ISSN: 1538-7445

Wang SY, Peng L, Li CP, Li AP, Zhou JW, Zhang ZD, Liu QZ. (2008). Genetic variants of the XRCC7 gene involved in DNA repair and risk of human bladder cancer. *Int J Urol*, Vol.15, No.6 (June 2008):, pp.534–539, ISSN: 1442-2042

Wenshan He, Sijia Luo, Tao Huang, Jinghua Ren, Xiaoling Wu, Jun Shao. Qingyao Zhu. (2011). The Ku70 −1310C/G promoter polymorphism is associated with breast cancer susceptibility in Chinese Han population. *Mol Biol Rep*, (May 2011), n.d.

Wiebauer K, Jiricny J. (1990). Mismatch-specific thymine DNA glycosylase and DNA polymerase beta mediate the correction of G.T mispairs in nuclear extracts from human cells. *Proc Natl Acad Sci USA*, Vol.87, No.15 (August 1990), pp.5842–5845

Wilson DM 3rd, Simeonov A. (2010). Small molecule inhibitors of DNA repair nuclease activities of APE1. *Cell Mol Life Sci*, Vol.67, No.21 (November 2010), pp. 3621-3631, ISSN: 1420-682X

Winsey SL, Haldar NA, Marsh HP, Bunce M, Marshall SE, Harris AL, Wojnarowska F, Welsh KI. (2000). A variant within the DNA repair gene XRCC3 is associated with the development of melanoma skin cancer. *Cancer Res*, Vol.60, No.20 (Octombrie 2000), pp.5612–5616, ISSN: 1538-7445

Wood RD. (1989). Repair of pyrimidine dimer ultraviolet light photoproducts by human cell extracts. Biochemistry, Vol.28, No.21 (October 1989), pp.8287–8292, ISSN: 0006-2960

Wu CN, Liang SY, Tsai CW, Bau DT. (2008). The role of XRCC4 in carcinogenesis and anticancer drug discovery. *Recent Pat Anticancer Drug Discov*, Vol.3, No.3 (November 2008), pp.209–219, ISSN: 1574-8928

Xing DY, Tan W, Song N, Lin DX. (2001). Ser326Cys polymorphism in hOGG1 gene and risk of esophageal cancer in a Chinese population. *Int J Cancer*, Vol.95, No.3 (May 2001), pp.140–143, ISSN: 1097-0215

Yasbin RE. (2002). DNA repair mechanism and Mutagenesis, In: *Modern Microbial Genetics*, Second Edition. Streips UN, Yasbin RE, 24-46, Wiley-Liss Inc, ISBN: 0-471-22197-X, New York, USA.

Yeh YC, Chang DY, Masin J, Lu AL. (1991). Two nicking enzyme systems specific for mismatch-containing DNA in nuclear extracts from human cells. *J Biol Chem*, Vol.266, No.10 (April 1991), pp.6480–6484, ISSN: 0021-9258

Yu JJ. (2009). Unlocking the Molecular Mechanisms of DNA Repair and Platinum Drug Resistance in Cancer Chemotherapy. *Current Drug Therapy*, Vol 4, No 1 (January 2009) , pp.19-28, ISSN: 1574-8855

Yu Z, Chen J, Ford BN, Brackley ME, Glickman BW. (1999). Human DNA repair systems: an overview. *Environ Mol Mutagen*, Vol.33, No.1 (February 1999), pp.3–20, ISSN: 0893-6692

6

Acute Promyelocytic Leukemia: A Model Disease for Targeted Cancer Therapy

Emma Lång and Stig Ove Bøe
Oslo University Hospital, Oslo,
Norway

1. Introduction

Acute promyelocytic leukemia (APL) is a distinct subtype of acute myeloid leukemia (AML) characterized by a severe bleeding tendency, accumulation of abnormal promyelocytes in the bone marrow and a reciprocal t(15;17) chromosomal translocation that fuses the gene encoding the promyelocytic leukemia protein (PML) to that encoding retinoic acid receptor alpha (RARA) (de Thé & Chen, 2010). During the past 30 years two therapeutic drugs have been introduced into the clinic that have dramatically improved the treatment outcome of this disease (Wang & Chen, 2008). The first of these components was all-trans retinoic acid (ATRA), a vitamin A derivative that significantly increased clinical remission and improved the 5-years disease-free survival rates from below 40% to more than 80% (Huang et al., 1988). The second drug was arsenic trioxide (ATO), a component that was discovered to be remarkably effective in treating APL as a single agent (Sun et al., 1992). Today, most hospitals employ ATRA in combination with chemotherapy as frontline therapy, while ATO is being used for refractory or relapsed patients. Recent clinical studies have also revealed a positive synergistic effect between the two drugs, suggesting that future therapy of newly diagnosed patients may involve a combination of the two reagents (Estey et al., 2006; Hu et al., 2009; Shen et al., 2004; Wang et al., 2004).

The success of using ATRA and ATO in APL therapy appears to be linked to the ability of these drugs to interact with the fusion oncoprotein PML/RARA, which is produced by the APL-associated t(15;17) translocation, and that causes the disease. ATRA contacts a ligand binding domain present within the RARA moiety of this chimeric protein and promotes differentiation of APL cells along the granulocyte linage (Huang et al., 1988). ATO, on the other hand, has recently been shown to bind one or more cysteine rich motifs within the PML protein (Jeanne et al., 2010; Zhang et al., 2010) and contributes to the cure of APL through a mechanism that involves eradication of leukemic-initiating cells (LICs) (Nasr et al., 2008; Ito et al., 2008; Zheng et al., 2007).

Due to the success of using ATRA and ATO in the clinic, and because of the ability of these drugs to promote clinical remission through a direct contact with PML/RARA, APL has become one of the most attractive model diseases for the development of targeted cancer therapy. The APL cure offers a proof of principle that a cancer can be cured through targeted inactivation of an oncoprotein, and it provides a rationale for the development of novel therapeutic strategies that target fusion oncoproteins produced by chromosomal translocations. In this chapter we will summarize the current knowledge of the biological properties of PML, RARA and PML/RARA with particular emphasis on tumorigenesis in APL patients and the molecular mechanisms that underlie the response to ATRA and ATO.

2. APL treatment – a historical perspective

2.1 The discovery of ATRA-based APL therapy

APL was first characterized as a distinct clinical entity in 1957 (Hillestad, 1957). Throughout the 1950s and 1960s, this disease had a 100% mortality rate and no effective treatment options. In 1973, chemotherapy by the topoisomerase inhibitor daunorubicin was shown to have some curative effect, yielding a complete remission (CR) rate of 55% (Bernard et al., 1973), and in the early eighties induction therapy based on anthracyclins (daunorubicin, idarubicin among others) and the nucleocide analogue cytosine arabinoside (Ara-C) was found to yield CR rates of up to 80% in newly diagnosed patients (Cunningham et al., 1989; Sanz et al., 1988). However, the patients frequently suffered from one of the inherent drawbacks with induction therapy, namely the release of coagulation factors from dead leukemic cells, causing severe bleedings and increased risk of fatal outcome (Cordonnier et al., 1985; Drapkin et al., 1978; Ruggero et al., 1977). Consequently, most APL patients required intensive platelet and fibrinogen support, and based on the criterion of 5-years disease-free survival (DFS), only 35-45% of the cases were cured (Fenaux et al., 2007). The focus on APL therapy changed in 1978, as it became clear that leukemic cells undergo terminal differentiation upon treatment with differentiating-inducing agents, such as ATRA, Ara-C and 13-cis retinoic acid (Breitman et al., 1981; Degos et al., 1985; Gold et al., 1983; Koeffler et al., 1985; Sachs, 1978). Such differentiation therapy showed an advantage over induction therapy, with respect to incidences of severe bleedings, and led to reduced mortality rates. In 1985, the first attempt to treat APL patients with ATRA was made with promising results, but the percentage of patients with 5-years DFS was still relatively low (less than 50%) (Huang et al., 1987; Huang et al., 1988). Subsequently, optimization trials, combining ATRA with chemotherapy, raised the CR rates up to 90-95% and the 5-years DFS to 86% (Wang & Chen, 2008). In addition, the combination of ATRA and chemotherapy, which currently represents standard frontline APL therapy, helped reducing retinoic acid syndrome (RAS), a potentially fatal side effect caused by induction therapy and manifested in a burst of inflammatory cytokines released from malignant promyelocytes (de Botton et al., 2003; Fenaux et al., 1999; Sanz et al., 1999; Tallman et al., 1997).

2.2 The discovery of ATO-based APL therapy

Arsenic, in the form of arsenic trioxide (ATO), was first described as an agent that possesses antileukemic properties in the year 1878. In this study, Fowler's solution, a solution of ATO in potassium bicarbonate, was shown to dramatically reduce the number of white blood cells in a patient with chronic myelogenous leukemia (CML) (Cutler & Bradford, 1878). Subsequently, this remedy was used as a primary antileukemic agent until the discovery of radiation therapy in the early 20th century (Forkner & Scott, 1931; Kwong & Todd, 1997). In the 1970s, ATO reappeared as a therapeutic agent for APL as Chinese researchers showed that ailing-1, a mixture of ATO and crude herbal extracts, was effective in the treatment of both de novo as well as relapsed cases (Shen et al., 1997; Sun et al., 1992; Zhang et al., 1996). Additional clinical studies showed that ATO, as a single agent, caused complete remission in up to 90% of patients and reduced the relapse rate for high risk patients (Niu et al., 1999; Shen et al., 1997). A research group in the United States confirmed these preliminary studies and further showed that ATO treatment induced partial differentiation of leukemic cells, caspase activation and subsequently apoptosis (Soignet *et al.*, 1998).

2.3 Present and future APL therapy

Currently, ATRA in combination with chemotherapy is being employed as frontline therapy for APL, whereas ATO primarily is being used for treatment of cases that are resistant to ATRA or patients suffering from frequent relapses. However, several clinical trials are now assessing the synergistic effect of combining ATRA and ATO with and without chemotherapy. These trials are conducted mainly on the basis of successful studies in animal models, showing a positive effect of ATRA/ATO combinations in APL mice (Jing *et al.*, 2001; Lallemand-Breitenbach *et al.*, 1999). The main conclusion so far from the ongoing clinical studies is that newly diagnosed patients are likely to benefit from ATRA/ATO combination treatment in addition to low-dose chemotherapy (Estey *et al.*, 2006; Hu *et al.*, 2009; Shen *et al.*, 2004; Wang *et al.*, 2004).

3. The mechanism of PML, RARA and PML/RARA

3.1 The role of PML/RARA in APL pathogenesis

The molecular hallmark of APL is the t(15;17) chromosomal translocation that expresses the fusion oncoprotein PML/RARA. While this genetic aberration is identified in more than 97% of all APL cases, the remaining patients diagnosed with this disease harbor variant translocations that all involve the *RARA* gene in fusion with alternative partners such as the genes encoding promyelocytic leukemia zinc finger (*PLZF*) (Chen *et al.*, 1993), nucleophosmin (*NPM*) (Redner *et al.*, 1996), nuclear matrix associated (*NUMA*) (Wells *et al.*, 1997), or signal transducer and activator of transcription 5b (*STAT5B*) (Arnould *et al.*, 1999). The most compelling evidence that PML/RARA alone can contribute directly to APL development comes from studies in mice showing that expression of this oncoprotein as a transgene leads to development of an APL–like disease. However, these experiments also show that a relatively long latency period is required prior to onset of disease, suggesting the involvement of acquired genetic aberrations in addition to the t(15;17) translocation (Brown *et al.*, 1997; Grisolano *et al.*, 1997).

3.2 The function of PML

The first component of the PML/RARA fusion, the PML protein, is a tumor suppressor (Bernardi *et al.*, 2006; Salomoni & Pandolfi, 2002; Trotman *et al.*, 2006) that functions in multiple cellular processes, including apoptosis (Wang *et al.*, 1998), differentiation (Ito *et al.*, 2008), DNA repair (Bøe *et al.*, 2006; Dellaire *et al.*, 2006a), senescence (Ferbeyre *et al.*, 2000; Pearson *et al.*, 2000), angiogenesis (Bernardi *et al.*, 2006) and virus defence (Everett & Maul, 1994). The human *PML* gene is located on chromosome 15, consists of nine exons and produces several alternatively spliced protein isoforms designated PML I through VII. All of these PML variants contain an identical tripartite (TRIM) motif in their N-terminal region, and a C-terminus that varies due to alternative splicing (Borden, 2002; Fagioli *et al.*, 1992; Jensen *et al.*, 2001; Jul-Larsen *et al.*, 2010; Reymond *et al.*, 2001). The TRIM motif, which comprises a RING finger, two B-boxes and a predicted coiled coil domain, has been shown to be important for PML multimerization, a feature responsible for one of the most striking properties of this protein, namely the ability to generate nuclear structures termed PML nuclear bodies (PML NBs) (Lallemand-Breitenbach & de The, 2010). These bodies are highly dynamic and change their morphology and biochemical composition in a cell cycle-dependent manner. For example, during entry into mitosis, several PML NB resident components, including Daxx, Sp100 and SUMO, are lost concomitant with formation of PML NB aggregates called mitotic assemblies of PML proteins (MAPPs), whereas transition from mitosis to G1-phase coincides with exclusion of PML NBs from the progeny nuclei and complex formation with nucleoporins and microtubule filaments to form cytoplasmic assemblies of PML and nucleoporins (CyPNs) (Chen et al., 2008; Dellaire et al., 2006b; Jul-Larsen et al., 2009). Although, PML NBs have the capacity to recruit a large number of different protein components, PML is the only protein so far that has been shown to be required for their formation. For this reason, it is widely assumed that the ability to assemble these cellular compartments represents an integral part of PML biogenesis. It still remains, however, to clearly define the molecular mechanism involved in PML NB assembly and function.

3.3 The function of RARA
The second fusion partner, RARA, is a ligand binding transcription factor that contains a DNA binding motif in its central region and a retinoid binding domain at the C-terminus. To generate an active protein complex, this nuclear receptor forms a heterodimer with the RXR family of transcription factors. Upon direct binding to a RA responsive element (RARE) within the regulatory region of a target gene, RARA/RXR complexes promote transcriptional silencing by recruiting co-repressor proteins such as NCOR1, SMRT and histone deacetylase to the promoter-binding complexes. In the presence of physiological concentrations of ligand (i.e. retinoids), a conformational change occurs within the RARA/RXR heterodimer that leads to dissociation of co-repressors and concomitant recruitment of histone acetylases and components of the basic transcription machinery, thus transforming the protein complex from a gene silencer to a gene activator (Bastien & Rochette-Egly, 2004). RARA regulates several genes involved in myeloid progenitor cell differentiation, including c-myc (Bentley & Groudine, 1986; Gowda et al., 1986), C/EBPβ (Duprez et al., 2003), C/EBPε (Park et al., 1999) and PU.1 (Mueller et al., 2006), suggesting an important role of this protein in blood cell maturation.

3.4 The function of PML/RARA
Upon fusion between PML and RARA, the variable C-terminus of the PML protein is lost, whereas the constant N-terminal TRIM motif generally remains intact. In the case of RARA, fusion to PML leads to loss of the first 50 to 60 N-terminal amino acids, a deletion that does not appear to affect the DNA and ligand binding activities of this protein (de Thé et al., 1991). Thus, PML/RARA retains the powerful protein-protein interaction domain of the PML protein, whereas the variable isoform-specific region is replaced by the trans-activating functions of RARA (Fig. 1.).
One of the gained PML/RARA functions that is thought to contribute largely to APL development is the ability of this chimeric protein to form stable transcription repression complexes that are irresponsive to physiological concentrations of retinoids. As a consequence, gene promoters that are targeted by PML/RARA become constitutively repressed, an observation that has led to the general assumption that this oncoprotein causes a block in blood cell differentiation through transcriptional inhibition of key genes

involved in hematopoietic maturation. Consistent with a role in gene repression, PML/RARA has also been shown to recruit the histone methyl transferase SUV39H1 (Carbone *et al.*, 2006), members of the polycomb repressive complex 2 (PRC2) (Villa *et al.*, 2007) and DNA methyltransferases (DNMTs) (Di Croce *et al.*, 2002), proteins that are known to induce a repressive chromatin structure. In addition to increased repressor activity, the PML/RARA fusion also appears to possess a considerable expanded repertoire of target genes compared to the normal RARA protein. This notion is supported by *in vitro* binding studies showing that PML/RARA has a broader and more relaxed DNA binding specificity compared to RARA (Hauksdottir & Privalsky, 2001; Kamashev *et al.*, 2004), and by a genome wide screen revealing a wide range of PML/RARA target genes (Hoemme *et al.*, 2008). The altered DNA binding and transcription repression properties of PML/RARA are partially due to the ability of this chimeric protein to form homodimeres through protein-protein interactions mediated by the TRIM motif of PML (Jansen *et al.*, 1995; Perez *et al.*, 1993). In addition, this chimeric protein has also been shown to form functional complexes with other transcription factors such as RXR and Daxx, a feature that may further contribute to the expanded promoter binding capacity (Zeisig *et al.*, 2007; Zhu *et al.*, 2005; Zhu *et al.*, 2007).

PML/RARA is also thought to contribute to malignant transformation and development of APL through inhibition of PML tumor suppressor functions. A dominant negative effect of PML/RARA on this protein is evident by studies demonstrating disruption of nuclear PML bodies into a dispersed microspeckled pattern in cells expressing this oncoprotein (Dyck *et al.*, 1994; Koken *et al.*, 1994; Weis *et al.*, 1994). Interestingly, while disruption of PML NBs by PML/RARA in the nucleus is evident, this oncoprotein readily assembles into MAPPS and CyPNs, the mitotic and cytoplasmic versions of PML NBs, respectively (Jul-Larsen *et al.*, 2009). The disruption of PML NBs in the nucleus may reflect the role of this oncoprotein in repression of gene activity.

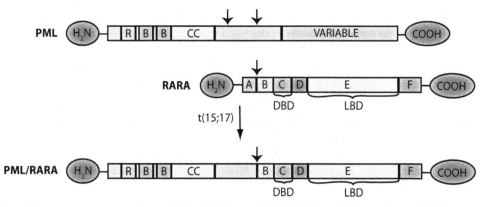

Fig. 1. Structural organization of PML, RARA and PML/RARA. PML contains a RING domain (R), two B boxes (B), a coiled coil (CC) and a variable C-terminus. RARA consists of six regulatory domains (A-F), of which domain C and E harbor the DNA binding domain (DBD) and the ligand binding domain (LBD), respectively. The t (15;17) translocation produces PML/RARA, which retains the N-terminal PML motifs as well as RARA DNA and ligand binding activity. Arrows indicate protein breakpoints.

While PML/RARA is constantly expressed in more than 97% of all APL patients, the reciprocal fusion protein RARA/PML, which contains the N-terminus of RARA and variable lengths of the PML C-terminus, is identified in only 70-80% of the cases (Alcalay *et al.*, 1992; Grimwade *et al.*, 1996). Not much is known about the role of this protein in the pathogenesis of APL. However, one study has described a possible link between RARA/PML fusion gene deletions and resistance to ATRA-based therapy (Subramaniyam *et al.*, 2006).

4. The mechanism of ATRA and ATO-mediated APL therapy

4.1 The mechanism of ATRA-based APL therapy

Phenotypically, pharmacological concentrations of ATRA lead to effective differentiation of immature APL cells to terminally differentiated granulocytes. From a therapeutic point of view this may be beneficial since the immature malignant cells progress from being highly proliferative and long-lived to arrested and short-lived. In addition, *in vitro* cell culture experiments have shown that ATRA-induced differentiation also coincides with activation of apoptosis (Altucci *et al.*, 2001; Grignani *et al.*, 1998; Martin *et al.*, 1990). The relative contribution of apoptotic cell death versus increased turnover of mature granulocytes to ATRA-induced clearance of tumorigenic cells is not clear. Although ATRA appears to be highly effective in clearing the bulk of proliferative tumor cells, a residual population of cells with detectable t(15;17) translocation almost invariably persist following treatment with this reagent alone, a feature that probably explains the additional need for chemotherapy in order to achieve complete remission (Chen *et al.*, 1991; Chomienne *et al.*, 1990; Huang *et al.*, 1988; Zhu *et al.*, 1995).

At the molecular level, therapeutic doses of ATRA reverse the differentiation block caused by PML/RARA through a direct interaction with the ligand binding site present on the RARA moiety. As for normal RARA, the ligand-receptor interaction induces a change in the PML/RARA protein structural conformation, which leads to release of transcription repressors and subsequent activation of the basal transcription machinery. Coincident with transcription activation, ATRA also induces recruitment of the proteasome to the ligand binding transcription activation domain AF2 of RARA, and subsequent proteasome-dependent degradation (Kopf *et al.*, 2000; Zhu *et al.*, 1999). A protein that has been proposed to participate in this pathway is the ubiquitin-activating enzyme E1-like (UBE1L) protein, which itself represents one of the ATRA-induced proteins (Kitareewan *et al.*, 2002). ATRA-mediated degradation appears to affect RARA and PML/RARA equally well and may be functionally linked to transcription activation, since mutations in RARA that impairs its DNA binding activity also inhibits ATRA-mediated catabolism (Zhu *et al.*, 1999). The relative contribution of transcriptional activation, differentiation and degradation on therapy remains to be fully elucidated.

4.2 The mechanism of ATO-based APL therapy

Compared to ATRA, ATO has a more limited ability to induce terminal differentiation of APL cells. *In vitro* studies using cultured cells have revealed a dose-dependent effect of this drug on differentiation and apoptosis (Chen *et al.*, 1997). At high concentrations (0.5-2.0 µM) ATO induced cell death by apoptosis, while at low concentrations (0.1-0.25 µM) this drug caused partial differentiation of APL cells along the granulocyte linage (Cai *et al.*, 2000; Chen *et al.*, 1997). The results from these experiments appear to be in good agreement with studies demonstrating ATO-induced partial differentiation and apoptosis in APL patients or animal models, where the effective serum concentrations of ATO generally ranges from 0.1 to 1.0 µM (Chen *et al.*, 1997; Lallemand-Breitenbach *et al.*, 1999). Interestingly, ATO-mediated differentiation has been shown to become dramatically enhanced in the presence of cyclic adenosine monophosphate (cAMP). The mechanism responsible for this synergistic effect was proposed to be the combined effect of ATO-induced PML/RARA degradation and cAMP-mediated inhibition of cell cycle progression (Guillemin *et al.*, 2002; Zhu *et al.*, 2002).

At the molecular level, ATO exerts its therapeutic effect on APL in part by initiating a cascade of biochemical alterations that primarily affect the PML moiety of PML/RARA. Firstly, the presence of arsenic in the cell culture medium has been shown to increase PML and PML/RARA multimerization, an effect that is manifested by decreased solubility of these proteins upon preparation of cell lysates and reduced mobility within PML NBs as determined by analysis of GFP-tagged PML in living cells (Jeanne *et al.*, 2010; Zhang *et al.*, 2010). Concomitant with increased aggregation, PML becomes extensively SUMOylated on at least three different lysine residues. All of the three different SUMO isoforms, including SUMO1, 2 and 3, appear to participate in this reaction, and both mono and poly-SUMOylation events have been reported (Lallemand-Breitenbach *et al.*, 2001; Lallemand-Breitenbach *et al.*, 2008; Muller *et al.*, 1998; Tatham *et al.*, 2008). Subsequent to SUMOylation, a protein called RNF4 binds SUMOylated residues on PML in order to catalyze poly-ubiquitination, a modification that directs PML and PML/RARA to the proteasome for degradation (Lallemand-Breitenbach *et al.*, 2008; Tatham *et al.*, 2008). Recently, a direct interaction between PML and ATO, that potentially triggers this SUMO-mediated degradation pathway, was mapped to cysteine residues located in the TRIM and B-box motifs of PML (Jeanne *et al.*, 2010; Zhang *et al.*, 2010).

In addition to affecting differentiation of leukemic cells, recent studies have also implicated ATO in clearance of leukemic-initiating cells (LICs), a small population of malignantly transformed cells with stem cell characteristics that frequently are refractory to cancer therapeutic drugs. Consistent with this, PML/RARA expression has been reported to support properties of self-renewal of LICs (Wojiski *et al.*, 2009), and certain characteristics of promyelocytic phenotypes provide the basic properties for the development of APL-initiating LICs (Guibal *et al.*, 2009). Furthermore, a recent study demonstrated LIC clearance in association with ATO-induced PML/RARA degradation by a mechanism that appeared to be uncoupled from the observed cell differentiation (Nasr *et al.*, 2008; Shao *et al.*, 1998). In addition, ATO has been reported to cause increased proliferation of LICs in a chronic myelogenous mouse model, hence sensitizing otherwise therapy-insensitive leukemic cells to Ara-C-based treatment (Ito *et al.*, 2008; Ito *et al.*, 2009).

The proapoptotic activity of ATO is not specific for APL cells (Akao *et al.*, 1998; Bachleitner-Hofmann *et al.*, 2001; Ishitsuka *et al.*, 1998; Perkins *et al.*, 2000; Rousselot *et al.*, 1999; Wang *et al.*, 1996; Zhang *et al.*, 1998; Zheng *et al.*, 1999), although non-APL tumor cells have been shown to be less sensitive to this drug (Huang *et al.*, 1999). ATO induces apoptosis by downregulation of the antiapoptotic protein Bcl-2, leading to a disturbance in the regulated balance between pro- and antiapoptotic proteins (Akao *et al.*, 1998; Chen *et al.*, 1996; Zhang *et al.*, 1998). In addition, ATO increases radioactive oxygen species (ROS) production in malignant cells. As a consequence, this drug leads to disruption of the mitochondrial membrane potential, followed by cytochrome c release, caspase activation and subsequent apoptotic cell death (Jing *et al.*, 1999).

4.3 The synergy between ATRA and ATO

While ATRA and ATO on their own are known to be effective in curing APL, it is also becoming increasingly clear that treatment regiments based on a combination of the two drugs leads to a quicker clinical remission, a more effective clearance of leukemic cells and a significantly longer period of relapse free survival (Estey et al., 2006; Hu et al., 2009; Shen et al., 2004; Wang et al., 2004). This synergistic effect may result due to the ability of both these drugs to cause PML/RARA degradation, a parameter that appears to be critical for the success of APL therapy. In addition, the combined effect of ATO and ATRA may also result due to the ability of the two agents to act on separate targets, both of which are important for disease remission. For example, ATO may be effective in eradicating self-renewable LICs through stimulated PML/RARA degradation, while ATRA represents a more effective differentiating agent, and hence may lead to a more complete clearance of undifferentiated APL cells.

5. Therapy-induced degradation of PML/RARA

ATRA and ATO-induced therapy of APL may be connected to the ability of these drugs to induce PML/RARA catabolism (Fig. 2.). In agreement with this, reduced PML/RARA expression can be observed in both ATRA and ATO-treated cells, and the two drugs synergize both for their ability to induce oncoprotein degradation as well as for their capacity to promote clinical remission (Hu et al., 2009; Nasr et al., 2008; Shen et al., 2004). An important role of protein degradation for effective APL therapy is also supported by experiments in mice. For example, treatment of an APL mouse model with the proteasome inhibitor bortezomid led to reduced degradation of PML/RARA and concomitant resistance to ATRA and ATO-based therapy (Nasr et al., 2008). In addition, PML/RARA mutated in critical SUMOylation target sites, were found to be more resistant to ATO-mediated degradation compared to unmodified PML/RARA (Lallemand-Breitenbach et al., 2001; Lallemand-Breitenbach et al., 2008).

In addition to proteasome-dependent degradation induced by ATRA and ATO, PML/RARA has also been shown to be amenable for degradation by the lysosome-dependent degradation pathway autophagy (Isakson et al., 2010; Klionsky, 2007). This degradation mechanism appears to play a major role both for basal turnover as well as for therapy-induced catabolism of PML/RARA. Indeed, pharmacological inhibitors of autophagy were found to completely prevent ATRA and ATO-stimulated degradation of PML/RARA expressed in the APL cell line NB4 (Isakson et al., 2010). In contrast to proteasome-dependent degradation, autophagy-mediated proteolyses of PML/RARA appears to be independent of a direct interaction between the drugs and the target protein. Instead, ATRA and ATO seem to stimulate autophagy in APL cells primarily through a mechanism that involves the mammalian target of rapamycin (mTOR) and Unc-51-like kinase 1 (ULK1) (Bøe & Simonsen, 2010; Isakson et al., 2010). Furthermore, PML/RARA is highly aggregation prone and therefore a good substrate for this degradation pathway (Isakson et al., 2010; Lallemand-Breitenbach et al., 2001). Aggregates of PML/RARA may form during the process of protein synthesis. In agreement with this, synthesis of PML/RARA has been shown to be associated with endoplasmatic reticulum stress, a feature indicative of aberrant folding during protein synthesis (Khan et al., 2004).

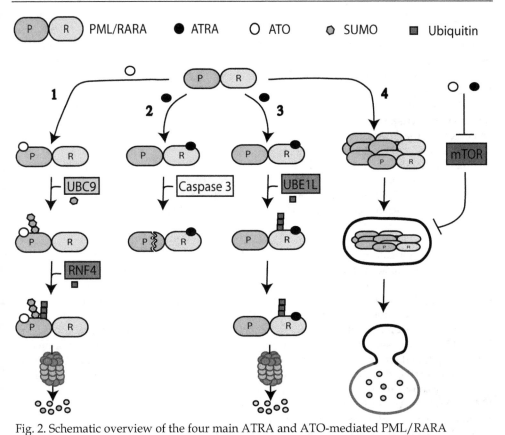

Fig. 2. Schematic overview of the four main ATRA and ATO-mediated PML/RARA degradation pathways: 1. ATO-induced proteasome-dependent degradation, 2. ATRA-induced caspase cleavage, 3. ATRA-induced proteasome-dependent degradation, 4. ATRA/ATO-induced autophagy-mediated degradation.

Two different types of proteases have also been implicated in PML/RARA proteolysis. First, PML/RARA has been shown to be susceptible to a caspase 3-like activity expressed in APL cells and that becomes induced by the presence of ATRA (Nervi et al., 1998). The second protease shown to be involved is neutrophil elastase, a myeloid specific serine protease that is maximally expressed in promyelocytes (Lane & Ley, 2003). The contribution of this protease to APL development is unclear since one study showed enhanced penetrance of PML/RARA in a neutrophil elastase defective mice (Lane & Ley, 2003), while another demonstrated decreased tumorigenesis in a mouse model expressing a neutrophil elastase cleavage defective PML/RARA protein (Uy et al., 2010).

PML turnover has also been shown to be regulated by a pathway that involves direct phosphorylation by the casein kinase 2 (CK2) and subsequent ubiquitin-mediated degradation, a mechanism that was proposed to cause decreased PML tumor suppressor activity in lung cancer (Scaglioni et al., 2006). However, the significance of CK2-mediated PML phosphorylation in PML/RARA degradation and APL pathogenesis has not been elucidated.

6. The mechanism of APL therapy resistance

The second most common translocation associated with APL, the t(11;17) translocation that expresses PLZF/RARA fusion instead of PML/RARA, is generally insensitive to ATRA and ATO-based therapy (Chen *et al.*, 1993; Licht *et al.*, 1995). The poor response of these patients to ATO add support to studies showing that this drug primarily target PML, which is absent in PLZF/RARA. In the case of the poor response to ATRA, on the other hand, the underlying mechanism has been hypothesized to be due to enhanced co-repressor activity conferred by the PLZF moiety of the PLZF-RARA fusion (Grignani *et al.*, 1998; He *et al.*, 1998; Lin *et al.*, 1998). However, the notion that PLZF/RARA is irresponsive to ATRA stimulation has been contradicted in more recent studies demonstrating ATRA-induced gene expression and differentiation also in PLZF/RARA expressing APL cells (Nasr *et al.*, 2008; Petti *et al.*, 2002; Rice *et al.*, 2009). Thus, further work is needed in order to fully understand the mechanism underlying the insensitivity of PLZF/RARA positive APL cells to ATRA.

Resistance to ATRA-mediated therapy is also seen in APL patients that have relapsed following the first clinical remission. Such acquired resistance may be caused by a number of different physiological factors, including increased catabolism, reduced cellular uptake, or increased cytoplasmic sequestration of the therapeutic drugs (Freemantle *et al.*, 2003; Gallagher, 2002). In addition, *in vitro* cell culture experiments, using the APL cell line NB4, have revealed mutations within the PML/RARA gene of subclones with acquired resistance to ATRA. Interestingly, several of these mutations were found clustered at/or near the ligand binding domain of RARA leading to defects in ATRA binding. Since these mutants generally retain their capacity to form complex with RXR and to bind DNA, they have been suggested to act as dominant inhibitors of wild type RARA (Duprez *et al.*, 2000; Kitamura *et al.*, 1997; Nason-Burchenal *et al.*, 1998; Rosenauer *et al.*, 1996; Shao *et al.*, 1997). Mutations in PML/RARA have also been identified in a subset of ATRA-relapsed patients, and these mutations were found to be variably associated with inactivation of ATRA binding (Ding *et al.*, 1998; Gallagher *et al.*, 2006; Imaizumi *et al.*, 1998; Marasca *et al.*, 1999; Takayama *et al.*, 2001; Zhou *et al.*, 2002). Interestingly, one study identified mutations within the intact PML locus of APL patients with ATRA-resistance and poor prognosis (Gurrieri *et al.*, 2004).

Recently, PML/RARA mutations have also been discovered in two APL cases with poor response to ATO (Goto *et al.*, 2011). In both cases, the mutations were located within the second B-box motif of the PML protein. Since the amino acids affected by these mutations were close to a cysteine-rich region, previously proposed to bind ATO (Jeanne *et al.*, 2010), the authors of this paper hypothesized that these mutations may affect interactions between this drug and PML/RARA. Alternatively, the mutated protein may have defects in oligomerization, since the B-box domains are known to function in PML multimerization. Combined, the PML/RARA mutations that have been identified in ATRA and/or ATO–resistant APL cells support the notion that these drugs interact with separate moieties of the fusion protein to induce clinical remission.

7. Perspectives

During the past 30 years, APL has progressed from a deadly disease to a highly curable malignancy. In addition, the advances that have been made in understanding the pathology and cure of APL at the molecular level have led to the emergence of a highly attractive model disease for the development of targeted cancer therapy. For example, the case of APL clearly demonstrates the therapeutic effectiveness of targeting a defined oncoprotein, and since recurrent translocations and expression of fusion oncoproteins similar to that of PML/RARA is a common trait also among other types of cancers (including leukemias and sarcomas), a large number of malignancies, in addition to APL, may benefit from similar targeted therapies. Thus, it will be important to continue identifying therapeutic concepts that contribute to the success of APL therapy and to modulate these concepts for treatment of other cancers.

Since both ATRA and ATO have been shown to exert their therapeutic effects through interactions with specific regions of the PML/RARA oncoprotein, it may be assumed that these drugs will be effective only against APL. However, one should also keep in mind that the ability of ATRA and ATO to mediate cure of APL is regarded as a rather fortuitous discovery and not merely as a result of rational therapeutic design. For this reason, these drugs are likely to have other yet unidentified cellular targets, beside the APL-associated fusion portion, that are important for effective treatment. Evidence for this comes from one of the studies mentioned above showing that both ATRA and ATO-stimulated autophagic degradation of PML/RARA through a mTOR-dependent pathway that does not seem to involve direct interactions between drugs and the oncoprotein (Isakson et al., 2010). In addition, it is also becoming increasingly clear that ATO has the potential to cure a subset of cancers that don't express PML/RARA. For example, induced clearance of LICs has been demonstrated both in PML/RARA positive as well as PML/RARA negative leukemic cells (Ito et al., 2008; Nasr et al., 2008). Furthermore, a phase II clinical study was recently published that showed promising results of using ATO in combination with interferon alpha and zidovudine for treatment of patients with chronic adult T cell leukemia (Kchour et al., 2009), and finally, this drug was found to sensitize glucocorticoid-resistant acute lymphoblastic leukemia cells to dexamethasone (Bornhauser et al., 2007). Thus, it is likely that APL for many years to come will continue to represent an important model disease for targeted and non-targeted effects of ATRA and ATO, while increased understanding of the molecular pathways involved may lead to discoveries of new therapies that are applicable for other types of cancers.

8. Acknowledgements

The work in our laboratory is funded by the Research Council of Norway, The Norwegian Cancer society and South-Eastern Norway Regional Health Authority.

9. References

Akao, Y., Mizoguchi, H., Kojima, S., Naoe, T., Ohishi, N. & Yagi, K. (1998). Arsenic induces apoptosis in B-cell leukaemic cell lines in vitro: activation of caspases and down-regulation of Bcl-2 protein. *British Journal of Haematology* 102, 1055-1060.

Alcalay, M., Zangrilli, D., Fagioli, M., Pandolfi, P. P., Mencarelli, A., Lo Coco, F., Biondi, A., Grignani, F. & Pelicci, P. G. (1992). Expression pattern of the RAR alpha-PML fusion gene in acute promyelocytic leukemia. *Proc Natl Acad Sci U S A* 89, 4840-4844.

Altucci, L., Rossin, A., Raffelsberger, W., Reitmair, A., Chomienne, C. & Gronemeyer, H. (2001). Retinoic acid-induced apoptosis in leukemia cells is mediated by paracrine action of tumor-selective death ligand TRAIL. *Nature Medicine* 7, 680-686.

Arnould, C., Philippe, C., Bourdon, V., Gr goire, M. J., Berger, R. & Jonveaux, P. (1999). The signal transducer and activator of transcription STAT5b gene is a new partner of retinoic acid receptor alpha in acute promyelocytic-like leukaemia. *Human Molecular Genetics* 8, 1741-1749.

Bachleitner-Hofmann, T., Gisslinger, B., Grumbeck, E. & Gisslinger, H. (2001). Arsenic trioxide and ascorbic acid: synergy with potential implications for the treatment of acute myeloid leukaemia? *British Journal of Haematology* 112, 783-786.

Bastien, J. & Rochette-Egly, C. (2004). Nuclear retinoid receptors and the transcription of retinoid-target genes. *Gene* 328, 1-16.

Bentley, D. L. & Groudine, M. (1986). A block to elongation is largely responsible for decreased transcription of c-myc in differentiated HL60 cells. *Nature* 321, 702-706.

Bernard, J., Weil, M., Boiron, M., Jacquillat, C., Flandrin, G. & Gemon, M. F. (1973). Acute promyelocytic leukemia: results of treatment by daunorubicin. *Blood* 41, 489-496.

Bernardi, R., Guernah, I., Jin, D. & other authors (2006). PML inhibits HIF-1alpha translation and neoangiogenesis through repression of mTOR. *Nature* 442, 779-785.

Borden, K. L. (2002). Pondering the promyelocytic leukemia protein (PML) puzzle: possible functions for PML nuclear bodies. *Molecular & Cellular Biology* 22, 5259-5269.

Bornhauser, B. C., Bonapace, L., Lindholm, D., Martinez, R., Cario, G., Schrappe, M., Niggli, F. K., Schafer, B. W. & Bourquin, J. P. (2007). Low-dose arsenic trioxide sensitizes glucocorticoid-resistant acute lymphoblastic leukemia cells to dexamethasone via an Akt-dependent pathway. *Blood* 110, 2084-2091.

Breitman, T. R., Collins, S. J. & Keene, B. R. (1981). Terminal differentiation of human promyelocytic leukemic cells in primary culture in response to retinoic acid. *Blood* 57, 1000-1004.

Brown, D., Kogan, S., Lagasse, E., Weissman, I., Alcalay, M., Pelicci, P. G., Atwater, S. & Bishop, J. M. (1997). A PMLRARalpha transgene initiates murine acute promyelocytic leukemia. *Proceedings of the National Academy of Sciences U S A* 94, 2551-2556.

Bøe, S. O., Haave, M., Jul-Larsen, A., Grudic, A., Bjerkvig, R. & Lonning, P. E. (2006). Promyelocytic leukemia nuclear bodies are predetermined processing sites for damaged DNA. *Journal of Cell Science* 119, 3284-3295.

Bøe, S. O. & Simonsen, A. (2010). Autophagic degradation of an oncoprotein. *Autophagy* 6, 964-965.

Cai, X., Shen, Y. L., Zhu, Q. & other authors (2000). Arsenic trioxide-induced apoptosis and differentiation are associated respectively with mitochondrial transmembrane potential collapse and retinoic acid signaling pathways in acute promyelocytic leukemia. *Leukemia* 14, 262-270.

Carbone, R., Botrugno, O. A., Ronzoni, S., Insinga, A., Di Croce, L., Pelicci, P. G. & Minucci, S. (2006). Recruitment of the histone methyltransferase SUV39H1 and its role in the oncogenic properties of the leukemia-associated PML-retinoic acid receptor fusion protein. *Molecular & Cellular Biology* 26, 1288-1296.

Chen, G. Q., Zhu, J., Shi, X. G. & other authors (1996). In vitro studies on cellular and molecular mechanisms of arsenic trioxide (As2O3) in the treatment of acute promyelocytic leukemia: As2O3 induces NB4 cell apoptosis with downregulation of Bcl-2 expression and modulation of PML-RAR alpha/PML proteins. *Blood* 88, 1052-1061.

Chen, G. Q., Shi, X. G., Tang, W. & other authors (1997). Use of arsenic trioxide (As2O3) in the treatment of acute promyelocytic leukemia (APL): I. As2O3 exerts dose-dependent dual effects on APL cells. *Blood* 89, 3345-3353.

Chen, Y. C., Kappel, C., Beaudouin, J., Eils, R. & Spector, D. L. (2008). Live cell dynamics of promyelocytic leukemia nuclear bodies upon entry into and exit from mitosis. *Molecular biology of the cell* 19, 3147-3162.

Chen, Z., Brand, N. J., Chen, A., Chen, S. J., Tong, J. H., Wang, Z. Y., Waxman, S. & Zelent, A. (1993). Fusion between a novel Kruppel-like zinc finger gene and the retinoic acid receptor-alpha locus due to a variant t(11;17) translocation associated with acute promyelocytic leukaemia. *The EMBO Journal* 12, 1161-1167.

Chen, Z. X., Xue, Y. Q., Zhang, R. & other authors (1991). A clinical and experimental study on all-trans retinoic acid-treated acute promyelocytic leukemia patients. *Blood* 78, 1413-1419.

Chomienne, C., Ballerini, P., Balitrand, N., Daniel, M. T., Fenaux, P., Castaigne, S. & Degos, L. (1990). All-trans retinoic acid in acute promyelocytic leukemias. II. In vitro studies: structure-function relationship. *Blood* 76, 1710-1717.

Cordonnier, C., Vernant, J. P., Brun, B. & other authors (1985). Acute promyelocytic leukemia in 57 previously untreated patients. *Cancer* 55, 18-25.

Cunningham, I., Gee, T. S., Reich, L. M., Kempin, S. J., Naval, A. N. & Clarkson, B. D. (1989). Acute promyelocytic leukemia: treatment results during a decade at Memorial Hospital. *Blood* 73, 1116-1122.

Cutler, E. G. & Bradford, E. H. (1878). Action of iron, cod-liver oil, and arsenic on the globular richness of the blood. *American Journal of Medical Sciences* 75, 74-84.

de Botton, S., Chevret, S., Coiteux, V. & other authors (2003). Early onset of chemotherapy can reduce the incidence of ATRA syndrome in newly diagnosed acute promyelocytic leukemia (APL) with low white blood cell counts: results from APL 93 trial. *Leukemia* 17, 339-342.

de Thé, H., Lavau, C., Marchio, A., Chomienne, C., Degos, L. & Dejean, A. (1991). The PML-RAR alpha fusion mRNA generated by the t(15;17) translocation in acute promyelocytic leukemia encodes a functionally altered RAR. *Cell* 66, 675-684.

de Thé, H. & Chen, Z. (2010). Acute promyelocytic leukaemia: novel insights into the mechanisms of cure. *Nature Reviews Cancer* 10, 775-783.

Degos, L., Castaigne, S., Tilly, H., Sigaux, F. & Daniel, M. T. (1985). Treatment of leukemia with low-dose ara-C: a study of 160 cases. *Seminars in Oncology* 12, 196-199.

Dellaire, G., Ching, R. W., Ahmed, K., Jalali, F., Tse, K. C., Bristow, R. G. & Bazett-Jones, D. P. (2006a). Promyelocytic leukemia nuclear bodies behave as DNA damage sensors whose response to DNA double-strand breaks is regulated by NBS1 and the kinases ATM, Chk2, and ATR. *The Journal of cell biology* 175, 55-66.

Dellaire, G., Eskiw, C. H., Dehghani, H., Ching, R. W. & Bazett-Jones, D. P. (2006b). Mitotic accumulations of PML protein contribute to the re-establishment of PML nuclear bodies in G1. *Journal of cell science* 119, 1034-1042.

Di Croce, L., Raker, V. A., Corsaro, M. & other authors (2002). Methyltransferase recruitment and DNA hypermethylation of target promoters by an oncogenic transcription factor. *Science* 295, 1079-1082.

Ding, W., Li, Y. P., Nobile, L. M., Grills, G., Carrera, I., Paietta, E., Tallman, M. S., Wiernik, P. H. & Gallagher, R. E. (1998). Leukemic cellular retinoic acid resistance and missense mutations in the PML-RARalpha fusion gene after relapse of acute promyelocytic leukemia from treatment with all-trans retinoic acid and intensive chemotherapy. *Blood* 92, 1172-1183.

Drapkin, R. L., Gee, T. S., Dowling, M. D., Arlin, Z., McKenzie, S., Kempin, S. & Clarkson, B. (1978). Prophylactic heparin therapy in acute promyelocytic leukemia. *Cancer* 41, 2484-2490.

Duprez, E., Benoit, G., Flexor, M., Lillehaug, J. R. & Lanotte, M. (2000). A mutated PML/RARA found in the retinoid maturation resistant NB4 subclone, NB4-R2, blocks RARA and wild-type PML/RARA transcriptional activities. *Leukemia* 14, 255-261.

Duprez, E., Wagner, K., Koch, H. & Tenen, D. G. (2003). C/EBPbeta: a major PML-RARA-responsive gene in retinoic acid-induced differentiation of APL cells. *Embo J* 22, 5806-5816.

Dyck, J. A., Maul, G. G., Miller, W. H., Jr., Chen, J. D., Kakizuka, A. & Evans, R. M. (1994). A novel macromolecular structure is a target of the promyelocyte-retinoic acid receptor oncoprotein. *Cell* 76, 333-343.

Estey, E., Garcia-Manero, G., Ferrajoli, A., Faderl, S., Verstovsek, S., Jones, D. & Kantarjian, H. (2006). Use of all-trans retinoic acid plus arsenic trioxide as an alternative to chemotherapy in untreated acute promyelocytic leukemia. *Blood* 107, 3469-3473.

Everett, R. D. & Maul, G. G. (1994). HSV-1 IE protein Vmw110 causes redistribution of PML. *The EMBO journal* 13, 5062-5069.

Fagioli, M., Alcalay, M., Pandolfi, P. P., Venturini, L., Mencarelli, A., Simeone, A., Acampora, D., Grignani, F. & Pelicci, P. G. (1992). Alternative splicing of PML transcripts predicts coexpression of several carboxy-terminally different protein isoforms. *Oncogene* 7, 1083-1091.

Fenaux, P., Chastang, C., Chevret, S. & other authors (1999). A randomized comparison of all transretinoic acid (ATRA) followed by chemotherapy and ATRA plus chemotherapy and the role of maintenance therapy in newly diagnosed acute promyelocytic leukemia. The European APL Group. *Blood* 94, 1192-1200.

Fenaux, P., Wang, Z. Z. & Degos, L. (2007). Treatment of acute promyelocytic leukemia by retinoids. *Current Topics in Microbiology & Immunology* 313, 101-128.

Ferbeyre, G., de Stanchina, E., Querido, E., Baptiste, N., Prives, C. & Lowe, S. W. (2000). PML is induced by oncogenic ras and promotes premature senescence. *Genes & development* 14, 2015-2027.

Forkner, C. E. & Scott, T. F. M. (1931). Arsenic as a therapeutic agent in chronic myelogenous leukemia. *Journal of the American Medical Association* 97, 3-5.

Freemantle, S. J., Spinella, M. J. & Dmitrovsky, E. (2003). Retinoids in cancer therapy and chemoprevention: promise meets resistance. *Oncogene* 22, 7305-7315.

Gallagher, R. E. (2002). Retinoic acid resistance in acute promyelocytic leukemia. *Leukemia* 16, 1940-1958.

Gallagher, R. E., Schachter-Tokarz, E. L., Zhou, D. C. & other authors (2006). Relapse of acute promyelocytic leukemia with PML-RARalpha mutant subclones independent of proximate all-trans retinoic acid selection pressure. *Leukemia* 20, 556-562.

Gold, E. J., Mertelsmann, R. H., Itri, L. M., Gee, T., Arlin, Z., Kempin, S., Clarkson, B. & Moore, M. A. (1983). Phase I clinical trial of 13-cis-retinoic acid in myelodysplastic syndromes. *Cancer Treatment Reports* 67, 981-986.

Goto, E., Tomita, A., Hayakawa, F., Atsumi, A., Kiyoi, H. & Naoe, T. (2011). Missense mutations in PML-RARA critical for the lack of responsiveness to arsenic trioxide treatment. *Blood.*

Gowda, S. D., Koler, R. D. & Bagby, G. C., Jr. (1986). Regulation of C-myc expression during growth and differentiation of normal and leukemic human myeloid progenitor cells. *The Journal of clinical investigation* 77, 271-278.

Grignani, F., De Matteis, S., Nervi, C. & other authors (1998). Fusion proteins of the retinoic acid receptor-alpha recruit histone deacetylase in promyelocytic leukaemia. *Nature* 391, 815-818.

Grimwade, D., Howe, K., Langabeer, S. & other authors (1996). Establishing the presence of the t(15;17) in suspected acute promyelocytic leukaemia: cytogenetic, molecular and PML immunofluorescence assessment of patients entered into the M.R.C. ATRA trial. M.R.C. Adult Leukaemia Working Party. *Br J Haematol* 94, 557-573.

Grisolano, J. L., Wesselschmidt, R. L., Pelicci, P. G. & Ley, T. J. (1997). Altered myeloid development and acute leukemia in transgenic mice expressing PML-RAR alpha under control of cathepsin G regulatory sequences. *Blood* 89, 376-387.

Guibal, F. C., Alberich-Jorda, M., Hirai, H. & other authors (2009). Identification of a myeloid committed progenitor as the cancer-initiating cell in acute promyelocytic leukemia. *Blood* 114, 5415-5425.

Guillemin, M. C., Raffoux, E., Vitoux, D. & other authors (2002). In vivo activation of cAMP signaling induces growth arrest and differentiation in acute promyelocytic leukemia. *Journal of Experimental Medicine* 196, 1373-1380.

Gurrieri, C., Nafa, K., Merghoub, T. & other authors (2004). Mutations of the PML tumor suppressor gene in acute promyelocytic leukemia. *Blood* 103, 2358-2362.

Hauksdottir, H. & Privalsky, M. L. (2001). DNA recognition by the aberrant retinoic acid receptors implicated in human acute promyelocytic leukemia. *Cell Growth Differ* 12, 85-98.

He, L. Z., Guidez, F., Tribioli, C., Peruzzi, D., Ruthardt, M., Zelent, A. & Pandolfi, P. P. (1998). Distinct interactions of PML-RARalpha and PLZF-RARalpha with co-repressors determine differential responses to RA in APL. *Nature Genetics* 18, 126-135.

Hillestad, L. K. (1957). Acute promyelocytic leukemia. *Acta Medica Scandinavica* 159, 189-194.

Hoemme, C., Peerzada, A., Behre, G. & other authors (2008).Chromatin modifications induced by PML-RARÎ± repress critical targets in leukemogenesis as analyzed by ChIP-Chip, pp. 2887-2895.

Hu, J., Liu, Y. F., Wu, C. F. & other authors (2009). Long-term efficacy and safety of all-trans retinoic acid/arsenic trioxide-based therapy in newly diagnosed acute promyelocytic leukemia. *Proceedings of the National Academy of Sciences U S A* 106, 3342-3347.

Huang, M. E., Ye, Y. C., Chen, S. R. & other authors (1987). All-trans retinoic acid with or without low dose cytosine arabinoside in acute promyelocytic leukemia. Report of 6 cases. *Chinese Medical Journal (Engl)* 100, 949-953.

Huang, M. E., Ye, Y. C., Chen, S. R., Chai, J. R., Lu, J. X., Zhoa, L., Gu, L. J. & Wang, Z. Y. (1988). Use of all-trans retinoic acid in the treatment of acute promyelocytic leukemia. *Blood* 72, 567-572.

Huang, X. J., Wiernik, P. H., Klein, R. S. & Gallagher, R. E. (1999). Arsenic trioxide induces apoptosis of myeloid leukemia cells by activation of caspases. *Medical Oncology* 16, 58-64.

Imaizumi, M., Suzuki, H., Yoshinari, M. & other authors (1998). Mutations in the E-domain of RAR portion of the PML/RAR chimeric gene may confer clinical resistance to all-trans retinoic acid in acute promyelocytic leukemia. *Blood* 92, 374-382.

Isakson, P., Bjørås, M., Bøe, S. O. & Simonsen, A. (2010). Autophagy contributes to therapy-induced degradation of the PML/RARA oncoprotein. *Blood* 116, 2324-2331.

Ishitsuka, K., Hanada, S., Suzuki, S. & other authors (1998). Arsenic trioxide inhibits growth of human T-cell leukaemia virus type I infected T-cell lines more effectively than retinoic acids. *British Journal of Haematology* 103, 721-728.

Ito, K., Bernardi, R., Morotti, A. & other authors (2008). PML targeting eradicates quiescent leukaemia-initiating cells. *Nature* 453, 1072-1078.

Ito, K., Bernardi, R. & Pandolfi, P. P. (2009). A novel signaling network as a critical rheostat for the biology and maintenance of the normal stem cell and the cancer-initiating cell. *Current Opinion in Genetics & Development* 19, 51-59.

Jansen, J. H., Mahfoudi, A., Rambaud, S., Lavau, C., Wahli, W. & Dejean, A. (1995). Multimeric complexes of the PML-retinoic acid receptor alpha fusion protein in acute promyelocytic leukemia cells and interference with retinoid and peroxisome-proliferator signaling pathways. *Proceedings in the National Academy of Sciences U S A* 92, 7401-7405.

Jeanne, M., Lallemand-Breitenbach, V., Ferhi, O. & other authors (2010). PML/RARA oxidation and arsenic binding initiate the antileukemia response of As2O3. *Cancer Cell* 18, 88-98.

Jensen, K., Shiels, C. & Freemont, P. S. (2001). PML protein isoforms and the RBCC/TRIM motif. *Oncogene* 20, 7223-7233.

Jing, Y., Dai, J., Chalmers-Redman, R. M., Tatton, W. G. & Waxman, S. (1999). Arsenic trioxide selectively induces acute promyelocytic leukemia cell apoptosis via a hydrogen peroxide-dependent pathway. *Blood* 94, 2102-2111.

Jing, Y., Wang, L., Xia, L., Chen, G. Q., Chen, Z., Miller, W. H. & Waxman, S. (2001). Combined effect of all-trans retinoic acid and arsenic trioxide in acute promyelocytic leukemia cells in vitro and in vivo. *Blood* 97, 264-269.

Jul-Larsen, A., Grudic, A., Bjerkvig, R. & Bøe, S. O. (2009). Cell-cycle regulation and dynamics of cytoplasmic compartments containing the promyelocytic leukemia protein and nucleoporins. *Journal of Cell Science* 122, 1201-1210.

Jul-Larsen, A., Grudic, A., Bjerkvig, R. & Bøe, S. O. (2010). Subcellular distribution of nuclear import-defective isoforms of the promyelocytic leukemia protein. *BMC Molecular Biology* 11, 89.

Kamashev, D., Vitoux, D. & De The, H. (2004). PML-RARA-RXR oligomers mediate retinoid and rexinoid/cAMP cross-talk in acute promyelocytic leukemia cell differentiation. *Journal of Experimental Medicine* 199, 1163-1174.

Kchour, G., Tarhini, M., Kooshyar, M. M. & other authors (2009). Phase 2 study of the efficacy and safety of the combination of arsenic trioxide, interferon alpha, and zidovudine in newly diagnosed chronic adult T-cell leukemia/lymphoma (ATL). *Blood* 113, 6528-6532.

Khan, M. M., Nomura, T., Chiba, T., Tanaka, K., Yoshida, H., Mori, K. & Ishii, S. (2004). The fusion oncoprotein PML-RARalpha induces endoplasmic reticulum (ER)-associated degradation of N-CoR and ER stress. *Journal of Biological Chemistry* 279, 11814-11824.

Kitamura, K., Kiyoi, H., Yoshida, H., Saito, H., Ohno, R. & Naoe, T. (1997). Mutant AF-2 domain of PML-RARalpha in retinoic acid-resistant NB4 cells: differentiation induced by RA is triggered directly through PML-RARalpha and its down-regulation in acute promyelocytic leukemia. *Leukemia* 11, 1950-1956.

Kitareewan, S., Pitha-Rowe, I., Sekula, D., Lowrey, C. H., Nemeth, M. J., Golub, T. R., Freemantle, S. J. & Dmitrovsky, E. (2002). UBE1L is a retinoid target that triggers PML/RARalpha degradation and apoptosis in acute promyelocytic leukemia. *Proceedings in the National Academy of Sciences U S A* 99, 3806-3811.

Klionsky, D. J. (2007). Autophagy: from phenomenology to molecular understanding in less than a decade. *Nature Reviews Molecular Cell Biology* 8, 931-937.

Koeffler, H. P., Hirji, K. & Itri, L. (1985). 1,25-Dihydroxyvitamin D3: in vivo and in vitro effects on human preleukemic and leukemic cells. *Cancer Treatment Reports* 69, 1399-1407.

Koken, M. H., Puvion-Dutilleul, F., Guillemin, M. C. & other authors (1994). The t(15;17) translocation alters a nuclear body in a retinoic acid-reversible fashion. *The EMBO Journal* 13, 1073-1083.

Kopf, E., Plassat, J. L., Vivat, V., de The, H., Chambon, P. & Rochette-Egly, C. (2000). Dimerization with retinoid X receptors and phosphorylation modulate the retinoic acid-induced degradation of retinoic acid receptors alpha and gamma through the ubiquitin-proteasome pathway. *Journal of Biological Chemistry* 275, 33280-33288.

Kwong, Y. L. & Todd, D. (1997). Delicious poison: arsenic trioxide for the treatment of leukemia. *Blood* 89, 3487-3488.

Lallemand-Breitenbach, V., Guillemin, M. C., Janin, A., Daniel, M. T., Degos, L., Kogan, S. C., Bishop, J. M. & de The, H. (1999). Retinoic acid and arsenic synergize to eradicate leukemic cells in a mouse model of acute promyelocytic leukemia. *Journal of Experimental Medicine* 189, 1043-1052.

Lallemand-Breitenbach, V., Zhu, J., Puvion, F. & other authors (2001). Role of promyelocytic leukemia (PML) sumolation in nuclear body formation, 11S proteasome recruitment, and As2O3-induced PML or PML/retinoic acid receptor alpha degradation. *Journal of Experimental Medicine* 193, 1361-1371.

Lallemand-Breitenbach, V., Jeanne, M., Benhenda, S. & other authors (2008). Arsenic degrades PML or PML-RARalpha through a SUMO-triggered RNF4/ubiquitin-mediated pathway. *Nature Cell Biology* 10, 547-555.

Lallemand-Breitenbach, V. & de The, H. (2010). PML nuclear bodies. *Cold Spring Harbor Perspectives in Biology* 2, a000661.

Lane, A. A. & Ley, T. J. (2003). Neutrophil elastase cleaves PML-RARalpha and is important for the development of acute promyelocytic leukemia in mice. *Cell* 115, 305-318.

Licht, J. D., Chomienne, C., Goy, A. & other authors (1995). Clinical and molecular characterization of a rare syndrome of acute promyelocytic leukemia associated with translocation (11;17). *Blood* 85, 1083-1094.

Lin, R. J., Nagy, L., Inoue, S., Shao, W., Miller, W. H., Jr. & Evans, R. M. (1998). Role of the histone deacetylase complex in acute promyelocytic leukaemia. *Nature* 391, 811-814.

Marasca, R., Zucchini, P., Galimberti, S., Leonardi, G., Vaccari, P., Donelli, A., Luppi, M., Petrini, M. & Torelli, G. (1999). Missense mutations in the PML/RARalpha ligand binding domain in ATRA-resistant As(2)O(3) sensitive relapsed acute promyelocytic leukemia. *Haematologica* 84, 963-968.

Martin, S. J., Bradley, J. G. & Cotter, T. G. (1990). HL-60 cells induced to differentiate towards neutrophils subsequently die via apoptosis. *Clinical & Experimental Immunology* 79, 448-453.

Mueller, B. U., Pabst, T., Fos, J., Petkovic, V., Fey, M. F., Asou, N., Buergi, U. & Tenen, D. G. (2006). ATRA resolves the differentiation block in t(15;17) acute myeloid leukemia by restoring PU.1 expression. *Blood* 107, 3330-3338.

Muller, S., Matunis, M. J. & Dejean, A. (1998). Conjugation with the ubiquitin-related modifier SUMO-1 regulates the partitioning of PML within the nucleus. *The EMBO Journal* 17, 61-70.

Nason-Burchenal, K., Allopenna, J., Begue, A., Stehelin, D., Dmitrovsky, E. & Martin, P. (1998). Targeting of PML/RARalpha is lethal to retinoic acid-resistant promyelocytic leukemia cells. *Blood* 92, 1758-1767.

Nasr, R., Guillemin, M. C., Ferhi, O. & other authors (2008). Eradication of acute promyelocytic leukemia-initiating cells through PML-RARA degradation. *Nature Medicine* 14, 1333-1342.

Nervi, C., Ferrara, F. F., Fanelli, M. & other authors (1998). Caspases mediate retinoic acid-induced degradation of the acute promyelocytic leukemia PML/RARalpha fusion protein. *Blood* 92, 2244-2251.

Niu, C., Yan, H., Yu, T. & other authors (1999). Studies on treatment of acute promyelocytic leukemia with arsenic trioxide: remission induction, follow-up, and molecular monitoring in 11 newly diagnosed and 47 relapsed acute promyelocytic leukemia patients. *Blood* 94, 3315-3324.

Park, D. J., Chumakov, A. M., Vuong, P. T., Chih, D. Y., Gombart, A. F., Miller, W. H., Jr. & Koeffler, H. P. (1999). CCAAT/enhancer binding protein epsilon is a potential retinoid target gene in acute promyelocytic leukemia treatment. *The Journal of clinical investigation* 103, 1399-1408.

Pearson, M., Carbone, R., Sebastiani, C. & other authors (2000). PML regulates p53 acetylation and premature senescence induced by oncogenic Ras. *Nature* 406, 207-210.

Perez, A., Kastner, P., Sethi, S., Lutz, Y., Reibel, C. & Chambon, P. (1993). PMLRAR homodimers: distinct DNA binding properties and heteromeric interactions with RXR. *The EMBO Journal* 12, 3171-3182.

Perkins, C., Kim, C. N., Fang, G. & Bhalla, K. N. (2000). Arsenic induces apoptosis of multidrug-resistant human myeloid leukemia cells that express Bcr-Abl or overexpress MDR, MRP, Bcl-2, or Bcl-x(L). *Blood* 95, 1014-1022.

Petti, M. C., Fazi, F., Gentile, M. & other authors (2002). Complete remission through blast cell differentiation in PLZF/RARalpha-positive acute promyelocytic leukemia: in vitro and in vivo studies. *Blood* 100, 1065-1067.

Redner, R. L., Rush, E. A., Faas, S., Rudert, W. A. & Corey, S. J. (1996). The t(5;17) variant of acute promyelocytic leukemia expresses a nucleophosmin-retinoic acid receptor fusion. *Blood* 87, 882-886.

Reymond, A., Meroni, G., Fantozzi, A. & other authors (2001). The tripartite motif family identifies cell compartments. *The EMBO Journal* 20, 2140-2151.

Rice, K. L., Hormaeche, I., Doulatov, S. & other authors (2009). Comprehensive genomic screens identify a role for PLZF-RARalpha as a positive regulator of cell proliferation via direct regulation of c-MYC. *Blood* 114, 5499-5511.

Rosenauer, A., Raelson, J. V., Nervi, C., Eydoux, P., DeBlasio, A. & Miller, W. H., Jr. (1996). Alterations in expression, binding to ligand and DNA, and transcriptional activity of rearranged and wild-type retinoid receptors in retinoid-resistant acute promyelocytic leukemia cell lines. *Blood* 88, 2671-2682.

Rousselot, P., Labaume, S., Marolleau, J. P., Larghero, J., Noguera, M. H., Brouet, J. C. & Fermand, J. P. (1999). Arsenic trioxide and melarsoprol induce apoptosis in plasma cell lines and in plasma cells from myeloma patients. *Cancer Research* 59, 1041-1048.

Ruggero, D., Baccarani, M., Guarini, A. & other authors (1977). Acute promyelocytic leukemia: results of therapy and analysis of 13 cases. *Acta Haematologica* 58, 108-119.

Sachs, L. (1978). Control of normal cell differentiation and the phenotypic reversion of malignancy in myeloid leukaemia. *Nature* 274, 535-539.

Salomoni, P. & Pandolfi, P. P. (2002). The role of PML in tumor suppression. *Cell* 108, 165-170.

Sanz, M. A., Jarque, I., Martin, G. & other authors (1988). Acute promyelocytic leukemia. Therapy results and prognostic factors. *Cancer* 61, 7-13.

Sanz, M. A., Martin, G., Rayon, C. & other authors (1999). A modified AIDA protocol with anthracycline-based consolidation results in high antileukemic efficacy and reduced toxicity in newly diagnosed PML/RARalpha-positive acute promyelocytic leukemia. PETHEMA group. *Blood* 94, 3015-3021.

Scaglioni, P. P., Yung, T. M., Cai, L. F., Erdjument-Bromage, H., Kaufman, A. J., Singh, B., Teruya-Feldstein, J., Tempst, P. & Pandolfi, P. P. (2006). A CK2-dependent mechanism for degradation of the PML tumor suppressor. *Cell* 126, 269-283.

Shao, W., Benedetti, L., Lamph, W. W., Nervi, C. & Miller, W. H., Jr. (1997). A retinoid-resistant acute promyelocytic leukemia subclone expresses a dominant negative PML-RAR alpha mutation. *Blood* 89, 4282-4289.

Shao, W., Fanelli, M., Ferrara, F. F. & other authors (1998). Arsenic trioxide as an inducer of apoptosis and loss of PML/RAR alpha protein in acute promyelocytic leukemia cells. *Journal of the National Cancer Institute* 90, 124-133.

Shen, Z. X., Chen, G. Q., Ni, J. H. & other authors (1997). Use of arsenic trioxide (As2O3) in the treatment of acute promyelocytic leukemia (APL): II. Clinical efficacy and pharmacokinetics in relapsed patients. *Blood* 89, 3354-3360.

Shen, Z. X., Shi, Z. Z., Fang, J. & other authors (2004). All-trans retinoic acid/As2O3 combination yields a high quality remission and survival in newly diagnosed acute promyelocytic leukemia. *Proceedings in the National Academy of Sciences U S A* 101, 5328-5335.

Soignet, S. L., Maslak, P., Wang, Z. G. & other authors (1998). Complete remission after treatment of acute promyelocytic leukemia with arsenic trioxide. *New England Journal of Medicine* 339, 1341-1348.

Subramaniyam, S., Nandula, S. V., Nichols, G., Weiner, M., Satwani, P., Alobeid, B., Bhagat, G. & Murty, V. V. (2006). Do RARA/PML fusion gene deletions confer resistance to ATRA-based therapy in patients with acute promyelocytic leukemia? *Leukemia* 20, 2193-2195.

Sun, H. D., Ma, L., Hu, X. C. & Zhang, T. D. (1992). Ai-Lin 1 treated 32 cases of acute promyelocytic leukemia. *Chinese Journal of Integrated Chinese Western Medicine* 12, 170-172.

Takayama, N., Kizaki, M., Hida, T., Kinjo, K. & Ikeda, Y. (2001). Novel mutation in the PML/RARalpha chimeric gene exhibits dramatically decreased ligand-binding activity and confers acquired resistance to retinoic acid in acute promyelocytic leukemia. *Experimental hematology* 29, 864-872.

Tallman, M. S., Andersen, J. W., Schiffer, C. A. & other authors (1997). All-trans-retinoic acid in acute promyelocytic leukemia. *New England Journal of Medicine* 337, 1021-1028.

Tatham, M. H., Geoffroy, M. C., Shen, L., Plechanovova, A., Hattersley, N., Jaffray, E. G., Palvimo, J. J. & Hay, R. T. (2008). RNF4 is a poly-SUMO-specific E3 ubiquitin ligase required for arsenic-induced PML degradation. *Nature Cell Biology* 10, 538-546.

Trotman, L. C., Alimonti, A., Scaglioni, P. P., Koutcher, J. A., Cordon-Cardo, C. & Pandolfi, P. P. (2006). Identification of a tumour suppressor network opposing nuclear Akt function. *Nature* 441, 523-527.

Uy, G. L., Lane, A. A., Welch, J. S., Grieselhuber, N. R., Payton, J. E. & Ley, T. J. (2010). A protease-resistant PML-RAR{alpha} has increased leukemogenic potential in a murine model of acute promyelocytic leukemia. *Blood* 116, 3604-3610.

Villa, R., Pasini, D., Gutierrez, A. & other authors (2007). Role of the polycomb repressive complex 2 in acute promyelocytic leukemia. *Cancer Cell* 11, 513-525.

Wang, G., Li, W., Cui, J. & other authors (2004). An efficient therapeutic approach to patients with acute promyelocytic leukemia using a combination of arsenic trioxide with low-dose all-trans retinoic acid. *Journal of Hematology & Oncology* 22, 63-71.

Wang, T. S., Kuo, C. F., Jan, K. Y. & Huang, H. (1996). Arsenite induces apoptosis in Chinese hamster ovary cells by generation of reactive oxygen species. *Journal of Cellular Physiology* 169, 256-268.

Wang, Z. G., Ruggero, D., Ronchetti, S., Zhong, S., Gaboli, M., Rivi, R. & Pandolfi, P. P. (1998). PML is essential for multiple apoptotic pathways. *Nature Genetics* 20, 266-272.

Wang, Z. Y. & Chen, Z. (2008). Acute promyelocytic leukemia: from highly fatal to highly curable. *Blood* 111, 2505-2515.

Weis, K., Rambaud, S., Lavau, C., Jansen, J., Carvalho, T., Carmo-Fonseca, M., Lamond, A. & Dejean, A. (1994). Retinoic acid regulates aberrant nuclear localization of PML-RAR alpha in acute promyelocytic leukemia cells. *Cell* 76, 345-356.

Wells, R. A., Catzavelos, C. & Kamel-Reid, S. (1997). Fusion of retinoic acid receptor alpha to NuMA, the nuclear mitotic apparatus protein, by a variant translocation in acute promyelocytic leukaemia. *Nature Genetics* 17, 109-113.

Wojiski, S., Guibal, F. C., Kindler, T., Lee, B. H., Jesneck, J. L., Fabian, A., Tenen, D. G. & Gilliland, D. G. (2009). PML-RARalpha initiates leukemia by conferring properties of self-renewal to committed promyelocytic progenitors. *Leukemia* 23, 1462-1471.

Zeisig, B. B., Kwok, C., Zelent, A., Shankaranarayanan, P., Gronemeyer, H., Dong, S. & So, C. W. (2007). Recruitment of RXR by homotetrameric RARalpha fusion proteins is essential for transformation. *Cancer Cell* 12, 36-51.

Zhang, P., Wang, S. Y. & Hu, X. H. (1996). Arsenic trioxide treated 72 cases of acute promyelocytic leukemia. *Chinese Journal of Hematology* 17, 58-62.

Zhang, W., Ohnishi, K., Shigeno, K., Fujisawa, S., Naito, K., Nakamura, S., Takeshita, K., Takeshita, A. & Ohno, R. (1998). The induction of apoptosis and cell cycle arrest by arsenic trioxide in lymphoid neoplasms. *Leukemia* 12, 1383-1391.

Zhang, X. W., Yan, X. J., Zhou, Z. R. & other authors (2010). Arsenic trioxide controls the fate of the PML-RARalpha oncoprotein by directly binding PML. *Science* 328, 240-243.

Zheng, J., Deng, Y. P., Lin, C., Fu, M., Xiao, P. G. & Wu, M. (1999). Arsenic trioxide induces apoptosis of HPV16 DNA-immortalized human cervical epithelial cells and selectively inhibits viral gene expression. *International Journal of Cancer* 82, 286-292.

Zheng, X., Seshire, A., Ruster, B., Bug, G., Beissert, T., Puccetti, E., Hoelzer, D., Henschler, R. & Ruthardt, M. (2007). Arsenic but not all-trans retinoic acid overcomes the aberrant stem cell capacity of PML/RARalpha-positive leukemic stem cells. *Haematologica* 92, 323-331.

Zhou, D. C., Kim, S. H., Ding, W., Schultz, C., Warrell, R. P., Jr. & Gallagher, R. E. (2002). Frequent mutations in the ligand-binding domain of PML-RARalpha after multiple relapses of acute promyelocytic leukemia: analysis for functional relationship to response to all-trans retinoic acid and histone deacetylase inhibitors in vitro and in vivo. *Blood* 99, 1356-1363.

Zhu, J., Shi, X. G., Chu, H. Y., Tong, J. H., Wang, Z. Y., Naoe, T., Waxman, S., Chen, S. J. & Chen, Z. (1995). Effect of retinoic acid isomers on proliferation, differentiation and PML relocalization in the APL cell line NB4. *Leukemia* 9, 302-309.

Zhu, J., Gianni, M., Kopf, E., Honore, N., Chelbi-Alix, M., Koken, M., Quignon, F., Rochette-Egly, C. & de The, H. (1999). Retinoic acid induces proteasome-dependent degradation of retinoic acid receptor alpha (RARalpha) and oncogenic RARalpha fusion proteins. *Proceedings in the National Academy of Sciences U S A* 96, 14807-14812.

Zhu, J., Zhou, J., Peres, L., Riaucoux, F., Honore, N., Kogan, S. & de The, H. (2005). A sumoylation site in PML/RARA is essential for leukemic transformation. *Cancer Cell* 7, 143-153.

Zhu, J., Nasr, R., Peres, L. & other authors (2007). RXR is an essential component of the oncogenic PML/RARA complex in vivo. *Cancer Cell* 12, 23-35.

Zhu, Q., Zhang, J. W., Zhu, H. Q. & other authors (2002). Synergic effects of arsenic trioxide and cAMP during acute promyelocytic leukemia cell maturation subtends a novel signaling cross-talk. *Blood* 99, 1014-1022.

7

Apoptosis and Apoptosis Modulators in Myeloid Leukemia

Maha Abdullah and Zainina Seman
University Putra Malaysia
Malaysia

1. Introduction

Acute myeloid leukemia (AML) is one of the most common types of leukemia in adults (American Cancer Society, 2010) however overall survival rate remain poor despite advancement in treatment modality.

Since the last 50 years, systemic chemotherapy has greatly improved outcome in many types of cancers. The use of continuous infusion Arabinosylcytosine (Ara-C) combined with another agent, usually an anthracycline or anthracenedione, the "3+7" regimen, has been the backbone of induction therapy for AML cases (Yates et al., 1973). An attempt to add other drugs (Preisler et al., 1987) and intensification of the Ara-C dose (Schiller et al., 1992; Weick et al., 1996) to this approach has achieved some degree of success. Currently more work is attempted at improving patient outcome by intensifying the doses of anthracyclines (Lowenberg et al., 2010a) or by adding targeted therapies like gemtuzumabozogamicin (Lowenberg et al., 2010b; Nabhan et al., 2005).

For consolidation therapy, the use of Ara-C with or without other agents has been employed to maintain remission and cure. Allogeneic hematopoietic cell transplantation (HCT) based on initial cytogenetic (Cornelissen et al., 2007; Koreth et al., 2009) and molecular studies (Castaigne et al., 2004) have been proposed as an alternative consolidation therapies.

Induction therapy aims to produce complete remission (CR) defined as a marrow with less than 5% blast, a neutrophil count greater than $1000/mm^3$ and a platelet count greater than $100,000/mm^3$ (Cheson et al., 2003). Majority of younger patients (65-75%) will achieve CR after receiving induction treatment while CR in elderly group is much lower (40-50%).

Patients who do not respond to induction treatment display chemotherapy resistance (Estey et al., 1996). In trials done by the Southwest Oncology Group (SWOG), resistant disease was found in about 33% (patients younger than 56) out of 404 patients' enrolled into the studies, 62% for patients in between 56-65 year old, 61% for patients between 66-75 years old and 57% for age more than 75 year old (Frederick et al., 2006).

Resistance is also common at relapse (Estey et al., 1996). Relapse itself could be due to resistance to treatment in a subgroup of leukaemic cells which survived induction therapy despite CR. Patients usually relapse within two to three years after achieving CR.

2. Multi-drug resistance protein as a mechanism of drug resistance

Development of drug resistance is a major problem in AML therapy. It will eventually occur in most haematological malignancies treated with chemotherapy. Classically, drug resistance is divided into extrinsic and intrinsic (Jean-Pierre et al., 2003). Extrinsic resistance (host factors) refers to the inability of the drug to reach the tumour cell. It occurs when the bioavailability of the oral form varies from patient to patient like poor absorption resulting in low serum levels.

Intrinsic (cellular) resistance is due to properties of the tumour cell. It can be classified as simple resistance, when cells are resistant to only one particular drug, or as multidrug resistance (MDR) when cross resistance is observed among chemotherapeutic drugs with different biochemical targets. Multidrug resistance is more common than simple resistance and it can be due to several mechanisms. The most common pharmacological mechanism involved is due to an active efflux of drugs from the tumour cells or enhanced drug metabolism which prevented the drug from reaching its target in the nucleus.

The most important protein described in MDR cells is P-glycoprotein (P-gp), a transmembrane energy-dependent drug efflux pump, which is most efficient at transporting naturally occurring substances. It is encoded by the MDR1/ABCB1 gene and belongs to a superfamily of ABC (ATP binding cassette) transporters. P-gp expression in AML at initial presentation has been reported to be 20% to 40% (Motoji T et al., 2000). Increase in P-gp expression in leukaemic cells causes reduced intracellular concentration of cytotoxic drugs. There are many drugs used in AML that are transported by P-gp including anthracyclines and anthracenediones like daunorubicin and mitoxantrone, the vinca alkaloids (vincristine and vinblastine) and the epipodophyllotoxins (etoposide and teniposide).

Other ABC transport proteins that have been implicated in MDR include the multi-drug resistance associated proteins (MRP1/ABCC1) and the breast cancer resistance protein (BCRP/ABCG2). All these proteins are not unique to drug resistance cells but expressed in tissue with excretory and secretory functions. However, many studies have found that overexpression of these proteins correlate with poor treatment response (Damiani et al., 2010; Bendarra et al., 2005).

A non-ABC protein, found widely expressed in P-gp negative multidrug resistant cancer cell termed initially as lung resistance related protein (LRP) and now known as major vault protein (MVP) also has been implicated in drug resistance mechanism (Izquierdo et al., 1996; Huh et al., 2006). This protein is involved in bidirectional transportation of a variety of substrates between nucleus and cytoplasm. It is present in many cells and seems to be upregulated in cancer cells and has been found to be an adverse prognostic factor in AML (Styczynski et al., 2007). The expression of P-gp (Leith et al., 1999), MRP and LRP in AML was also found to correlate with advanced age (>60 years) and high white cell count (van delHeuvel et al., 2007). It also correlates with high risk of relapse (Daniela et al., 2007).

There have been extensive trials conducted on AML therapy to circumvent drug resistance like reversion of P-gp, targeted agents against DNA replication and repair, cell cycling and apoptosis.

With the extensive knowledge on P-gp efflux mechanism and its contribution to drug resistance in AML, quinine and cyclosporine were tested to reverse the P-gp action. However, these substances did not significantly improve the response rate in AML (Eric et al., 2003; Solary et al., 1996; Liu et al., 1998; Tallman et al., 1995). Combination of tetrandrine, a potent inhibitor of the MDR-1 efflux pump, with induction therapy also showed no significant difference in response between P-gp positive and P-gp negative patients (Wen et al., 2006). Nevertheless, an early study revealed by using P-gp reversal modulators, the emergence of drug resistance could be prevented (Futscher et al., 1996). However, a recent randomized phase III trial involving 302 newly diagnosed AML patients, evaluated the effect of P-gp inhibitor valspodar (PSC-833) showed no difference in overall disease survival (Jonathan et al., 2010). Similar result was obtained in another phase III randomized trial involving poor risk AML patients when valspodar was added in the induction therapy (Peter et al., 2004)

3. Molecular 'signatures' in AML

AML is characterized by a high degree of heterogeneity with respect to chromosome abnormalities, gene mutations and expression of multiple genes. The heterogeneous nature of AML has significant clinical impact as there are marked differences in survival following intensive chemotherapy (explained in detail elsewhere in this book). The World Health Organization (WHO) classifies AML by cytogenetics, morphology, immunophenotype and clinical features (Swerdlow et al., 2008). Diagnostic karyotype emerges as the most significant prognostic factor as determined in multivariable analyses that take into account age, type of AML (de novo or secondary) and presenting white blood cell count (WBC), and accordingly provides the framework for current risk stratified treatment approaches (Grimwade, 2007). Nevertheless as cytogenetic and molecular genetic aberrations are not mutually exclusive the expression of downstream target genes that encode proteins involved in complex biologic networks are affected (Mrozek et al., 2009) and may alter predictability of standard prognostic markers. Microarray genome-wide gene-expression profiling (GEP) and microRNA-expression profiling assays have revealed AML signatures and may be readily applicable for diagnosis and outcome class prediction in AML (Mrozek et al., 2009). Many of the molecules involved are known mediators of signal transduction pathways and apoptosis.

4. Apoptotic molecules in AML

Apoptosis occurs principally via two separate yet interlinked signaling mechanisms: the extrinsic pathway, activated by proapoptotic receptor signals at the cellular surface (members of tumor necrosis factor, TNF, family), and the intrinsic pathway (members of Bcl-2 family), activated by mitochondrial signals from within the cell. These pathways converge through "effector" caspases, which orchestrate the apoptotic program. Nevertheless, each requires different initiation caspases to begin the process. The *extrinsic* pathway is activated by engagement of death receptors on the cell membrane. The death receptors involved in the extrinsic apoptotic pathway belong to the TNF receptor superfamily that include Fas (CD95 or Apo1), TNFR1 (TNF receptor 1), death receptor 3 (DR3/Wsl-1/APO-3/TRAMP/LARD), death receptor 4 (DR4/TRAIL–R1), death receptor 5 (DR5/TRAIL–R2) and DR6. These receptors are characterized by an intracellular death domain. There are also decoy receptors (i.e. DcR1 and DcR2) that contain no death domain or a truncated death domain and can bind ligand but cannot signal. Therefore, these decoy receptors function as antagonists to inhibit death ligand/death receptor–induced apoptosis. Binding of ligands, such as FasL, tumor necrosis factor-alpha (TNF-alpha) and TNF-related apoptosis-inducing ligand (TRAIL) to their respective membrane receptors Fas, TNF-R and

TRAIL-R induces trimerization of the receptors and recruitment of adaptor proteins such as the Fas-associated death domain (FADD) to the death domain. This then recruits procaspase-8 which then leads to the formation of the oligomeric death-induced signaling complex (DISC). DISC in turn promotes activation of caspase-8 and a cascade of other caspase enzymes that culminates with cell death (reviewed in Elrod and Sun, 2008).

The *intrinsic* pathway is triggered by various extracellular and intracellular stresses, including growth factor deprivation, DNA damage, oncogene induction, hypoxia and cytotoxic drugs. Cellular signals originated by various mechanisms by these different stresses converge on a cellular target represented by mitochondria. Mitochondrial membrane permeability is controlled by pro-apoptotic (Bax, Bak, Bad, Bid, Bim, Bmf, NOXA, PUMA, Bok, Bcl-G, Bfk) and anti-apoptotic (Bcl-2, Bcl-L, Mcl-1, Bcl-w, A1) members of the Bcl-2 family, inducing or preventing heterodimerization of pro-apoptotic members. A series of biochemical events is induced that lead to damage of the outer mitochondrial membrane, with the consequent release of cytochrome c and other pro-apoptotic molecules, such as Smac/DIABLO, from the inner membrane into the cytosol enabling the formation of the apoptosome, a large molecular complex formed by cytochrome c, apoptotic protease activating factor 1 (APAF-1) and caspase-9, and massive activation of caspases. These proteins all play crucial roles for cell survival and the loss of any of these proteins causes major deregulation of survival of some cell types (reviewed in Ashkenazi and Herbst, 2008).

Dysregulation of apoptosis plays an important role in the development of a variety of human pathologies, including cancer and particularly leukemia. The evasion of programmed cell death has been regarded as one of the six essential alterations in cellular physiology that dictate the growth of cancer cells and is a hallmark of virtually all cancers. Moreover, tumors that have alterations in proteins involved in cell death signaling are very frequently resistant to chemotherapy and are difficult to treat with chemotherapeutic agents that primarily act by inducing apoptosis (Testa et al., 2007).

Fas, DR4 and DR5 are generally expressed in both normal and malignant cells. An examination of patients with de novo AML revealed Fas was expressed on eight of nine (89%) patients tested (Tourneur et al., 2004). Another study showed expression of Fas on 62% of 29 AML patients (Min et al., 2004). Fas mutation was observed in 4/28 CML cases and none of the six AML cases tested (Rozenfeld-Granot et al., 2001). DR4 and DR5 mutations detected in cancers including chronic myelogenous leukemia were very low (0–10.6%) (Liu et al., 2005). On the other hand, DR4 and DR5 receptors were positive in 20 (69%) and 29 (100%) patients, respectively. This study also showed, relapse-free survival was significantly prolonged in patients with CD95-positive AML cells compared with patients with CD95-negative AML cells (73% versus 38% at 3 years; p = 0.047) using univariate analysis (Min et al., 2004). This was however not supported by another study on 99 AML patients where multivariate analysis showed no correlation with overall survival and disease free survival (Brouwer et al., 2001).

Three ligands (TNF-α, FasL and TRAIL) of the TNF-family and their respective four receptors (TNF-R1, Fas, TRAIL-R1 and TRAIL-R2) are potentially important as anti-cancer therapeutics. The demonstration that TNF-α selectively kills tumor cells but not normal cells, set it up for the first molecules to be studied. Unfortunately, marked pro-inflammatory effects precluded its systemic administration (Buzzoni and Butler, 1996). Fas was also excluded as agonistic antibodies triggering Fas activation was highly hepatotoxic causing death in mouse models (Ogasarawa et al., 1993). In contrast, TRAIL and agonistic anti-

TRAIL-R1/TRAIL-R2 antibodies appear to be well tolerated *in vivo*. TRAIL/Apo-2L exhibited potent anti-tumor activity and induces little cytotoxic effects in immunodeficient mice xenograft models implanted with several human tumor cell lines (Ashkenazi et al., 1999). However, the *in vivo* half-life of the TRAIL-ligand is very short (<4 minutes) (Kelley et al., 2001). Agonistic TRAIL-R1 and TRAIL-R2 antibodies do not bind to TRAIL decoy receptors, TRAIL-R3 and TRAIL-R4, which are frequently expressed on the membrane of tumor cells.

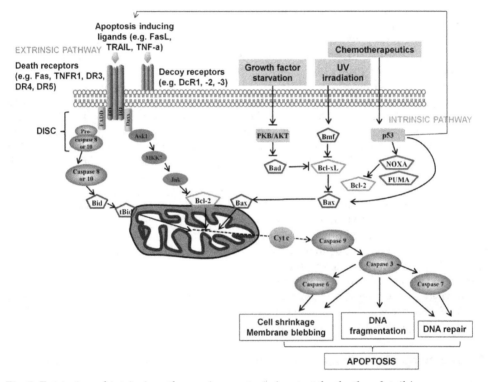

Fig. 1. Extrinsic and intrinsic pathways in apoptosis (see text for further details).

Antisense therapies involved the use of sequences of single-stranded DNA to complement and bind specific coding regions on mRNA hence forming DNA–mRNA which is then degraded by a ribonuclease, therefore gene expression and translation are prevented. Most widely studied were with XIAP (X-linked inhibitor of apoptosis) and antiapoptotic proteins Bcl-2.

Sufficient evidence exists to show that Bcl-2 was overexpressed in AML patients and predictive of worst outcome (Campos et al., 1993; Andreef and Konopleva, 2002). It seemed conceivable that Bcl-2 downregulation might lower the apoptotic threshold of leukemic cells and, through this mechanism, favor response to chemotherapy. Much success has been achieved. A phase I study using oblimersen, an antisense to Bcl-2, added during induction and then consolidation therapy, in elderly AML patients, induced remission in 14/27 patients, of which seven relapsed within 12.6 months (Marcucci et al., 2005); In a multicenter phase II trial, 12/39 relapsed AML patients treated with oblimersen and gentuzamab (anti-

CD33) achieved complete remission of which 10/12 survived for more than 6 months (Moore et al., 2004).

XIAP binds and inhibits caspases 3, 7, and 9, mediators of the apoptotic cascade. Downregulation of XIAP using multiple approaches (e.g., antisense, RNAi, knock-out animals and cell lines, immuno-depletion) in vitro and in vivo conditions resulted in increased caspase activation and/or cell death. Antitumor activity was also observed with the use of second generation anti-sense compound, AEG35156, in xenograft models of cancer (Lacasse et al., 2005) Results from clinical trials however, have been variable. While one study on five phase 1 (12–350mg/m2 AEG35156) and eight phase 2 (350 mg/m2 AEG35156) patients showed increased apoptotic cells and increase response (Bing et al., 2011) another study on 27 patients randomized to receive high dose Ara-C and idarubicin with or without AEG35156 (650 mg) found a lower overall response rate in the group which received the anti-XIAP drug (Schimmer et al., 2011).

The analysis of Mcl-1 protein expression in AML showed great heterogeneity, but the levels of the protein do not seem to correlate with response to standard chemotherapy (Kaufmann et al., 1998). Bad and Bcl-xL have been shown to be expressed in normal and leukemic hematopoietic precursor cells. Immature hematopoietic cells do not express Bcl-2 but do express Bcl-xL. CD34 positive cells express Bcl-2, Bcl-xL and Bad. Bcl-2 expression is higher on CD34 positive cells than on AML cells. Phosphorylated Bad was expressed in AML (Andreef et al., 1999).

Potential abnormalities of the various initiator caspases in AML have been explored. Levels of caspase-8, caspase-2 and caspase-3 are heterogeneous in AML. AML with an immature phenotype (i.e., M0 and M1 AML) predominantly express caspase-8L (Mohr et al., 2005).The significance of caspases as prognostic indicators in AML are unclear as current reports are still controversial may be due to the different format of molecules examined (Svingen et al., 2000; Estrov et al., 1998; Holleman et al., 2005).

Expression of pro- and anti-apoptotic molecules continues to be studied in AML to correlate its mutated state, expression, activity or methylated state with treatment outcome (Testa et al., 2007). At present, the prognostic utility of measurements of pro- and antiapoptotic molecules for predicting clinical outcome and response to chemotherapy is uncertain.

5. Drug modulation of signaling, differentiation and apoptotic pathways

The study of cancer cell biology in predicting treatment outcome cannot stop at the presentation stage as cells continue to be modified by the microenvironment and are ultimately subjected to chemotherapy. While remarkable progress have been achieved in targeted therapies, for most tumors chemo- or radiotherapy is likely to remain in the near future. Both chemo- and radiotherapy are designed to kill cancer cells by damaging nuclear DNA. DNA damage triggers the DNA damage response (DDR) which have three critical goals: (i) halting cell cycle progression and division to prevent transfer of DNA damage to progeny cells; (ii) increasing accessibility of the damage sites to- and engagement of- the DNA damage repair machinery, and (iii) triggering apoptosis to exterminate cells whose damaged DNA cannot successfully be repaired (reviewed in Darzynkiewicz et al., 2009).

Chemotherapeutic drugs such as cisplatin, mitomycin, methotrexate, mitoxantrone, adriamycin, and bleomycin induce Fas expression in human cancer cells, primarily through a p53–dependent mechanism (Muller et al., 1998). Adriamycin, etoposide, Ara–C, cisplatin and camptosar were shown to induce the expression of DR4 and DR5 or only DR5 expression, through either p53-dependent, or p53-independent mechanisms (Wu et al., 1997; Guan et al., 2001; Sheikh et al., 1998). Etoposide was shown to induce DR5 expression in human acute leukemia cells (Wen et al., 2000).

To complete induction of cell death, chemotherapeutic drugs have to suppress survival mediators in activated signaling pathways. Paclitaxel treatment of transfected MDA MB-435 human breast carcinoma cell line was observed to downregulate phosphorylated Akt (Klos et al., 2003). Nevertheless, chemotherapy induction of cell death is not equal in all cells. Adriamycin produced differential responses in Akt phosphorylation and kinase activity in a panel of breast cancer cell lines. While MCF7, MDA468 and T47D cells showed a dose dependent increase in p-Akt levels; in contrast, SKBR3 and MDA231 cells showed a dose-dependent decrease and no or minimal change was detected in MDA361, MDA157 and BT474 cells (Li et al., 2005). The diversity in response may also be predictive of a heterogeneity in treatment outcome.

Other signaling molecules are activated by chemotherapeutic drugs leading to cell death. Ara-C induced apoptosis in HL-60 cell lines through the activation of p38 (Stadheim et al., 2000). Adriamycin was shown to activate Jnk in a T cell leukemia cell line (Yu et al., 1999). Leukemia cell lines (TF-1 and K562) primed for apoptosis were also revealed to stimulate Jnk and p38 phosphorylation (Tucker et al., 2004)

Certain cytokines have apoptotic activity. TNF-alpha and IFN-gamma induced the expression of DR5 in a number of cancer cell lines (Meng and El-Deiry, 2000). IFN-gamma had differential effect on induction of death receptors in colon carcinoma cell lines. While it raised the levels of CD95 membrane 6 – 8-fold, it had no effect on the TRAIL-receptors (DR4, DR5, DcR1 and DcR2) (van Geelan et al., 2003). Interferon-alpha was also reported to increase DR5 expression in human hepatoma (Shigeno et al., 2003).

In contrast some cytokines exert protective effect from chemotherapeutic drug induced cell death, decreasing the effectiveness of cancer radiotherapy and chemotherapy. Normal hematopoietic cells, like other normal cell types, die by the process of apoptosis when deprived of viability inducing cytokines that include colony stimulating factors (CSFs) and various other cytokines. Induction of apoptosis by cancer chemotherapy such as vincristine, adriamycin, methotrexate and Ara-C was suppressed by IL (interleukin)-6, IL-3, granulocyte-CSF (G-CSF), granulocyte-monocyte CSF (GM-CSF) and IFN-gamma in myeloid leukemia cells (reviewed in Lotem and Sachs, 2002). These cytokines upregulate pro-survival molecules such as Bcl-2 [IL-2, IL-3, stem cell factor (SCF), IFN-gamma], Bcl-xL [IL-3, IL-6, IL-7, IL15, GM-CSF, IFN-gamma and erythropoietin (EPO)] and other apoptosis suppressing genes such as Survivin (Carter et al., 2001), X-linked inhibitor of apoptosis protein (XIAP) and cellular inhibitor of apoptosis 2 (cIAP2) (Digicylioglu and Lipton, 2001) that are caspase inhibitors and FLICE-like inhibitory protein (FLIP), that may disrupt the ability of cell surface molecules such as Fas to activate apoptosis (Kovalovich et al., 2001) Some myeloid leukemic cells are autonomous and do not require an exogenous source of cytokines for viability (Griffin and Lowenberg,1986), while others do. Thus, it is possible to suppress leukemia not only by cytotoxic agents or by induction of terminal differentiation, but also by decreasing the in vivo supply of apoptosis suppressing cytokines or the response of leukemic cells to these cytokines (reviewed in Sachs, 1996).

A characteristic abnormality of leukemia cells is that they are blocked at an early stage of their development. Myeloid leukemic cells however can be induced to differentiate to non dividing mature granulocytes and macrophages by different cytokines, including cytokine independent myeloid leukemic cells that were induced to differentiate with IL-6. Different myeloid leukemic clones however have different blocks and ability to undergo differentiation by cytokines. Our own work on in vitro cultured AML blasts exhibited different degrees of spontaneous apoptosis. Univariate analysis of 13 AML patients revealed blasts with lower levels of cell viability after 72h culture was significantly correlated with a longer disease free survival . Within a smaller number of samples (n=7) we observed blasts with lower levels of cell viability were associated with reduced levels CD34 and higher levels of CD16, indicating an increased level of cell differentiation (Maha et al., 2008). The observations may indicate an abnormal developmental program in leukemic cells which may be reprogrammed epigenetically by appropriate differentiation inducing cytokines. Constitutive expression of transcription factors such as c-myc, c-myb and E2F1 (Gonda and Metcalf, 1984; Blatt et al., 1992; Melamed et al., 1993) as well as others such as the homeobox gene Hox B8 (Hox 2.4) (Blatt et al., 1992) or GATA-1 (Tanaka et al., 2000), disrupted the ability of cells to undergo cytokine induced differentiation (reviewed in Lotem and Sachs, 2002)

Cytokines as a differentiation treatment against leukemia however has been disappointing. Hematopoietic leukemia cell lines of myeloid origin such as K562, U937, HL-60, CS-1, KG-1, MUTZ-3, or ex vivo AML or chronic myeloid leukemia (CML) blasts were modestly permissive to induction of in vitro differentiation by EPO, G-CSF, GM-CSF, IL-4, IL-6, SCF, or synergistic combinations of several cytokines (Leung et al., 2005; Koss et al., 1996; Goliaei et al. 1998; Kamano et al., 1994; Kamijo et al., 1990). A niche for hematopoietic cytokines in differentiation therapy exists in the treatment of congenital neutropenia disorder. The administration of G-CSF to patients has overcome a block of myeloid differentiation leading to a substantial prolongation of their survival (Berliner, 2008).

Clinically, differentiation therapy has been most successful in acute promyelocytic leukemia (APL) using all-trans-retinoic acid (ATRA) as the inducer. This targeted APL cells carrying the chromosomal translocation between chromosomes 15 and 17 [t(15;17)(q22;q21)]. Subsequently, APL therapy was improved with the combination regimen of ATRA with cytotoxic chemotherapy. Currently, complete remission rates of up to 90% to 95% are achievable using ATRA/ATO (arsenic trioxide) and anthracycline-based chemotherapy (Niu et al., 1999; Soignet et al., 2001; Raffoux et al., 2003; Ghavamzadeh et al., 2006; Mathews et al., 2006; Estey et al., 2006; Sanz et al., 2008).

Another targeted treatment with tyrosine kinase inhibitor (TKI) imatinib for the treatment of CMLalso achieved better success. Gefinitib and erlotinib which inhibit the intracellular tyrosine kinase activity of epidermal growth factor receptor (EGFR), induce a differentiation program in myeloid leukemia cells that corresponds to neutrophil maturation (Stegmaier et al., 2005; Boehrer et al., 2008a; Boehrer et al., 2008b).

These results together emphasize further not only the heterogeneity of leukemias but also complexity of host-cancer interaction and its influence on outcome in survival and also during induction of cell death.

6. In vivo drug induced molecular profiles: Potential predictor of drug resistance

The in vivo molecular changes in acute myeloid leukemia cells early after start of conventional genotoxic chemotherapy are incompletely understood, and it is not known if early molecular modulations reflect clinical response. As increasing evidence is proposing tumor-host mechanisms as important for effective chemotherapy, there is an immediate need to investigate these issues in vivo in human cancer (Oyan et al., 2009)

For that purpose, blasts from patients undergoing chemotherapy were collected as a 'natural' and rich source to study response of these cells to the myriad of signals they were subjected to. Even though cells undergo cell death, as white blood cell counts may decline at early stages of chemotherapy, very low percentages of apoptotic cells were detected. Oyan et al. (2009) comparing treated ('3+7', idarubicin + Ara-C) with untreated AML cells from seven patients, observed upregulation of 113 genes (23 of unknown function) at early time points (2 – 4 hours) and 108 genes at late time points (18 – 24 hours). Among the 113 genes a substantial number (31 genes) were related to the tumor suppressor p53 (Oyan et al., 2009). p53 is implicated to affect a variety of cellular processes, the most undisputed roles of p53 are to induce growth arrest and to induce apoptosis (Bates and Vousden, 1996). p53 is the most commonly mutated gene in a variety of human cancers (Greenblatt et al., 1994). In AML however, mutations of p53 are rare, occurring in approximately 5% to 10% (Fenaux et al., 1992) but in these cases it correlates with worse outcome (Wattel et al., 1994). Wild-type p53 appears to change the balance in expression of apoptosis-inducing versus apoptosis-suppressing genes in favor of the former and thus induce apoptosis.

In tune with the above, a significant increase in gene expression of the apoptosis facilitators PUMA and Bax and a decrease in the Bcl-2 /Bax ratio as well as Bcl-2 /PUMA were observed for most of the AML samples. The mRNA profile of three other pro-apoptotic mediators Bad , Bak1 and Bim did not change significantly during the first hours, but the level of gene expression varied across patients. Altogether five tumor necrosis factor-related receptor genes were modulated 2-4 h after induction therapy (Oyan et al., 2009).

Induction of ligand to death receptor during chemotherapy was also supported by Devemy et al. (2001) who observed increased TNF transcripts in treated AML cells. We also studied molecular changes in paired AML samples at diagnosis and during chemotherapy (Ara-C + daunorubicin). We showed increased TNF-alpha was significantly higher in chemo-sensitive patients. Thus, expression of TNF-alpha early during chemotherapy may be a marker to predict good treatment outcome. In chemo-resistant cases, a higher, though not significant, percentage of cases expressed IL-1beta and IL-18 (Maha et al., 2009).

We observed a significantly higher percentage of chemo-responsive AML patients with blasts cells increased for the expression of IL-6. This was consistent with Devemy et al (2001) who reported that increase of IL-6 transcripts during remission induction therapy of AML patients was accompanied by a fall in blood count and bone marrow cellularity. The role of cytokines in the induction of cell differentiation is well established. Oyan et al (2009) also observed several receptors expressed on monocytic/macrophage lineage cells were upregulated, probably related to chemotherapy induced differentiation of the leukemic cells. Thus, induction of cytokines expression in drug responsive AML patients may be due to induction of cell differentiation.

Comparing blasts profiles before and during early chemotherapy also revealed upregulation of genes potentially involved in interaction between AML blasts and the host microenvironment. Chemokine receptors CXCR4 and CX3CR1 were upregulated in the late phase after start of chemotherapy indicating intention to home into a microenvironment that favours their growth and survival. This supports the hypothesis that the host response in chemotherapy is crucial for persistent remission (Oyan et al., 2009).

We further examined activation of signaling molecules in AML blasts. Chemotherapy increased the percentage of cases showing phosphorylation of the Akt molecules and Forkhead transcription factor (FKHR) but no significant differences were observed between chemo-resistant and chemo-sensitive cases. We however, observed a significantly higher percentage of chemo-resistant cases showing phosphorylation and inactivation of the pro-apoptotic Bad molecule. A higher percentage of chemo-sensitive cases were phosphorylated for p38, and Jnk (Maha et al., 2009). In summary, we were able to show in chemo-sensitive cases, chemotherapy stimulated IL-6, induced apoptosis by up-regulating TNF-alpha and downregulated phosphorylated Bad. In reverse, in chemo-resistant cases, cells survived by maintaining high levels of phosphorylated Bad maybe through protective role of IL-1b and IL-18 cytokines (Maha et al., 2009).

Most anticancer drugs exert their effects by the induction of apoptosis and/or interfering with cell cycle progression. Often these drugs give rise to specific patterns of cell death and cell cycle arrest that vary according to the drug used and the molecular status of the target cell. Simple in vitro methods may aid in this investigation. Drug cytotoxicity and sensitivity of individual tumor samples was demonstrated by combining cytochrome c and propidium iodide staining of DNA content and detected on flowcytometry. This method elucidated mitochondrial resistance mechanisms which may prove useful in identifying the apoptosis-sensitive cell cycle phase for a given tumor sample/anticancer drug combination. It offers the opportunity to design personalized drug regimens and to identify new combined treatment modalities (Mohr et al., 2004).

7. Conclusion

The heterogeneity in AML continues to elude the best methods to characterize them. Genome and proteome-wide analysis has further revealed complexity in the makeup of the leukemic cell. The rapid advancement in targeted therapies implied the urgent need for alternative therapy and the readiness of the community to embrace it. Nevertheless so far, combinatorial medicine still holds out as the best option for successful treatment. If targeted therapies remain the way forward it will eventually bank deeply on the ability to identify molecular signatures in the individual leading to the establishment of personalized medicine.

In the meantime, the mechanisms in leukemogenesis, drug resistance and relapse remain an area of much research. From cell biology to cytogenetics to molecular defects to signaling pathways, all have contributed to a better understanding of cancer biology. New knowledge in epigenetics and microRNA remain to be elucidated.

Current diagnostic and prognostication are based on the assumption that the phenotype of the leukemic cell is static and thus definitive. There is much evidence that suggest otherwise. Activation of oncogenes leads to constitutive expression of signal transduction pathways involved in cell survival and anti-apoptotic activities. These pathways are multiple and made up of a myriad of molecules that are receptive to the environment. The host-cancer microenvironment is a dynamic microcosm of interacting signals and cascading molecules that constantly respond to stimuli in the surrounding to find a balance that maintains survival. In the course of treatment, blast cells are exposed to DNA damaging cytotoxic agents which trigger a gamut of other signaling mediators to exert the opposite effect. It would appear that a struggle ensues in which the strength of the victor determines whether the blast cell would maintain life or be pushed off-balance and replaced with a new profile signaling cell death. This new phenotype corresponded to a sensitive response to chemotherapy. On the other hand, cells may strengthen on pro-survival features which corresponded with resistance to chemotherapy. A few reports, including ours, are lending support to this hypothesis.

Unsurprisingly, chemotherapy-induce phenotype is not confined purely to either a survival or an apoptosis profile but a complex mix of conflicting signals to survive or die in addition to triggers to shut down cell proliferation, induce terminal differentiation or activate inflammatory responses. Thus, further elucidation of these profiles would involve assignment of each of the modulated molecule to its rightful pathway.

The immaturity feature in leukemias will undoubtedly be a factor that will further compound the heterogeneity in results obtained. An example is the striking correlations found between lower Bax/Bcl-2 ratio and higher progenitor marker expression, such as CD34, CD117 and CD133 antigens, confirming the link between this apoptotic index and the maturation pathways (Del Principe et al., 2005). Attempts to induce cell death by triggering death receptors has so far achieved mix results with the use of TNF-alpha, Fas ligands and the tumor necrosis factor-related apoptosis-inducing ligand (TRAIL) (i.e., DR4 and DR5). These molecules also selectively kill cancer cells while sparing normal cells (reviewed in Elrod and Sun, 2008). These results indicate a preferential expression of specific death receptors on different tissues.

Selection of lab methods for prognostication depends on the ability to identify lineage, maturation stages, genetic aberrations and activated signal transduction pathways. This feat may include the difficult task of combining surface markers, cytokines (secreted proteins) and phosphorylated proteins (unstable intracellular proteins) in the same tube on the same platform such as flowcytometry. Furthermore many of these proteins such as TNF-a, IL-6, p38 and Jnk have dual function of pro-survival and pro-apoptosis capabilities depending on the stimulating conditions cells are exposed to at that period of time. Precise markers will be required to differentiate these situations. Altogether, all of these add up to an interesting and exciting field of research for the immediate future.

8. References

[1] American Cancer Society. Cancer facts & figures 2010. American Cancer Society Web site. http://www.cancer.org. Accessed June 29, 2010.

[2] Andreeff M, Jiang S, Zhang X, Konopleva M, Estrov Z, Snell VE et al. Expression of Bcl-2 related genes in normal and AML progenitors: changes induced by chemotherapy and retinoic acid. Leukemia 1999; 11: 1881–1892.

[3] Andreef M, Konopleva M. Mechanisms of drug resistance in AML. Cancer Treat Res 2002;112: 237-262.

[4] Ashkenazi A, Herbst RS. To kill a tumor cell: the potential of proapoptotic receptor agonists. J Clin Invest. 2008 Jun;118(6):1979-1990.

[5] Ashkenazi A, Pai RC, Fong S, Leung S, Lawrence DA, Marsters SA, et al. Safety and antitumor activity of recombinant soluble Apo2 ligand. J Clin Invest 1999;104:155-162.

[6] Bates, S., and Vousden, K. H. p53 in signaling checkpoint arrest or apoptosis. Curr. Opin. Genet. Dev. 1996; 6: 1-7.

[7] Bazzoni F, Butler B. The tumor necrosis factor ligand and receptor families N Engl J Med 1996;334: 1717-1725.

[8] Berliner N. Lessons from congenital neutropenia: 50 years of progress in understanding myelopoiesis. *Blood*. 2008;111:5427–5432.

[9] Bing ZC, Duncan HM, Stephen JM, et al. XIAP antisense oligonucleotide (AEG35156) achieves target knockdown and induces apoptosis preferentially in CD34+38 cells in a phase 1/2 study of patients with relapsed/refractory AML. Apoptosis;2011: 16:67–74.

[10] Blatt C, Lotem J and Sachs L. Inhibition of specific pathways of myeloid cell differentiation by an activated Hox-2.4 homeobox gene. Cell Growth Differ. 1992; 3, 671-676.

[11] Boehrer S, Ades L, Galluzzi L, et al. Erlotinib and gefitinib for the treatment of myelodysplastic syndrome and acute myeloid leukemia: a preclinical comparison. *BiochemPharmacol*. 2008a;76:1417–1425.

[12] Boehrer S, Ades L, Braun T, et al. Erlotinib exhibits antineoplastic off-target effects in AML and MDS: a preclinical study. *Blood*. 2008b;111:2170–2180.

[13] Byrd JC, Mrozek K, Dodge RK, et al. Pretreatment cytogenetic abnormalities are predictive of induction success, cumulative incidence of relapse, and overall survival in adult patients with de novo acute myeloid leukemia: results from Cancer and Leukemia Group B (CALGB 8461). Blood. 2002;100:4325–4336.

[14] Campos L, Rouault JP, Sabido O. High expression of bcl-2 protein in acute myeloid leukemia cells is associated with poor response to chemotherapy. Blood 1993;81: 3091-3096.

[15] Carter BZ, Miella M, Altieri DC and Andreef M. Cytokine-regulated expression of survivin in myeloid leukemia. Blood. 2001; 97, 2784-2790.

[16] Castaigne S, Chevret S, Archimbaud E, et al. Randomized comparison of double induction and timed-sequential induction to a "37" induction in adults with AML: long-term analysis of the Acute Leukemia French Association (ALFA) 9000 study. Blood. 2004;104:2467-2474.

[17] Cheson B, Bennett J, Kopecky K et al. Revised recommendations of the International Working Group for diagnosis, standardization of response criteria, treatment outcomes, and reporting standards for therapeutic trials in acute myeloid leukemia, J ClinOncol. 2003;21:4642–4649.

[18] Cornelissen JJ, van Putten WL, Verdonck LF, et al. Results of a HOVON/SAKK donor versus no-donor analysis of myeloablative HLA-identical sibling stem cell transplantation in first remission acute myeloid leukemia in young and middle-aged adults: benefits for whom? Blood. 2007;109:3658 –3666.

[19] Damiani D, Tiribelli M, Michelutti A et al. Fludarabine-based induction therapy does not overcome the negative effect of ABCG2 (BCRP) over-expression in adult acute myeloid leukemia patients. Leuk Res. 2010;34(7):942-945.

[20] Daniela D, Mario T, Donatella R et al. The role of MDR-related proteins in the prognosis of adult acute myeloid leukaemia (AML) with normal karyotype. HematolOncol 2007; 25: 38–43.

[21] Darzynkiewicz Z, Traganos F, Wlodkowic D. Impaired DNA damage response--an Achilles' heel sensitizing cancer to chemotherapy and radiotherapy. Eur J Pharmacol. 2009;625(1-3):143-150.

[22] Del Principe MI, Del Poeta G, Venditti A, Buccisano F, Maurillo L, Mazzone C, Bruno A, Neri B, IrnoConsalvo M, Lo Coco F,Amadori S. Apoptosis and immaturity in acute myeloid leukemia. Hematology. 2005;10(1):25-34.

[23] Devemy E, Li B, Tao M et al. Poor prognosis acute myelogenousleukemia: 3 — biological and molecular biological changes during remission induction therapy. Leuk Res 2001; 25(9):783-791.

[24] Digicaylioglu M and Lipton SA. Erythropoietin-mediated neuroprotection involves cross-talk between Jak2 and NF-kappaBsignalling cascades. Nature. 2001; 412, 641 - 647.

[25] Dohner H, Estey EH, Amadori S, et al. Diagnosis and management of acute myeloid leukemia in adults: recommendations from an international expert panel, on behalf of the European LeukemiaNet. Blood. 2010;115:453- 474

[26] Dufour A, Schneider F, Metzeler KH, et al. Acute myeloid leukemia with biallelic CEBPA gene mutations and normal karyotype represents a distinct genetic entity associated with a favorable clinical outcome. J ClinOncol. 2010;28:570 -577.

[27] Eric S, Bernard D, Lydia C et al. Quinine as a multidrug resistance inhibitor: a phase 3 multicentric randomized study in adult de novo acute myelogenousleukemia. Blood.2003;102:1202-1210.

[28] Estey E, Kornblau S, Pierce S et al. A stratification system for evaluating and selecting therapies in patients with relapsed or primary refractory acute myeloid leukaemia. Blood 1996;88:756.

[29] Estey E, Garcia-Manero G, Ferrajoli A, et al. Use of all-trans retinoic acid plus arsenic trioxide as an alternative to chemotherapy in untreated acute promyelocyticleukemia. Blood. 2006;107:3469-3473.

[30] Estrov Z, Thall PF, Talpaz M, Estey EH, Kantarjian HM, Harris D, et al. Caspase 2 and caspase 3 protein levels as predictors of survival in acute myelogenousleukaemia.Blood 1998; 92:3090-3097.

[31] Falini B, Mecucci C, Tiacci E, et al. Cytoplasmic nucleophosmin in acute myelogenousleukemia with a normal karyotype. N Engl J Med. 2005;352:254 -266.

[32] Fenaux P, Preudhomme C, Quiquandon I, et al. Mutations of the p53 gene in acute myeloid leukaemia. Br J Haematol. 1992;80:178-183.

[33] Frederick R A, Holly G, David R H, et al. Age and acute myeloid leukemia. Blood. 2006 107: 3481-3485.

[34] Futscher BW, Foley NE, Gleason-Guzman MC, Meltzer PS, Sullivan DM, Dalton WS. Verapamil suppresses the emergence of P-glycoproteinmediated multi-drug resistance. Int J Cancer. 1996;66:520-525.

[35] Ghavamzadeh A, Alimoghaddam K, Ghaffari SH, et al. Treatment of acute promyelocyticleukemia with arsenic trioxide without ATRA and/or chemotherapy. Ann Oncol. 2006;17:131-134.

[36] Gibson BE, Wheatley K, Hann IM, et al. Treatment strategy and long-term results in paediatric patients treated in consecutive UK AML trials. Leukemia. 2005;19:2130-2138.

[37] Goliaei B, Deizadji A. Effects of hyperthermia and granulocyte-macrophage colony-stimulating factor on the differentiation of human leukemic cell line U937. Leuk Res. 1998;22:705-710.

[38] Gonda TJ and Metcalf D. Expression of myb, myc and fos proto-oncogenes during the differentiation of a murine myeloid leukaemia. Nature. 1984; 310, 249- 251.

[39] Greenblatt, M. S., Benneu, W. P., Hollstein, M., and Harris, C. C. Mutations in the p53 tumorsuppressorgene: clues to cancer etiology and molecular pathogenesis. Cancer Res. 1994; 54: 4855-4878.

[40] Griffin JD and Lowenberg B. (1986).Clonogenic cells in acute myeloblastic leukemia. Blood. 1986; 68, 1185-1195

[41] Grimwade D. Impact of cytogenetics on clinical outcome in AML. In: Karp JE, ed. Acute MyelogenousLeukemia. Totowa, New Jersey: Humana Press; 2007:177-192.

[42] Grimwade D, Hills RK. Independent prognostic factors for AML outcome.Hematology Am SocHematolEduc Program. 2009:385-395.

[43] Grimwade D, Hills RK, Moorman AV, et al. Refinement of cytogenetic classification in acute myeloid leukemia: determination of prognostic significance of rare recurring chromosomal abnormalities amongst 5,876 younger adult patients treated in the UK Medical Research Council trials. Blood. 2010;116:354-365.

[44] Guan B, Yue P, Clayman GL, Sun SY. Evidence that the death receptor DR4 is a DNA damage–inducible, p53–regulated gene. J Cell Physiol 2001; 188:98–105.

[45] Holleman A, Den Boer M, Kazemeier KM, Beverloo HB, Von Bergh A, Janka-Schaub GE, et al. Decreased PARP and procaspase-2 protein levels are associated with cellular drug resistance in childhood lymphoblastic leukemia. Blood 2005;106:1817-1823.

[46] Huh HJ, Park CJ, Jang S et al. Prognostic significance of multidrug resistance gene 1 (MDR1), multidrug resistance-related protein (MRP) and lung resistance protein (LRP) mRNA expression in acute leukemia. J Korean Med Sci. 2006 Apr;21(2):253-258.

[47] Izquierdo M, Scheffer G, Flens M et al. Major vault protein LRP-related multidrug resistance. Eur J Cancer. 1996;32A:979-984.

[48] Jean-Pierre M, Ollivier L. Drug resistance in acute leukaemia and reversion. Turk J Med Sci. 2003;33:271-279.

[49] Jonathan EK, Stephen LG, Guido M et al. P-glycoprotein inhibition using valspodar (PSC-833) does not improve outcomes for patients younger than age 60 years with newly diagnosed acute myeloid leukemia: Cancer and Leukemia Group B study 19808. Blood 2010 116: 1413-1421.

[50] Kamano H, Tanaka T, Ohnishi H, et al. Effects of the antisense myb expression on hemin- and erythropoietin-induced erythroid differentiation of K562 cells. BiochemMolBiol Int. 1994;34:85–92

[51] Kamijo R, Takeda K, Nagumo M, Konno K. Effects of combinations of transforming growth factor-beta 1 and tumor necrosis factor on induction of differentiation of human myelogenous leukemic cell lines. J Immunol. 1990;144:1311–1316.

[52] Kaufmann SH, Karp JE, Svingen PA, Kraiewski S, Burke PJ, Gore SD, Reed JC. Elevated expression of the apoptotic regulator Mcl-1 at the time of leukemic relapse. Blood 1998;91: 991-1000.

[53] Kelley S, Harris L, Xie D, DeForge L, Totpal K, Bussiere J, et al. Preclinical studies to predict the disposition of Apo2L/tumor necrosis factor-related apoptosis-inducing ligand in humans: characterization on in vivo efficacy, pharmacokinetics, and safety. J PharmacolExpTher 2001;299: 31-38.

[54] Klos KS, Zhou X, Lee S, Zhang L, Yang W, Nagata Y, Yu D. Combined trastuzumab and paclitaxel treatment better inhibits ErbB-2-mediated angiogenesis in breast carcinoma through a more effective inhibition of Akt than either treatment alone. Cancer. 2003;98(7):1377-1385.

[55] Koreth J, Schlenk R, Kopecky KJ, Honda S, Sierra J, Djulbegovic BJ, Wadleigh M, DeAngelo DJ, Stone RM, Sakamaki H, Appelbaum FR, Döhner H, Antin JH, Soiffer RJ, Cutler C. Allogeneic stem cell transplantation for acute myeloid leukemia in first complete remission: systematic review and meta-analysis of prospective clinical trials. JAMA. 2009;301(22):2349-2361.

[56] Koss A, Lucero G, Koziner B. Granulocyte-colony stimulating factor, granulocyte-macrophage colony stimulating factor and interleukin 4 induce differentiation in the U-937 human monocyticleukemia cell line. Leuk Lymphoma. 1996;22:163-171. follow. 186, color plate XIV-V.

[57] Kovalovich K, Li W, DeAngelis R, Greenbaum LE, Ciliberto G and Taub R. Interleukin-6 protects against Fas-mediated death by establishing a critical level of anti-apoptotic hepatic proteins FLIP, Bcl-2, and Bcl-xLJ. Biol. Chem. 2001; 276, 26605-26613.

[58] Krauter J, Wagner K, Schäfer I, Marschalek R, Meyer C, Heil G, Schaich M, EhningerG, Niederwieser D, Krahl R, Büchner T, Sauerland C, Schlegelberger B, Döhner K, DöhnerH,Schlenk RF, Ganser A. Prognostic factors in adult patients up to 60 years old with acute myeloid leukemia and translocations of chromosome band11q23: individual patient data-based meta-analysis of the German Acute Myeloid Leukemia Intergroup. J ClinOncol. 2009; 27(18):3000-3006.

[59] Lacasse EC, Kandimalla ER, Winocour P, et al. Application of XIAP antisense to cancer and other proliferative disorders: development of AEG35156/ GEM640. Ann N Y Acad Sci. 2005;1058:215-234.

[60] Lamba JK, Crews KR, Pounds SB, Cao X, Gandhi V, Plunkett W, Razzouk BI, Lamba V, Baker SD, Raimondi SC, Campana D, Pui CH, Downing JR, Rubnitz JE, Ribeiro RC. Identification of predictive markers of cytarabine response in AML by integrative analysis of gene-expression profiles with multiple phenotypes. Pharmacogenomics. 2011;12(3):327-339.

[61] Leith CP, Kopecky KJ, Chen IM, Eijdems L, Slovak ML, McConnell TS, Head DR, Weick J, Grever MR,Appelbaum FR, Willman CL. Frequency and clinical significance of the expression of the multidrug resistance proteins MDR1/P-glycoprotein, MRP1, and LRP in acute myeloid leukemia: a Southwest Oncology Group Study. Blood. 1999;94(3):1086-99.

[62] Leung KN, Mak NK, Fung MC. Cytokines in the differentiation therapy of leukemia: from laboratory investigations to clinical applications.Crit Rev Clin Lab Sci. 2005;42(5-6):473-514.

[63] Li X, Lu Y, Liang K, Liu B, Fan Z. Differential responses to doxorubicin-induced phosphorylationand activation of Akt in human breast cancer cells. Breast Cancer Res. 2005;7(5):R589-597.

[64] Liu YJ, Wheatley K, Rees J et al. Comparison of two chemotherapy regimen with or without cyclosporine A in relapse/refractory acute myeloid leukaemia: result of the UK Medical Research Council AML-R Trial. Blood 1998;92:231a.

[65] Liu LG, Tanaka H, Ito K, Ito T, Sultana TA, Kyo T, Kimura A. Absence of gene mutation in TRAIL receptor 1 (TRAIL-R1) and TRAIL receptor 2 (TRAIL-R2) in chronic myelogenousleukemia and myelodysplastic syndrome, and analysis of mRNA Expressions of TRAIL and TRAIL-related genes in chronic myelogenousleukemia. ActaHaematol 2005; 113:113-123.

[66] Lowenberg, B., Ossenkoppele, G.J., van Putten, W.,etal.High dose daunorubicin in older patients with acute myeloid leukemia.NEng J Med. 2010a;361:1235-1248.

[67] Lowenberg B, Beck J, GrauxC,et al. Gemtuzumabozogamicin as postremission treatment in AML at 60 years of age or more: results of a multicenter phase 3 study. Blood. 2010b; 115: 2586-2591.

[68] Maha A, Cheong SK, Leong CF, Seow HF. Cell viability of acute myeloid leukaemia blasts in culture correlates with treatment outcome.Hematology. 2008;13(1):13-20.

[69] Maha A, Cheong SK, Leong CF, Seow HF. Molecular responses during chemotherapy in acute myeloid leukemias in predicting poor-response to standard chemotherapy.Malays J Pathol. 2009 Dec;31(2):81-91.

[70] Marcucci G, Stock W, Dai G, Klisovic RB, Liu S, Klisovic MI, Blum W, Kefauver C, Sher DA, Green M,Moran M, Maharry K, Novick S, Bloomfield CD, Zwiebel JA, Larson RA, Grever MR, Chan KK, Byrd JC. Phase I study of oblimersen sodium, an antisense to Bcl-2, in untreated older patients with acute myeloid leukemia: pharmacokinetics, pharmacodynamics, and clinical activity. J Clin Oncol. 2005 May 20;23(15):3404-11.

[71] Mathews V, George B, Lakshmi KM, et al. Single-agent arsenic trioxide in the treatment of newly diagnosed acute promyelocyticleukemia: durable remissions with minimal toxicity. Blood.2006;107:2627-2632.

[72] Melamed D, Tiefenbrun N, Yarden A and Kimchi A. Interferons and interleukin-6 suppress the DNA-binding activity of E2F in growth-sensitive hematopoietic cells. Mol. Cell. Biol. 1993; 13, 5255-5265.

[73] Meng RD, El-Deiry WS. p53-independent upregulation of KILLER/DR5 TRAIL receptor expression by glucocorticoids and interferon-gamma. Exp Cell Res. 2001;262(2):154-169.

[74] Min YJ, Lee JH, Choi SJ, Chi HS, Lee JS, Kim WK, Lee KH. Prognostic significance of Fas (CD95) and TRAIL receptors (DR4/DR5) expression in acute myelogenousleukemia. Leukemia research 2004; 28:359-365.

[75] Mohr A, Zwacka RM, Debatin KM and Stahnke K. A novel method for the combined flow cytometric analysis of cell cycle and cytochrome c release. Cell Death and Differentiation (2004) 11, 1153-1154.

[76] Mohr A, Zwacka RM, Jarmy G, Buneker C, Schrezenmeier H, Dohner K, et al. Caspase-8L expression protects CD34+ hematopoietic progenitor cells and leukemic cells from CD95-mediated apoptosis. Oncogene 2005; 24:2421-2429.

[77] Moore LO, Seiter K, Kolitz JE, Stock W, Yu R, Frankel SR. Phase 2 study of oblimersen sodium (G31\39; Bcl-2 antisense; Gena sense) plus gentuzumabozogamicin (Myelotarg) in elderly patients with relapsed acute myeloid leukemia (AML). Blood 2004;104:247a.

[78] Motoji T, Motomura S, Wang YH. Multidrug resistance of acute leukemia and a strategy to overcome it. Int J Hematol 2000 Dec;72(4):418-24.

[79] Mrozek K, Radmachera MD, Bloomfield CD and Marcucci G. Molecular signatures in acute myeloid leukemia. CurrOpinHematol 16:64–69

[80] Muller M, Wilder S, Bannasch D, Israeli D, Lehlbach K, Li–Weber M, Friedman SL, Galle PR, Stremmel W, Oren M, Krammer PH. p53 activates the CD95 (APO–1/Fas) gene in response to DNA damage by anticancer drugs. J Exp Med 1998; 188:2033–2045.

[81] Nabhan C, Rundhaugen LM, Riley MB, et al. Phase II pilot trial of gemtuzumabozogamicin (GO) as first line therapy in acute myeloid leukemia patients age 65 or older. Leukemia Research.2005;29:53–57

[82] Niu C, Yan H, Yu T, et al. Studies on treatment of acute promyelocyticleukemia with arsenic trioxide: remission induction, follow-up, and molecular monitoring in 11 newly diagnosed and 47 relapsed acute promyelocyticleukemia patients. Blood. 1999;94:3315–3324.

[83] Nowak D, Stewart D, Koeffler HP. Differentiation therapy of leukemia: 3 decades of development. Blood. 2009;113(16):3655-3665.

[84] O'Donnell MR, Appelbaum FR, Coutre SE, et al. Acute myeloid leukemia: NCCN clinical practice guidelines in oncology, v.2.2010. National Comprehensive Cancer Network On-Line. http://wwwnccnorg. Accessed April 18, 2010.

[85] Ogasarawa J, Watanabe-Fukunaga R, Adachi M, Matsuzawa A, Kasugai T, Kita mura Y, et al. Lethal effect of the anti-Fas antibody in the mice. Nature 1993; 364: 806-809.

[86] Øyan AM, Anensen N, Bø TH, Stordrange L, Jonassen I, Bruserud Ø, Kalland KH, Gjertsen BT. Genes of cell-cell interactions, chemotherapy detoxification and apoptosis are induced during chemotherapy of acute myeloid leukemia.BMC Cancer. 2009; 9:77.

[87] Paschka P, Marcucci G, Ruppert AS, et al. Adverse prognostic significance of KIT mutations in adult acute myeloid leukemia with inv(16) and t(8;21): a Cancer and Leukemia Group B Study. J ClinOncol. 2006;24:3904 –3911.

[88] Peter L. Greenberg, Sandra J. Lee, Ranjana Advani, Martin S. Tallman, Branimir I. Sikic, Louis Letendre, Kathleen Dugan, Bert Lum, David L. Chin, Gordon Dewald, Elisabeth Paietta, John M. Bennett, and Jacob M. Rowe. Mitoxantrone, Etoposide, and Cytarabine With or Without Valspodar in Patients With Relapsed or Refractory Acute Myeloid Leukemia and High-Risk Myelodysplastic Syndrome: A Phase III Trial (E2995). J Clin Oncol 2004;22:1078-1086.

[89] Preisler H, Davis RB, Kirshner J, et al. Comparison of three remission induction regimens and two postinduction strategies for the treatment of acute nonlymphocyticleukemia: a cancer and leukemia group B study. Blood. 1987;69:1441–1449.

[90] Raffoux E, Rousselot P, Poupon J, et al. Combined treatment with arsenic trioxide and all-trans-retinoic acid in patients with relapsed acute promyelocyticleukemia. J ClinOncol. 2003;21:2326–2334.

[91] Rowe JM. Optimal induction and post-remission therapy for AML in first remission. Hematology Am SocHematolEduc Program. 2009:396-405.

[92] Rozenfeld-Granot   G, Toren   A, Amariglio   N, Brok-Simoni   F, Rechavi   G. Mutation analysis of the FAS and TNFR apoptotic cascade genes in hematological malignancies. Exp Hematol. 2001;29(2):228-33.

[93] Sachs L. The control of hematopoiesis and leukemia: from basic biology to the clinic. Proc. Natl. Acad. Sci. USA. 1996; 93, 4742- 4749.

[94] Sanz MA, Grimwade D, Tallman MS, et al. Guidelines on the management of acute promyelocyticleukemia: recommendations from an expert panel on behalf of the European LeukemiaNet. *Blood*. Prepublished on September 23, 2008.

[95] Schiller G, Gajewski J, Nimer S, et al. A randomized study of intermediate versus conventional-dose cytarabine as intensive induction for acute myelogenous leukaemia. Br J Haematol. 1992;81:170 –177.

[96] Schlenk RF, Dohner K, Krauter J, et al. Mutations and treatment outcome in cytogenetically normal acute myeloid leukemia. *N Engl J Med*. 2008;358:1909 –1918.

[97] Schnittger S, Kohl TM, Haferlach T, et al. KIT-D816 mutations in AML1-ETO-positive AML are associated with impaired event-free and overall survival. *Blood*. 2006;107:1791-1799.

[98] Sheikh MS, Burns TF, Huang Y, Wu GS, Amundson S, Brooks KS, FornaceJr AJ, el-Deiry WS. p53-dependent and -independent regulation of the death receptor KILLER/DR5 gene expression in response to genotoxic stress and tumor necrosis factor alpha. Cancer Res 1998; 58:1593-1598.

[99] Shigeno M, Nakao K, Ichikawa T, Suzuki K, Kawakami A, Abiru S, Miyazoe S, Nakagawa Y, Ishikawa H, Hamasaki K, Nakata K, Ishii N, Eguchi K. Interferon-alpha sensitizes human hepatoma cells to TRAIL-induced apoptosis through DR5 upregulation and NF-kappa B inactivation. Oncogene 2003; 22:1653-1662.

[100] Schimmer AD, Herr W, Hänel M, Borthakur G, Frankel A, Horst HA, Martin S, Kassis J, Desjardins P, Seiter K, Fiedler W, Noppeney R, Giagounidis A, Jacob C, Jolivet J, Tallman MS, Koschmieder S. Addition of AEG35156 XIAP Antisense Oligonucleotide in Reinduction Chemotherapy Does Not Improve Remission Rates in Patients With Primary Refractory Acute Myeloid Leukemia in a Randomized Phase II Study. Clin Lymphoma Myeloma Leuk. 2011;11(5):433-8.

[101] Solary E, Witz F, Caillot D, et al. Combination of quinine as a potential reversing agent with mitoxantrone and cytarabine for the treatment of acute leukemias: a randomized multicentric study. Blood. 1996;88:1198-1205.

[102] Soignet SL, Frankel SR, Douer D, et al. United States multicenter study of arsenic trioxide in relapsed acute promyelocyticleukemia. *J ClinOncol*. 2001;19:3852-3860.

[103] Stadheim TA, Saluta GR, Kucera GL. Role of c-Jun N-terminal kinase/p38 stress signaling in 1-beta-D-arabinofuranosylcytosine-induced apoptosis. BiochemPharmacol 2000; 59(4):407-418.

[104] Stegmaier K, Corsello SM, Ross KN, Wong JS, Deangelo DJ, Golub TR. Gefitinib induces myeloid differentiation of acute myeloid leukemia. *Blood*. 2005;106:2841-2848.

[105] Stelljes M, Beelen DW, Braess J, Sauerland MC, Heinecke A, Berning B, Kolb HJ, Holler E,Schwerdtfeger R, Arnold R, Spiekermann K, Müller-Tidow C, Serve HL, Silling G, HiddemannW,Berdel WE, Büchner T, Kienast J; German AML Cooperative Group (AMLCG). Allogeneic transplantation as post-remission therapy for cytogenetically high-risk acute myeloid leukemia: landmark analysis from a single prospective multicenter trial. Haematologica. 2011;96(7):972-979.

[106] Styczynski J, Wysocki m, Debski R et al. Predictive value of multidrug resistance proteins and cellular drug resistance in childhood relapsed acute lymphoblastic leukemia. J Cancer Res ClinOncol. 2007;133(11):875-93.

[107] Svingen PA, Karp JE, Kraiewski S, Mesner PW, Gore SD, Burke PJ, et al. Evaluation of Apaf-1 and procaspases-2, -3, -7, and -9 as potential prognostic markers in acute leukaemia. Blood 2000;96:3922-3931.

[108] Swerdlow SH, Campo E, Harris NL, et al, eds.WHO Classification of Tumours of Haematopoietic and Lymphoid Tissues. Lyon, France: IARC Press; 2008.

[109] Tallman MS, Lee S, SikicBl et al. Mitoxantrone, etoposide and cytarabine plus cyclosporine for patients with relapse or refractory acute myeloid leukaemia: an Eastern Cooperative Oncology Group pilot study. Cancer .1999;85:358-367.

[110] Tanaka H, Matsumura I, Nakajima K, Daino H, Sonoyama J, Yoshida H, Oritani K, Machii T, Yamamoto M, Hirano T and Kanakura Y. GATA-1 blocks IL-6-induced macrophage differentiation and apoptosis through the sustained expression of cyclin D1 and bcl-2 in a murine myeloid cell line M1. Blood. 2000; 95, 1264-1273.

[111] Testa U and Riccioni R. Deregulation of apoptosis in acute myeloid leukemia. Haematologica 2007; 92:81-94

[112] Tourneur L, Delluc S, Lévy V, Valensi F, Radford-Weiss I, Legrand O, Vargaftig J, BoixC,Macintyre EA, Varet B, Chiocchia G, Buzyn A. Absence or low expression of fas-associated protein with death domain in acute myeloid leukemia cells predicts resistance to chemotherapy and poor outcome. Cancer Res. 2004 Nov 1;64(21):8101-8108.

[113] Tucker SJ, Rae C, Littlejohn AF, Paul A, MacEwan DJ. Switching leukemia cell phenotype between life and death. ProcNatlAcadSci U S A 2004; 101(35):12940-5.

[114] Van del Heuvel E, van der Holt B, Burnette AK et al. CD34-related coexpression of MDR1 and BCRP indicates a clinically resistant phenotype in patients with acute myeloid leukemia (AML) of older age. Ann Hematol. 2007;86(5):329-337.

[115] van Geelen CM, de Vries EG, Le TK, van Weeghel RP, de Jong S. Differential modulation of the TRAIL receptors and the CD95 receptor in colon carcinoma cell lines. Br J Cancer. 2003;89(2):363-373.

[116] Vardiman JW, Thiele J, Arber DA, et al. The 2008 revision of the World Health Organization (WHO) classification of myeloid neoplasms and acute leukemia: rationale and important changes. *Blood.* 2009;114:937–951.

[117] Wattel E, Preudhomme C, Hecquet B, et al. p53 mutations are associated with resistance to chemotherapy and short survival in hematologic malignancies. Blood. 1994;84:3148-3157.

[118] Wen LX, Hui LS, Zhong FA et al. Combination of tetrandrine as a potential-reversing agent with daunorubicin, etoposide and cytarabine for the treatment of refractory and relapsed acute myelogenousleukemia. Leuk Res. 2006;30(4):407-413.

[119] Wen J, Ramadevi N, Nguyen D, Perkins C, Worthington E, Bhalla K. Antileukemic drugs increase death receptor 5 levels and enhance Apo-2L-induced apoptosis of human acute leukemia cells. Blood 2000; 96:3900-3906.

[120] Weick JK, Kopecky KJ, Appelbaum FR, et al. A randomized investigation of high-dose versus standard-dose cytosine arabinoside with daunorubicin in patients with previously untreated acute myeloid leukemia: a Southwest Oncology Group study. Blood. 1996;88:2841–2851.

[121] Wu GS, Burns TF, McDonald IIIrd ER, Jiang W, Meng R, Krantz ID, Kao G, Gan DD, Zhou JY, Muschel R, Hamilton SR, Spinner NB, Markowitz S, Wu G, el-Deiry WS. KILLER/DR5 is a DNA damage-inducible p53-regulated death receptor gene. Nat Genet. 1997; 17:141-143.

[122] Yates JW, Wallace HJ Jr, Ellison RR, Holland JF. Cytosine arabinoside (NSC-63878) and daunorubicin (NSC-83142) therapy in acute nonlymphocyticleukemia. Cancer Chemother Rep. 1973;57:485 - 488.

[123] Yu R, Shtil AA, Tan TH, Roninson IB, Kong AN. Adriamycin activates c-Jun N-terminal kinase in human leukemia cells: a relevance to apoptosis. Cancer Letter 1999; 107(1):73-81.

8

Role of Signaling Pathways in Acute Myeloid Leukemia

Maha Abdullah and Zainina Seman
Immunology Unit, Department of Pathology
Faculty of Medicine and Health Sciences
Universiti Putra Malaysia
Malaysia

1. Introduction

Acute myeloid leukemia (AML) is a cancer wherein dysregulated differentiation, uncontrolled growth and inhibition of apoptosis lead to accumulation of immature myeloid progenitor cells and progression of oncogenic expression (Lowenberg et al., 1999). AML is now seen to be initiated and maintained from a small, self-renewing population of leukemic stem cells (LSCs), which give rise to a progeny of more mature and highly cycling progenitors (colony forming unit-leukemia, CFU-L). CFU-Ls do not self-renew, however they are committed to proliferation and limited differentiation. By doing so, they originate a population of blast cells which constitute the majority of leukemic cells in both the bone marrow and peripheral blood of patients. The exact phenotype of LSCs is still debated, but they are comprised in the CD34+/CD38-/low population (Lane et al., 2009). CD34+/CD38+ leukemic cells were unable to initiate leukemia in immunodeficient mice. It should be noted that only about 50% of AML are able to initiate leukemia in NOD/SCID mice (Testa et al., 2007)

2. Leukemogenesis

The pathogenesis of leukemia may be explained by two classes of alterations of oncogenic genes as a result of chromosomal aberrations. *Class I* mutations confers a proliferative and/or survival advantage to the cells. The current list of known leukemogenic class I mutations consists of more than 10 different protein tyrosine kinases (PTK) that undergo constitutive activation either by being fused to different N-terminal partner proteins providing an oligomerization domain, or by activating mutations such as point mutations in their kinase domain or internal tandem repeats (length mutations) in the juxtamembrane domain (Flt3, Kit). Most of these alterations are associated with chronic myeloproliferative disorders such as chronic myeloid leukemia/chronic myelomonocytic leukemia (CML/CMML) or Philadelphia negative myeloproliferative disorders, except activating mutations of Flt3 and Kit which are found almost exclusively in acute leukemia. Flt3 ITD (internal tandem duplication) mutants constitutively activate MAPK, AKT and STAT5, leading to Pim-1 activation and Bcl-xL (B-cell lymphoma) hyperexpression (Minami et al., 2003; Kim et al., 2005). Extracellular c-Kit mutations resulted in c-Kit receptor hyperactivation in response to Kit ligand, with subsequent strong activation of MAPK and PI3K, while codon 816 c-Kit mutations induced constitutive STAT-3 activation and upregulation of Bcl-xL and c-myc (Schnittger et al., 2006)). Other class I alterations are gain of function mutations of the three main RAS isoforms (N-Ras, Ki-Ras, Ha-Ras) which are frequently seen in different myeloid malignancies (Beaupre and Kurzrock, 1999). N-Ras mutations lead to increased activity of the Ras pathway, resulting in increased proliferation and decreased apoptosis (Testa et al., 2007). Overexpression of *class I* mutations is generally sufficient to transform hematopoietic cells to growth-factor independence *in vitro* and to induce a lethal *leukemialike* myeloproliferative disorder in mice (Ilaria, 2004).

(Flt- FMS-Like Tyrosine Kinase 3, STAT- Signal Transducer and Activator of Transcription, MAPK-Mitogen-Activated Protein Kinase)

In contrast to class I mutations, there is a large group of genetic alterations mostly associated with acute leukemia, referred to as *class II* mutations, which impair differentiation of hematopoietic cells and subsequent apoptosis but do not directly provide proliferative and/or survival advantage. Many of them are loss of function mutations (either through fusion formation or point mutations) of transcriptional regulators that are critical for normal hematopoietic development and differentiation. Transcription factor fusion genes include CBF, RAR, MLL, HOX and CBP while loss of function mutations occur in AML1, CEBP/a, PU.1, GATA1 and IKAROS (reviewed in Chalandon and Schwaller, 2005). Via mediators of apoptosis, fusion proteins send anti-apoptotic signals that favor the preferential survival of leukemic cells:PML/RAR-α or CBF/SMMHC through the p53 pathway and AML1/ETO through the Bcl2-related pathway (Klampfer et al., 1996; Britos-bray et al., 1998; Pandolfi, 2001). PML/RARα fusion protein was also shown to exert an anti-apoptotic activity by downmodulating the expression of some death-inducing genes, such as TNF-R1 (Testa et al., 1998) and TRAIL-R1/-R2 (Ricioni et al., 2005). Nucleophosmin acts as a cellular p53 negative regulator to protect hematopoietic cells from stress-induced apoptosis (Lambert and Buckle, 2006). These mutations are usually not sufficient to mimic the human disease in transgenic mice since they do not readily induce a leukemia phenotype. However, after a long latency period, signs of myelodysplasia are often seen with a variable propensity to develop an immature and clonal hematologic disorder closely resembling human AML (reviewed in Chalandon and Schwaller, 2005). Additional mutations, occurring at the level of signal transduction molecules (the receptor tyrosine kinases Flt3 or c-Kit, NRas and Ki-Ras), are required for the generation of disease (reviewed in Testa et al., 2007). This hypothesis is supported by the analysis of unselected blood samples from neonates which showed that about 1% have class II genetic alterations that are detectable by PCR (Greaves et al., 2003). (CBF-core binding factor, RAR –retinoic acid receptor, MLL-mixed lineage leukemia, HOX-homeobox, CBP-CREB binding protein, CEBP/a-CCAAT/enhancer binding protein, PML-promyelocyte leukemia, SMMHC-smooth muscle myosin heavy chain, TRAIL-tumor necrosis factor–related apoptosis-inducing ligand)

In the same light, being a heterogeneous disease, relapsed AML is unlikely to emanate from one predominant mechanism; instead, there are likely to be multiple biologic factors at play that allow for clinical relapse to occur. These factors likely include multidrug resistance proteins, aberrant signal transduction pathways, survival of leukemia stem cells, microenvironmental interactions, and immune tolerance. Many conditions in the environment select for the development of these target mechanisms, ranging from chemotherapeutic modalities, to signal transduction inhibitors, to upregulation of antileukemic immune responses (reviewed in Lancet and Karp, 2009)

PTK involved	Fusion gene	Chromosomal aberration	Disease phenotype
A. Fusion genes			
ABL (9q34)	BCR/ABL	t(9;22)(q34;q11)	CML
(ABL1)	TEL/ABL	t(9;12)(q34;p13)	Atypical CML
ARG (1q24)	BCR/ARG	t(1;22)(q24;q11)	Atypical CML
(ABL2)	TEL/ARG	t(1;12)(q24;p13)	Atypical CML
PDGF R (5q33)	TEL/PDGF R	t(5;12)(q33;p13)	CMML, atypical CML
	HIP1/PDGF R	t(5;7)(q33;q11)	CMML, atypical CML
	RAB5/PDGF R	t(5;17)(q33;p13)	CMML, atypical CML
	H4/PDGF R	t(5;10)(q33;q21)	CMML,atypical CML
	Myomegalin/PDGF R	t(1;5)(q23;q33)	CMML,atypical CML
	CEV14/PDGF R	t(5;14)(q33;q32)	relapse AML
	NIN1/PDGF R	t(1;5)(q23;q33)	atypical CML
	HCMOGT/PDGF R	t(5;17)(q33;p11)	juvenile CMML
	TP53BP1/PDGF R	t(5;15)(q33;q22)	atypical CML
PDGF R (4q12)	BCR/PDGF R	t(4;22)(q12;q11)	Atypical CML
AK2 (9p24)	BCR/JAK2	t(9;22)(p24;q11)	CML, atypical CML
	TEL/JAK2	t(9;12)(p24;p13)	Atypical CML, ALL, AML
	PCM1/JAK2	t(8;9)(p21-22;p23-24)	Atypical CML, AML, ALL
TRKC (15q25)	TEL/TRKC	t(12;15)(p13;q25)	AML
GFR3 (4p16)	TEL/FGFR3	t(4;12)(p16;p13)	AML
FRK(6q21)	TEL/FRK	t(6;12)(q21;p13)	AML
B. Gain of function mutations			
FLT3 (13q12)	ITD (80%), activation loop kinase domain (15%)		AML
KIT (4q12)	JM region, activation loop kinase domain		AML
JAK2 (9p21)	JAK2 V617F mutation	9pLOH	PV, ET, myelofibrosis
C. Deregulated expression			
FLT3 (13q12)	Overexpression	MLL alterations	ALL/AML

CML: chronic myeloid leukemia; AML: acute myeloid leukemia; ALL: acute lymphoblastic leukemia; CMML: chronic myelomonocytic leukemia; EMS; ITD: internal tandem duplication; JM: juxtamembrane; PV: polycythemia vera; ET: essential thrombocythemia; LOH: loss of heterozygosity

Table 1. Deregulated protein tyrosine kinases in myeloid leukemias (taken from Chalandon and Schwaller, 2005)

3. Signal Transduction Pathways (STP)

Signal transduction is the primary means by which eukaryotic cells respond to external signals from their environment and coordinate complex cellular changes. Extracellular signal is transduced into the cell through ligand-receptor binding, followed by the activation of intracellular signaling pathways that involve a series of protein phosphorylation and dephosphorylation, protein-protein interaction, and protein-small molecules interaction (Liu and Zhou, 2004). Cytokines interact with cell-surface receptors initiating signaling cascades that promote cell growth and division, while inhibiting the pathways of apoptotic cell death. The JAK/STAT, Raf/ MEK/ERK and PI3K/Akt signaling pathways are activated by a variety of cytokines that function to potentiate or inhibit hematopoiesis. These include IL (interleukin)-3, IL-7, SCF (stem cell factor), G (granulocyte)-CSF, type I interferons (IFN) and TGF- (transforming growth factor)- beta (Steelman et al., 2004).

The phosphatidylinositol 3-kinase (PI3K)

PI3K /protein kinase B (Akt)/mammalian target of rapamycin (mTOR) (a family of lipid kinases) signaling cascade is crucial to many widely divergent physiological processes which include cell cycle progression, transcription, translation, differentiation, apoptosis, motility, and metabolism (Yuan and Cantley, 2008). The family of PI3K enzymes phosphorylates inositol lipids and comprises three different classes, I, II, and III. Phosphorylated phosphatidylinositol 3,4,5trisphosphate [PtdIns (3,4,5)P3] recruits to the plasma membrane pleckstrin homology (PH) domain-containing proteins, which include phosphoinositide-dependent protein kinase 1 (PDK1) and Akt. The phospholipid products of PI3K activate downstream targets, including PDK, Akt and PKC (Palmer et al., 1995; Toker et al., 1994; Nakanishi et al., 1993).

Class I PI3K is further classified as A [activated by receptor tyrosine kinases (RTKs), Ras, and G-protein coupled receptors (GPCRs)] and B (activated by GPCRs) subtype. Class IA and 1B PI3Ks are heterodimeric enzymes composed of a regulatory and of catalytic subunits (Martelli et al., 2010).

Phosphoinositide-dependent kinase (PDK)

PDK requires the phospholipid product of PI3K for activation. There are believed to be two members of the PDK family – PDK1 and PDK2. Association of Akt with phosphoinositides produces a conformational change allowing Ser473 to be phosphorylated by PDK1 (Scheid et al., 2002).

Protein kinase B (Akt)

Akt is a 57-kDa serine/threonine protein kinase central to cell signaling downstream of growth factors, cytokines, and other cellular stimuli. Activated Akt was originally isolated from cells of the leukemia and lymphoma prone AKR strain of mice (Staal, 1987). It comprises three highly conserved isoforms: Akt1/α, Akt2/β, and Akt3/γ which are functionally different (Staal, 1987; Nicolson and Anderson, 2002; Staal et al., 1988). Once Akt is recruited at the plasma membrane, its activation loop is phosphorylated on Thr308 by PDK1 while the mTOR complex 2 (mTORC2), activated by RTK, phosphorylates Ser473 in the Akt COOH-terminus. Full Akt activation requires both phosphorylation steps. Active Akt migrates to both the cytosol and the nucleus. Nuclear Akt may fulfill important anti-apoptotic roles. So far, over 100 Akt substrates have been identified (Manning and Cantley, 2007). Of these, about 40 which mediate the pleiotropic Akt functions have been characterized, including Bad, caspase-9, murine double minute 2 (MDM2), IκB kinase (IKK) α, proline-rich Akt substrate 40-kDa (PRAS40) 40, the Foxo family of Forkhead box-o transcription factors, apoptosis signal-regulated kinase 1 [ASK1, a negative regulator of pro-apoptotic c-Jun N-terminal kinase (JNK)], Raf, p27Kip1, p21Cip1, glycogen synthase kinase

3β (GSK3β). Each of these substrates has a key role in the regulation of cell survival and proliferation, either directly or through an intermediary.

The antiapoptotic effects of Akt occur through its phosphorylation of a wide variety of targets. The first antiapoptotic target identified was Bad, a member of the Bcl-2 family. Phosphorylation of Bad at S136 by Akt allows phosphorylated Bad to interact with 14-3-3 proteins, promoting cell survival (Datta et al., 1997; Andreeff et al., 1999). Interaction of Bad with 14-3-3 proteins inhibits the ability of Bad to interact with Bcl-2 and Bcl-xL. This allows Bcl-xL to bind to proapoptotic Bax molecules and prevent the formation of proapoptotic Bax homodimers. However, Bad is also phosphorylated on different sites by members of the Raf/MEK/ERK (S112) and PKA (S112, S155) pathways.

In human cells, Akt phosphorylates and inactivates caspase-9. Overexpression of Akt inhibits cytochrome c-induced activation of caspase-9 (Cardone et al., 1998). Phosphorylation of the Foxo family of transcription factors is also attributed to Akt (Biggs et al 1999); Brunet et al., 1999; Rena et al., 1999; Tang et al., 1999).This phosphorylation results in forkhead transcription factors translocation to the cytoplasm, thus inhibiting transcription of pro-apoptotic genes such as FasL (Brunet et al., 1999). Akt activates transcription of antiapoptotic genes through phosphorylation of IKK and regulation of nuclear factor-kappa B (NF-kB) (Ozes et al., 1999). Akt also promotes cell survival and cell cycle progression by its ability to phosphorylate MDM2 and GSK-3 (Fukumoto et al., 2001; Zhou et al., 2001). Once phosphorylated by Akt, MDM2 translocates to the nucleus and interacts with p300. p300 dissociates from p19ARF, resulting in the degradation of p53 and cell cycle progression. Akt phosphorylates GSK-3, inhibiting its activity. The decreased GSK-3 activity increases stability of catenin and enhances its association with lymphoid enhancer factor/T cell factor (LEF/TCF) (Fukumoto et al., 2001). The catenin–LEF/TCF complex increases transcription of proteins such as cyclin D1 and c-myc, promoting cell cycle progression (Fukumoto et al., 2001). Clearly, Akt can affect both cell cycle progression and apoptosis (reviewed in Steelman et al., 2004).

MTORC1 is a critical regulator of translation initiation and ribosome biogenesis and plays an evolutionarily conserved role in cell growth control (Wullschleger et al., 2006). The enhanced sensitivity of cancer cells and mouse tumor models exhibiting oncogenic activation of the PI3K-Akt pathway to mTORC1 inhibitors, such as rapamycin, illustrates the importance of mTORC1 activation downstream of Akt (Sabatini, 2006). One of the best-conserved functions of Akt is its role in promoting cell growth (i.e., an increase in cell mass). The predominant mechanism appears to be through activation of mTOR complex 1 (mTORC1 or the mTOR-raptor complex), which is regulated by both nutrients and growth factor signaling. mTORC1 signaling integrates environmental clues (growth factors, hormones, nutrients, stressors) and information from the cell metabolic status. Thus, mTORC1 controls anabolic processes for promoting protein synthesis and cell growth (Manning and Cantley, 2007).

Janus kinase/Signal Transducer and Activator of Transcription (JAK/STAT)

The JAK/STAT pathway consists of three families of genes: the JAK, or Janus family of tyrosine kinases, the STAT (signal transducers and activators of transcription) family and the CIS/SOCS family, which serves to downregulate the activity of the JAK/STAT pathway (Silvennoinen et al., 1993; Kisseleva et al., 2002; Krebs and Hilton, 2002; Fujitani et al., 1997). The JAK/STAT pathway involves signaling from the cytokine receptor to the nucleus. JAKs are stimulated by activation of a cytokine receptor. Stimulation of JAKs results in STAT transcription factor activity. JAKs are a family of large tyrosine kinases, having molecular weights in the range of 120–140 kDa (1130–1142 aa). Four JAKs (JAK1, JAK2, JAK3 and Tyk2) have been identified in mammals. JAK3 expression is limited to hematopoietic cells (Steelman et al., 2004).

The STAT gene family consists of seven proteins (STAT1,STAT2, STAT3, STAT4, STAT5a, STAT5b and STAT6). Upregulation of STAT3 is detected with high frequency inhuman cancer. STAT3 is activated not only by cytokine receptors, such as the receptor for the IL-6 family cytokines, but also growth receptor tyrosine kinases, such as the EGFR family including Her2/Neu, and non-receptor tyrosine kinases such as Src and Abl(Turkson et al., 1998), and is also activated in response to stimulation of G-protein-coupled receptors (GPCR) (Pelletier et al., 2003). Classically, the receptor stimulation by ligand induces STAT3 binding to phosphotyrosine residues of receptors through its SH2 domain and its phosphorylation on a critical tyr705 residue by the receptor itself, or by associated Janus kinase (JAK, Jak1–3, Tyk2) or Src family tyrosine kinases (Yu et al., 2004).

Ras/Raf/MAPK kinase/extracellular signal-regulated kinase pathway (Ras/Raf/MEK/ERK)

The Ras/Raf/MEK/ERK pathway is a central signal transduction pathway, which transmits signals from multiple cell surface receptors to transcription factors in the nucleus (Chang et al., 2003a; Chang et al., 2003b; Chang et al., 2003c). This pathway is frequently referred to as the MAP kinase pathway as MAPK stands for mitogen-activated protein kinase indicating that this pathway can be stimulated by mitogens, cytokines and growth factors. The pathway can be activated by Ras stimulating the membrane translocation of Raf. This pathway also interacts with many different signal transduction pathways including PI3K/Akt and JAK/STAT.

Ras is a small GTP-binding protein, which is the common upstream molecule of several signaling pathways including Raf/MEK/ERK, PI3K/Akt and RalEGF/Ral (Chang et al., 2003a; Chang et al., 2003b; Chang et al., 2003c). There are three different Ras family members: Ha-Ras, Ki-Ras and N-Ras. The Ras proteins show varying abilities to activate the Raf/MEK/ERK and PI3K/Akt cascades, as Ki-Ras has been associated with Raf/MEK/ERK while Ha-Ras is associated with PI3K/Akt activation.

The Raf protein family consists of A-Raf, B-Raf and Raf-1, which are involved in the regulation of proliferation, differentiation and apoptosis induced after cytokine stimulation (Blalock et al., 1999; Mercer et al., 2003; Naumann et al., 1007, Pritchard et al., 1996; Mercer et al., 2002).Raf-1 has many effects on the regulation of apoptosis. Some of these effects occur at the mitochondrial membrane and are independent of MEK and ERK activity. It was observed that overexpression of activated A-Raf abrogates the cytokine dependence of hematopoietic cells. Overexpression of B-Raf in Rat-1 cells results in decreased apoptosis due to inhibition of caspase activity. Raf-1 has important roles in apoptosis as it phosphorylates and inactivates Bad (Wang et al., 1996). Raf-1 phosphorylates and co-immunoprecipitates with Bcl-2, as well as regulates Bag and Bad expression, in BCR/ABL-expressing cells (Salomoni et al., 1998). The ability of Raf proteins to phosphorylate MEK1 varies from B-Raf, Raf-1, A-Raf. The ability of Raf to abrogate cytokine dependency is inversely proportional to their MEK1 activity, with A-Raf, Raf-1, B-Raf (McCubrey et al., 1998; Hoyle et al., 2000). Stimulation of Raf activates MEK1 and ERK resulting in phosphorylation of transcription factors, proliferation, and inhibition of apoptosis (Steelman et al., 2004).

Raf-1 is also phosphorylated by Akt which has been associated with inhibition of Raf-1 activity (Wojknowski et al., 1997; Rommel et al., 1999). CAMP-dependent protein kinase (PKA) inhibits Raf-1 (Wu et al., 1993; Schramm et al., 1994; Dumaz et al., 2002). Protein kinase C isoforms (a, b and g) stimulates Raf-1 activity (Sozeri t al., 1992). Raf-1 has been postulated to have important roles in cell cycle progression, activation of the p53 and NF-kB transcription factors and the prevention of apoptosis (reviewed in Steelman et al., 2004) Interactions between the Raf and PI3K/Akt pathways, or crosstalk, is an area of intense research Recently, it was demonstrated that it is more effective to inhibit the growth of Raf- and MEK1-transformed hematopoietic cells with inhibitors that target both the Raf/MEK/ERK and PI3K/Akt pathways (Navolanic et al., 2004).

MEK

MEK proteins are the primary downstream targets of Raf. The MEK family of genes consists of five genes: MEK1, MEK2, MEK3, MEK4 and MEK5. The structure of MEK consists of an amino-terminal negative regulatory domain and a carboxy-terminal MAP kinase-binding domain, which is necessary for binding and activation of ERKs (Huang et al., 1995; Tanoue et al., 2001; Crews et al., 1992). Deletion of the regulatory MEK1 domain results in constitutive MEK1 and ERK activation. Activated MEK1 could abrogate cytokine dependency of certain hematopoietic cells. Constitutive activity of MEK1 inhibits NF-kB transcription by negatively regulating p38MAPK activity (Carter et al., 2000).

ERK

The main physiological substrates of MEK are the members of the ERK (extracellular signal-regulated kinase) or MAPK (mitogen activated protein kinase) family of genes. The ERK family consists of four distinct groups of kinases: ERK, Jun amino terminal kinases (JNK1/2/3), p38MAPK (p38 a/b/g/d) and ERK5. In addition, there are ERK3, ERK4, ERK6, ERK7 and ERK8 kinases, which while related to ERK1 and ERK2 have different modes of activation, and their biochemical roles are not as well characterized. Downstream targets of ERK include the p90Rsk kinase and the CREB, c-Myc and other transcription factors. ERK and p90Rsk can enter the nucleus to phosphorylate transcription factors which can lead to their activation (reviewed in Steelman et al., 2004).

Nuclear factor kappa B (NFkB)

Cilloni et al. (2007) have presented a comprehensive review on NF-kB. NF-kB proteins are a small group of related and evolutionarily conserved proteins which in mammals consists of five members: Rel (c-Rel), RelA/p65, RelB, p50, and p52 (Ghosh et al., 1998; Hayden et al., 2004).In resting cells, NF-kB proteins arepredominantly cytoplasmic, associating with members of the inhibitory IkB family such as IkBa, IkBb and Ikbe (Ghosh et al., 1998).These interact with NF-kB through multiple ankyrin repeats and as a result inhibit its DNA binding activity. Two NF-kB activation pathways exist; the first is normally triggered in response to infections or exposure to pro-inflammatorycytokines that activate the IkB kinase (IKK) complex leading to phosphorylation-induced IkB degradation, the other pathway leads to selective activation of p52: RelB dimers. This pathway is triggered by certain membersof the tumor necrosis factor (TNF)cytokine family through selective activation of IKKa by the upstream kinase, NF-kappa B-inducing kinase (NIK).In response to many stimuli such as inflammatorycytokines, bacterial lipopolysaccharide, phorbol esters, viral infection or stress, IkB are phosphorylated on two critical serine residues (Senftleben et al., 2001).

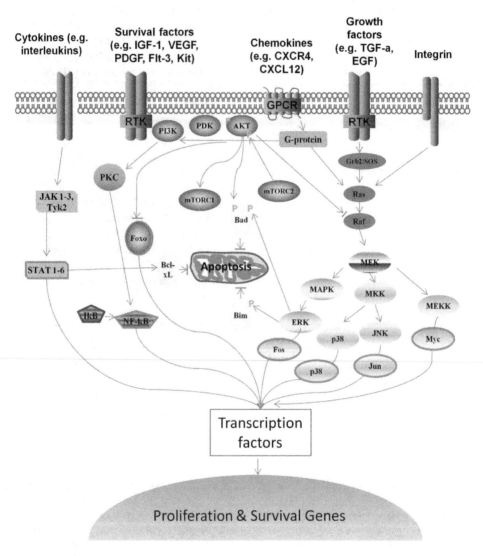

Fig. 1. Signal transduction pathways (refer text for details)

This modification triggers IkB ubiquitination and destruction via the 26Sproteasome degradation machinery. As a consequence, NF-kBis freed to enter the nucleus and regulate transcription of over 150 genes encoding cell adhesion molecules, cytokines, growth factors, components of the immune systems and anti-apoptotic genes such as FLIP (FLICE inhibitory protein), cIAPs (inhibitor of apoptosis), Bcl-2 and Bcl-xL (Aggarwall, 2004). It is also implicated in the regulation of cell proliferation by controlling D-type cyclins (Takebayashi et al., 2003).

The three main signaling pathways are kept in check by naturally occurring inhibitors or tumor suppressor proteins. For example, the JAK/STAT pathway has the SOCS/CIS family of proteins, which serve to limit its effects by a negative feedback pathway. The Raf/MEK/ERK pathway can be negatively regulated by the PI3K/Akt cascade as well as the MKP1 phosphatase, which inactivates phosphorylated ERK. The PI3K/Akt pathway has the PTEN and SHIP phosphatases, which serve to fine-tune its antiapoptotic effects (reviewed in Steelman et al., 2004).

4. Aberrant STP and drug resistance in AML

Genetic events that give rise to leukemic transformation occur through activation of components of receptor tyrosine kinase (RTK) signaling pathways (Liu and Zhou, 2004). These include fusion proteins or gene mutations such as seen with activated TEL-JAK, STAT5A and BCR-ABL. Transforming activity of oncogenic PTK is mediated by parallel activation of several downstream signaling pathways. Final downstream mediators of this complex signaling network are phosphoproteins that translocate to the nucleus and act as transcriptional regulators activating a distinct group of target genes. The oncogenic activity of a given PTK is mediated by several signaling pathways including JAK/STAT, Ras/MAPK, PI3K/AKT, or NF-kB.

Oncogenic activity severs dependence of transformed cell on external stimulation for survival. TEL-JAK fusion proteins contain the oligomerization domain of TEL and the tyrosine kinase domains of JAK1, JAK2, JAK3, or TYK2. These efficiently substitute for the survival and mitogenic signals controlled by IL-3, without concomitant activation of the IL-3 receptor. STAT5 are constitutively active in TEL-JAK2- and TEL-JAK1-expressing cells (Lacronique et al., 2000). The BCR-ABL oncogene produces an activated tyrosine kinase fusion protein and gain independence from IL-3 for cell growth (Mandanas et al., 1992). Activated forms of Ras, Raf, MEK, PI3K and Akt however, show significant differences in the ability to abrogate cytokine dependence (Steelman et al., 2004).

TEL/JAK2 isoforms, depending on the location of the breakpoints in the JAK2 gene, have been described in acute lymphoblastic leukemia of the B-cell type and atypical CML (Lacronique et al., 1997). Somatically acquired JAK2 mutation (V617F) was detected in 472/944 (50%) of patients with Ph-negative chronic myeloproliferative disorders [including polycythemia vera (PV), idiopathic myelofibrosis (IMF) and essential thrombocytosis (ET)] with predominance in PV (66%) followed by IMF (42%) and ET (26%) (Jones et al., 2005). Recent investigation of novel mutations in JAK2 revealed a higher incidence, ~99% and 55% in PV and ET, respectively (Tefferi, 2010).

Flt-3 mediates its proliferative and antiapoptotic effects through several signaling pathways including the STAT5, Ras/MAPK and PI3K/AKT pathways. Overexpression of Flt-3 was detected in 73% of AML and 78% of ALL patients (Nakao et al., 1996). Flt-3 *length mutations* (internal tandem duplications (ITD) in the juxtamembrane domain) (Nakao et al., 1996), is observed in more than 20% of adult and more than 10% of pediatric AML patients harbor an Flt-3-ITD (reviewed in Testa et al., 2007). In general, patients with mutant FLT3 show higher cell counts and decreased overall survival. Absence of the wild-type allele in patients with Flt-3-ITD predicted poor prognosis in 82 adult *de novo* AML cases with otherwise normal cytogenetics who received uniform high-dose therapy. Of the the 23 (28%) patients with Flt3-ITD, disease-free survival (DFS) was inferior (P = 0.03), yet overall survival (OS) was not different (P = 0.14) (Whitman et al., 2001). In cytogenetic normal AML patients aged > 60 years treated on Cancer and Leukemia Group B frontline trials, FLT3-ITD remained associated with shorter disease-free survival (P < .001; hazard ratio 2.10) and overall survival (P < .001; hazard Ratio 1.97) in multivariable analyses (Whitman et al., 2010). Flt3 kinase domain point mutants is mutated in about 35% of AML (Stirewalt et al., 2003). In a study of 481 patients, FLT3 mutation did not have an impact on event-free survival (EFS) in patients with CBF-AML (P = .84) and poor-risk AML (P = .37). However, while event-free survival was worse in the FLT3-internal tandem duplication (ITD) group (20 weeks vs 41 weeks; P < .00,001) this was not observed for the FLT3-tyrosine kinase domain (TKD) point mutation group (61 weeks vs 41 weeks; P = .15) (Santos et al., 2011).

The profiles of signal transduction that correlated with poor response to chemotherapy showed potentiated STAT5 and STAT3 phosphorylations as well as attenuated STAT1 phosphorylation following cytokine stimulation (Irish et al., 2004)

Ras mutations are frequently observed in certain hematopoietic malignancies including myelodysplastic syndromes, juvenile myelomonocytic leukemia and acute myeloid leukemia (Bartram et al., 1988; Flotho et al., 1999; Stirewalt et al., 2001). It has been shown to activate both the Raf/MEK/ERK and the PI3K/Akt pathways. Thus, mutations at Ras should theoretically activate both pathways simultaneously. Consequence of this activation may be the increased expression of growth factors that can potentially further activate this cascade by an autocrine loop. Many cytokine and growth factor gene promoters contain binding sites for transcription factors (Ets, Elk, Jun, Fos, CREB) whose activities are often activated by the Raf/MEK/ERK cascade (reviewed in Steelman et al., 2004).

There is increasing evidence that activation of the PI3K/AKT signaling pathway leading to downstream inactivation of Foxo transcription factors, activation of the mammalian target of rapamycin (mTOR), or induction of Skp2 (leading to degradation of the cell cycle inhibitor p27), plays a central role in transformation by several mutated PTK such as BCR/ABL, mutated FLT3 or KIT (Scheijen et al., 2004; Andreu et al., 2005). Emerging evidence suggests that activation of NF-kB involves crosstalk between the PI3K and Ras/MAPK pathways (Gelfanov et al., 2001; Kirchner et al., 2003). Several NF-kB target genes, such as cIAP1/cIAP2, Bcl-xL, or Mcl-1, are well-known inhibitors of apoptosis that may co-mediate the antiapoptotic effect of a constitutively activated PTK (Aichberger et al., 2005).

Expression of transcription factor fusions like AML1/ETO and PML/RARa in leukemic cells leads to induction of several genes associated with WNT signaling (Muller-Tidow et al., 2004). WNT signaling activation was found in a significant fraction of leukemic blasts from patients with AML-M0 (Zheng et al., 2004).

Other causes of PI3K/Akt/mTOR activation in AML may be the result of several factors, including low levels of PP2A, autocrine/paracrine secretion of growth factors such as IGF-1 and VEGF (reviewed in Martelli et al., 2010). Interactions between leukemic cells and bone marrow stromal cells through CXCR4 (a GPCR) which is abundantly expressed on leukemic cell surface where it is up-regulated by hypoxic conditions and its physiological ligand, (Fierro et al., 2009; Fiegl et al., 2009) CXCL12, produced by stromal cells, (Fiegl et al., 2009; Ayala et al., 2009) could result in PI3K/Akt/mTOR activation (Zeng et al., 2009). Furthermore, interactions between β1 integrins on AML cells and stromal fibronectin could lead to pathway activation, (Matsunaga et al., 2003; Matsunaga et al., 2008) possibly through up-regulation of integrin-linked kinase 1 (ILK1) which is involved in Akt phosphorylation on Ser473 in a PI3K-dependent manner in AML cells (Tabe et al., 2007).

PI3K/Akt/ mTOR pathway influences proliferation, survival, and drug resistance of AML cells.

From 50% to 80% of patients with AML display Akt phosphorylated on either Thr308 or Ser473 (or both) (Xu et al., 2003; Min et al., 2003). Univariate analysis of 146 AML patients revealed those with low levels of pAKT had somewhat better CR rates (60% versus 50%; P=0.21), longer median CR durations (71 versus 32 weeks; P=0.13), and statistically significant longer median survival times (59 versus 30 weeks; P=0.02) compared with those with high levels of pAKT. In another study, single analysis of Akt phosphorylated at threonine 308 (Thr308) and serine 473 (Ser473) showed AktThr308(high) patients had significantly shorter overall survival (11 vs 47 months; P=0.01), event-free survival (9 vs 26 months; P=0.005) and relapse-free survival (10 months vs not reached; P=0.02) than Thr308(low) patients. This was not observed for Akt Ser473 (Gallay et al., 2009). Poor prognosis of AML patients with elevated PI3K/Akt/mTOR signaling could be also related to the fact that this pathway controls the expression of the membrane ATP binding cassette (ABC) transporter, multidrug resistance-associated protein 1, associated with a lower survival rate (Tazzari et al., 2007; Schaich et al., 2005). Nevertheless, a more recent report has highlighted that constitutive activation of PI3K/Akt/mTOR signaling could be a favourable prognostic factor in de novo cases of AML. One hypothesis for the lower relapse rate in patients with enhanced PI3K/Akt/mTOR signaling is that it could drive immature leukemic cells (LSCs and CFU-L) into S phase, thus rendering them more susceptible to polychemotherapy (Tamburini et al., 2005)

The AKT pathway was among the signaling cascades whose simultaneous activation with other pathways, such as PKCα and ERK, was found to confer a poor prognosis in AML (Altman et al., 2011). Eventhough often mutated in human cancer, MMAC1/PTEN gene are infrequent as genetic aberrations in myeloid leukaemia (Aggerholm et al., 2000)

NF-kB has been found to be activated in CD34+/CD38– blast cells derived from patients with *de novo* AML (Guzman et al., 2001; Baumgartner et al., 2002). Leukemic stem cells residing in this population are quiescent or slowly cycling and therefore less sensitive to chemotherapy. They are therefore likely to be responsible for disease relapse and represent the target for future innovative therapies (Bonnett et al.,1997; Lowenberg et al., 1999; Jordan, 2002). Activation of NF-kB in leukemia patients has been well documented though NF-kB activation is not uniform among AML patients. Forty percent of AML patients evaluated presented with increased NF-kB DNA binding activity. These patients are characterized by increased white cell counts at diagnosis and increased blast percentages in the bone marrow suggesting a link between NF-kB and cell proliferation. In particular, cyclin D1, whose expression is regulated by NF-kB. Alternatively, NF-kB action could be due to the induction of genes coding for AML growth factors such as GM-CSF or granulocyte colony-stimulating factor (G-CSF) (Cilloni et al., 2007).

The majority of LSCs are quiescent and insensitive to traditional chemotherapeutic drugs. This latter feature explains, at least in part, the difficulties in eradicating this cell population by conventional polychemotherapy. Thus, novel therapeutic strategies for AML eradication should also target LSCs (Misaghian et al., 2009). In AML, aberrant activation of several signal transduction pathways strongly enhances the proliferation and survival of both LSCs and CFU-Ls (McCubrey et al., 2008; Steelman et al., 2008). Therefore, these signaling networks are attractive targets for the development of innovative therapeutic strategies in AML (Scholl et al., 2008).

5. Conclusion

Expression of STP proteins is heterogenous and of prognostic value in AML (Kornblau et al., 2009). These signaling pathways in AML may in the future help rationally select targeted therapies in individual patients (Foran, 2010). While current classification schemes have prognostic relevance they generally do not alter therapeutic recommendations. As knowledge of mutated genes in cancersim proves, our ability to treat patients afflicted with certain diseases will increase substantially. The genetic mutation may affect multiple signal transduction pathways. Targeting multiple pathways may be more efficacious as this approach may suppress or eliminate tumor growth at lower concentrations of the drugs than that required to inhibit growth by targeting a single pathway (Steelmanet al., 2004).

The heterogeneity in AML continues to elude the best methods to characterize them. Genome and proteome-wide analysis has further revealed complexity in the makeup of the leukemic cell. The rapid advancement in targeted therapies implied the urgent need for alternative therapy and the readiness of the community to embrace it. Nevertheless so far, combinatorial medicine still holds out as the best option for successful treatment. If targeted therapies remain the way forward it will eventually bank deeply on the ability to identify molecular signatures in the individual leading to the establishment of personalized medicine.

Novel array technologies enabled the analysis of numerous features at the level of DNA for gene copy number variation, mutations, methylation in addition to mRNA transcription and regulatory microRNA. Emerging technologies to assess protein expression and phosphorylation levels within cells e.g. cytokine and chemokine arrays to assess external forces acting on leukemic cells and phosphoproteins in apoptosis, cell-cycle, and signal-transduction pathways, are highly needed. Protein expression and posttranslational modifications, either alone or in concert with other profiling approaches, could provide independent or complementary information not captured by transcriptional profiles. Protein signature groups, with prognostic information distinct from cytogenetics may reveal underlying similarities indistinguishable by cytogenetics (Kornblau et al., 2009).

Quantitative flow cytometry appears well suited for identifying predictive markers in AML patients because it offers obvious advantages over other techniques (western blot, for example), including rapidness, a much lower number of cells required to perform the assay, and the possibility of identifying different subclones in the leukemic population by coimmunostaining with multiple antibodies to surface antigens (Martelli et al., 2010). The mechanisms in leukemogenesis, drug resistance and relapse remain an area of much research. From cell biology to cytogenetics to molecular defects to signaling pathways, all have contributed to a better understanding of the cancer. New knowledge in epigenetics and microRNA remain to be elucidated.

6. References

[1] Aggarwall BB. Nuclear factor-kB: the enemy within cancer. Cancer Cell 2004;6:203-208.

[2] Aggerholm A, Grønbaek K, Guldberg P, Hokland P. Mutational analysis of the tumour suppressor gene MMAC1/PTEN in malignant myeloid disorders.Eur J Haematol. 2000(2):109-113.

[3] Aichberger KJ, Mayerhofer M, Krauth MT, Skvara H, Florian S, Sonneck K, et al. Identification of mcl-1 as a BCR/ABL dependent target in chronic myeloid

leukemia (CML): evidence for cooperative antileukemic effects of imatinib and mcl-1 antisense oligonucleotides. Blood 2005;105:3303-3311.

[4] Andreeff M, Jiang S, Zhang X, Konopleva M, Estrov Z, Snell VE et al. Expression of Bcl-2 related genes in normal and AML progenitors: changes induced by chemotherapy and retinoic acid. Leukemia 1999; 11: 1881–1892

[5] Andreu EJ, Lledo E, Poch E, Ivorra C, Albero MP, Martinez-Climent JA, et al. BCR-ABL induces the expression of Skp2 through the PI3K pathway to promote p27Kip1 degradation and proliferation of chronic myelogenousleukemia cells. Cancer Res 2005;65:3264-3272.

[6] Altman JK, Sassano A, Platanias LC. Targeting mTOR for the treatment of AML. New agents and new directions.Oncotarget. 2011;2(6):510-517.

[7] Ayala F, Dewar R, Kieran M, Kalluri R. Contribution of bone microenvironment to leukemogenesis and leukemia progression. Leukemia 2009;23:2233–2241.

[8] Blalock WL, Weinstein-Oppenheimer C, Chang F, HoylePE,Wang XY, Algate PA et al. Signal transduction, cell cycle regulatory, and anti-apoptotic pathways regulated by IL-3 in hematopoietic cells: possible sites for intervention with antineoplastic drugs. Leukemia 1999; 13: 1109–1166.

[9] Bartram CR. Mutations in ras genes in myelocyticleukemias and myelodysplastic syndromes. Blood Cells 1988; 14:533–538.

[10] Baumgartner B, Weber M, Quirling M, Fischer C, Page S, Adam M, et al. Increased IkB kinase activity is associated with activated NF-kB in acute myeloid blasts. Leukemia 2002;12: 2062-2071.

[11] Bonnet D, Dick J. Human acute myeloid leukaemia is organized as a hierarchy that originates from a primitive hematopoietic cell. Nat Med 1997;3:730-737.

[12] Beaupre DM, Kurzrock R. RAS and leukemia: from basic mechanisms to gene directed therapy. J ClinOncol 1999; 17:1071-9.Greaves MF, Wiemels J. Origins of chromosome translocations in childhood leukaemia.Nat Rev Cancer 2003;3:639-649.

[13] Biggs III WH, Meisenhelder J, Hunter T, Cavenee WK, Arden KC. Protein kinase B/Akt-mediated phosphorylation promotes nuclear exclusion of the winged helix transcription factor FKHR1. ProcNatlAcadSci USA 1999; 96: 7421–7426.

[14] Britos-Bray M, Ramirez M, Cao W, Wang X, Liu PP, Civin CI, Friedman AD. CBF-SMMHC, expressed in M4eo acute myeloid leukaemia,reduces p53 induction and slows apoptosis in hematopoietic cells exposed to DNA-damaging agents. Blood 1998;92:4344-4352.

[15] Brunet A, Bonni A, Zigmond MJ, Lin MZ, Juo P, Hu LS et al. Akt promotes cell survival by phosphorylating and inhibiting a Forkhead transcription factor. Cell 1999; 96: 857–868.

[16] Cardone MH, Roy N, Stennicke HR, Salvesen GS, Franke TF, Stanbridge E et al. Regulation of cell death protease caspase-9 by phosphorylation. Science 1998; 282: 1318–1321.

[17] Carter AB, Hunninghake GW. A constitutive active MEK-ERK pathway negatively regulates NF-kappa B-dependent gene expression by modulating TATA-binding protein phosphorylation. J BiolChem 2000; 275: 27858–27864.

[18] Chalandon Y, Schwaller J. Targeting mutated protein tyrosine kinases and their signaling pathways in hematologic malignancies.Haematologica. 2005 Jul;90(7):949-968.

[19] Chang F, Lee JT, Navolanic PM, Steelman JG, Blalock WL, Franklin RA et al. Involvement of PI3K/Akt pathway in cell cycle progression, apoptosis, and neoplastic transformation: a target for cancer chemotherapy. Leukemia 2003a; 17: 590–603.

[20] Chang F, Steelman LS, Shelton JG, Lee JT, Navolanic PN, Blalock WL et al. Regulation of cell cycle progression and apoptosis by the Ras/Raf/MEK/ERK pathway. Int J Oncol 2003b; 22: 469–480.

[21] Chang F, Steelman LS, Lee JT, Shelton JG, Navolanic PM, Blalock WL et al. Signal transduction mediated by the Ras/Raf/MEK/ERK pathway from cytokine receptors to transcription factors: potential targeting for therapeutic intervention. Leukemia 2003c;17: 1263–1293.

[22] Cilloni D, Martinelli G, Messa F, Baccarani M, Saglio G. Nuclear factor kB as a target for new drug development in myeloid malignancies.Haematologica. 2007 Sep;92(9):1224-1229.

[23] Crews CM, Alessandrini A, Erikson RL. The primary structure of MEK, a protein kinase that phosphorylates the ERK gene product. Science 1992; 258: 478–480.

[24] Datta SR, Dudek H, Tao X, Masters S, Fu H, Gotoh Y et al. Akt phosphorylation of BAD couples survival signals to the cell intrinsic death machinery. Cell 1997; 91: 231–241.

[25] Dumaz N, Light Y, Marais R. Cyclic AMP blocks cell growth through Raf-1-dependent and Raf-1-independent mechanisms. Mol Cell Biol 2002; 22: 3717–3728.

[26] Fierro FA, Brenner S, Oelschlaegel U, Jacobi A, Knoth H, Ehninger G, Illmer T, Bornhauser M. Combining SDF-1/CXCR4 antagonism and chemotherapy in relapsed acute myeloid leukemia. Leukemia 2009;23:393–396.

[27] Fiegl M, Samudio I, Clise-Dwyer K, Burks JK, Mnjoyan Z, Andreeff M. CXCR4 expression and biologic activity in acute myeloid leukemia are dependent on oxygen partial pressure. Blood 2009;113:1504–1512.

[28] Flotho C, Valcamonica S, Mach-Pascual S, Schmahl G, Corral L, Ritterbach J et al. RAS mutations and clonality analysis in children with juvenile myelomonocyticleukemia (JMML).Leukemia 1999; 13: 32–37.

[29] Fujitani Y, Hibi M, Fukada T, Takahashi-Tezuka M, Yoshida H, Yamaguchi T et al. An alternative pathway for STAT activation that is mediated by the direct interaction between JAK and STAT. Oncogene 1997; 14: 751–761.

[30] Fukumoto S, Hsieh CM, Maemura K, Layne MD, Yet SF, Lee KH et al. Akt participation in the Wntsignaling pathway through Dishevelled. J BiolChem 2001; 276: 17479–17483.

[31] Gallay N, Dos Santos C, Cuzin L, Bousquet M, SimmonetGouy V, Chaussade C, Attal M, Payrastre B, Demur C, Recher C. The level of AKT phosphorylation on threonine 308 but not on serine 473 is associated with high-risk cytogenetics and predicts poor overall survival in acute myeloid leukaemia. Leukemia 2009;23:1029–1038.

[32] Gelfanov VM, Burgess GS, Litz-Jackson S, King AJ, Marshall MS, Nakshatri H, et al. Transformation of interleukin-3-dependent cells without participation of Stat5/bcl-xL: cooperation of akt with raf/erk leads to p65 nuclear factor kB mediated antiapoptosis involving c-IAP2. Blood 2001;98:2508-2517.

[33] GhoshS, May MJ, Kopp EB. NF-kB ad Rel proteins: evolutionary conserved mediators of immune responses. Annu Rev Immunol 1998; 16:225-60. 3. Hayden MS, Ghosh S. Signaling to NF-kB. Genes Dev 2004;18: 2195-2224.

[34] Guzman M, Neering S, Upchurch D,Grimes B, Howard DS, Rizzieri DA, et al. Nuclear factor kB is constitutivelyactivated in primitive human acute myelogenous leukaemia cells. Blood 2001;98:2301-2307.

[35] Hoyle PE, Moye PW, Steelman LS, Blalock WL, Franklin RA,Pearce M et al. Differential abilities of the Raf family of protein kinases to abrogate cytokine dependency and prevent apoptosis in murine hematopoietic cells by a MEK1-dependent mechanism. Leukemia 2000; 14: 642–656.

[36] Huang W, Kessler DS, Erikson RL. Biochemical and biological analysis of Mek1 phosphorylation site mutants. MolBiol Cell 1995; 6: 237–245.

[37] Ilaria RL Jr. Animal models of chronic myelogenous leukemia. Hematol Oncol Clin North Am. 2004;18:525-543.

[38] Irish JM, Hovland R, Krutzik PO, Perez OD, Bruserud Ø, Gjertsen BT, Nolan GP. Single cell profiling of potentiated phospho-protein networks in cancer cells.Cell. 2004 Jul 23;118(2):217-228.

[39] Jones AV, Kreil S, Zoi K, Waghorn K, Curtis C, Zhang L, Score J, Seear R, Chase AJ, Grand FH, White H, Zoi C, Loukopoulos D, Terpos E, Vervessou EC, Schultheis B, Emig M, Ernst T,Lengfelder E, Hehlmann R, Hochhaus A, Oscier D, Silver RT, Reiter A, Cross NC. Widespread occurrence of the JAK2 V617F mutation in chronicmyeloproliferative disorders. Blood. 2005;106(6):2162-2168.

[40] Jordan C. Unique molecular and cellular features of acute myelogenous leukaemia stem cells. Leukemia 2002;16:559-562.

[41] Kim KT, Baird K, Ahn JY, Meltzer P, Lilly M, Levis M, et al. Pim-1 is upregulated by constitutively activated FLT3 and plays a role in FLT3-mediated cell survival. Blood 2005;105:1759-177

[42] Kisseleva T, Bhattacharya S, Braunstein J, Schindler CW. Signaling through the JAK/STAT pathway, recent advances and future challenges. Gene 2002; 285: 1–24.

[43] Kirchner D, Duyster J, Ottmann O, Schmid RM, Bergmann L, Munzert G. Mechanisms of Bcr-Abl-mediated NFkB/Rel activation. ExpHematol 2003;31:504-511.

[44] Klampfer L, Zhang J, Zelenetz AO, Uchida H, Nimer SD. The AML1/ETO fusion protein activates transcription of BCL-2. ProcNatlAcadSci USA 1996;95:11863-11868.

[45] Kornblau SM, Womble M, Qiu YH, Jackson CE, Chen W, Konopleva M, Estey EH, Andreeff M. Simultaneous activation of multiple signal transduction pathways confers poor prognosis in acute myelogenousleukemia. Blood 2006;108:2358–2365.

[46] Kornblau SM, Tibes R, Qiu YH, Chen W, Kantarjian HM, Andreeff M, Coombes KR, Mills GB. Functional proteomic profiling of AML predicts response and survival. Blood 2009;113:154–164.

[47] Krebs DL, Hilton DJ. SOCS proteins: negative regulators of cytokine signaling. Stem Cells 2001; 19: 378–387.

[48] Lacronique V, Boureux A, Valle VD, Poirel H, Quang CT, Mauchauffe M, et al. A TEL-JAK2 fusion protein with constitutive kinase activity in human leukemia. Science 1997;278:1309-1312.

[49] Lacronique V, Boureux A, Monni R, Dumon S, Mauchauffé M, Mayeux P, Gouilleux F, Berger R,Gisselbrecht S, Ghysdael J, Bernard OA. Transforming properties of chimeric TEL-JAK proteins in Ba/F3 cells. Blood. 2000;95(6):2076-2083.

[50] Lambert B, Buckle M. Characterization of the interface between nucleophosmin (NPM) and p53:potential role in p53 stabilization. FEBS Lett 2006;6580:345-350.

[51] Lane SW, Scadden DT, Gilliland DG. The leukemic stem cell niche: current concepts and therapeutic opportunities. Blood 2009;114:1150-1157.

[52] Liu Y and Zhao H. A computational approach for ordering signal transduction pathway components from genomics and proteomics Data *BMC Bioinformatics* 2004, 5:158

[53] Lowenberg B, Downing J, Burnett A. Acute myeloid leukaemia. N Engl J Med 1999;341:1051-1062.

[54] Mandanas RA, Boswell HS, Lu L, Leibowitz D. BCR/ABL confers growth factor independence upon a murine myeloid cell line. Leukemia. 1992;6(8):796-800.

[55] Martelli AM, Evangelisti C, Chiarini F, McCubrey JA . The phosphatidylinositol 3-kinase/Akt/mTOR signaling network as a therapeutic target in acute myelogenous leukemia patients.Oncotarget. 2010 Jun;1(2):89-103.

[56] Matsunaga T, Takemoto N, Sato T, Takimoto R, Tanaka I, Fujimi A, Akiyama T, Kuroda H,Kawano Y, Kobune M, Kato J, Hirayama Y, et al. Interaction between leukemic-cell VLA-4 and stromal fibronectin is a decisive factor for minimal residual disease of acute myelogenousleukemia. Nat Med 2003;9:1158–65.

[57] Matsunaga T, Fukai F, Miura S, Nakane Y, Owaki T, Kodama H, Tanaka M, Nagaya T, Takimoto R, Takayama T, Niitsu Y. Combination therapy of an anticancer drug with the FNIII14 peptide of fibronectin effectively overcomes cell adhesion-mediated drug resistance of acute myelogenousleukemia. Leukemia 2008;22:353–360.

[58] McCubrey JA, Steelman LS, Hoyle PE, Blalock WL, Weinstein-Oppenheimer C, Franklin RA et al. Differential abilities of activated Rafoncoproteins to abrogate cytokine dependency, prevent apoptosis and induce autocrine growth factor synthesis in human hematopoietic cells. Leukemia 1998; 12:1903–1929.

[59] McCubrey JA, Abrams SL, Ligresti G, Misaghian N, Wong EW, Steelman LS, Basecke J, Troppmair J, Libra M, Nicoletti F, Molton S, McMahon M, et al. Involvement of p53 and Raf/MEK/ERK pathways in hematopoietic drug resistance. Leukemia 2008;22:2080–2090.

[60] Mercer K, Chiloeches A, Huser M, Kiernan M, Marais R, Pritchard C. ERK signalling and oncogene transformation are not impaired in cells lacking A-Raf. Oncogene 2002; 21: 347–355.

[61] Mercer KE, Pritchard CA. Raf proteins and cancer: B-Raf is identified as a mutational target. BiochimBiophysActa 2003; 1653: 25–40.

[62] Min YH, Eom JI, Cheong JW, Maeng HO, Kim JY, Jeung HK, Lee ST, Lee MH, Hahn JS, Ko YW. Constitutive phosphorylation of Akt/PKB protein in acute myeloid leukemia: its significance as a prognostic variable. Leukemia 2003;17:995-997.

[63] Minami Y, Yamamoto K, Kiyoi H, Ueda R, Saito H, Naoe T. Different antiapoptotic pathways between wild-type and mutated FLT3: insights into therapeutic targets in leukemia. Blood 2003;102:2969-2975.

[64] Misaghian N, Ligresti G, Steelman LS, Bertrand FE, Basecke J, Libra M, Nicoletti F, Stivala F, Milella M, Tafuri A, Cervello M, Martelli AM, et al. Targeting the leukemic stem cell: the Holy Grail of leukemia therapy. Leukemia 2009;23:25–42.

[65] Muller-Tidow C, Steffen B, Cauvet T, Tickenbrock L, Ji P, Diederichs S, et al. Translocation products in acute myeloidleukemia activate the Wntsignaling pathway in hematopoietic cells. Mol Cell Biol 2004;24:2890-2904.

[66] Nakao M, Yokota S, Iwai T, Kaneko H,Horiike S, Kashima K, et al. Internal tandem duplication of the flt3 gene found in acute myeloid leukemia. Leukemia 1996;10:1911-198.

[67] Naumann U, Eisenmann-Tappe I, Rapp UR. The role of Raf kinases in development and growth of tumors. Recent Results Cancer Res 1997; 143: 237–244.

[68] Navolanic PM, Lee JT, McCubrey JA. Docetaxol cytotoxicity is enhanced by inhibition of the Raf/MEK/ERK pathway. Cancer BiolTher 2004; 3: 29–30.

[69] Nicolson KM, Anderson NG. The protein kinase B/Aktsignaling pathway in human malignancy. Cell Signal 2002; 14: 381–395.

[70] Ozes ON, Mayo LD, Gustin JA, Pfeffer SR, Pfeffer LM, Donner DB. NF-kappaB activation by tumour necrosis factor requires the Akt serine–threonine kinase. Nature 1999; 401: 82–85.

[71] Pandolfi PP. Oncogenes and tumor suppressors in the molecular pathogenesis of acute promyelocytic leukaemia. Hum Mol Genet 2001;10:769-775.

[72] Pelletier S, Duhamel F, Coulombe P, Popoff MR, Meloche S. Rho family GTPases are required for activation of Jak/STAT signaling by G protein-coupled receptors. Mol Cell Biol. 2003; 23:1316–1333.

[73] Pritchard CA, Bolin L, Slattery R, Murray R, McMahon M. Post-natal lethality and neurological and gastrointestinal defects in mice with targeted disruption of the A-Raf protein kinase gene. CurrBiol 1996; 6: 614–617.

[74] Rena G, Guo S, Cichy SC, Unterman TG, Cohen P. Phosphorylation of the transcription factor forkhead family member FKHR by protein kinase B. J BiolChem 1999; 274: 17179–17183.

[75] Riccioni R, Pasquini L, Mariani G, Saulle E, Rossini A, Diverio D, et al. TRAIL decoy receptors mediate resistance of acute myelo id leukemia cells to TRAIL. Haematologica 2005; 90:612-624.

[76] Rommel C, Clarke BA, Zimmermann S, Nunez L, Rossman R, Reid K et al. Differentiation stage-specific inhibition of the Raf–MEK–ERK pathway by Akt. Science 1999; 286: 1738–1741.

[77] Sabatini, D.M. (2006). mTOR and cancer: insights into a complex relationship.Nat. Rev. Cancer 6, 729–734.

[78] Salomoni P, Wasik MA, Riedel RF, Reiss K, Choi JK, Skorski T et al. Expression of constitutively active Raf-1 in the mitochondria restores antiapoptotic and leukemogenic potential of a transformation-deficient BCR/ABL mutant. J Exp Med 1998; 187: 1995–2007.

[79] Santos FP, Jones D, Qiao W, Cortes JE, Ravandi F, Estey EE, Verma D, Kantarjian H, Borthakur G. Prognostic value of FLT3 mutations among different cytogenetic subgroups in acute myeloid leukemia. Cancer. 2011;117(10):2145-2155.

[80] Schaich M, Soucek S, Thiede C, Ehninger G, Illmer T. MDR1 and MRP1 gene expression are independent predictors for treatment outcome in adult acute myeloid leukaemia. Br J Haematol 2005;128:324–332.

[81] Scheijen B, Ngo HT, Kang H, Griffin JD. FLT3 receptors with internal tandem duplications promote cell viability and proliferation by signaling through Foxo proteins. Oncogene 2004;23:3338-3349.

[82] Schnittger S, Kohl TM, Haferlach T, Kern W, Hiddemann W, Spiekemann K, et al. KIT-816 mutations in AML1-ETO-positive AML are associated with impaired event-free and overall survival. Blood 2006;107:1790-1799.

[83] Scholl C, Gilliland DG, Frohling S. Deregulation of signaling pathways in acute myeloid leukemia. SeminOncol 2008;35:336–345.

[84] Schramm K, Niehof M, Radziwill G, Rommel C, Moelling K. Phosphorylation of c-Raf-1 by protein kinase A interferes with activation. BiochemBiophys Res Commun 1994; 201: 740–747.

[85] Senftleben U Cao Y, Xiao G, Greten FR, Krahn G, Bonizzi G, et al. Activation of IKKa of a second, evolutionary conserved NF-kBsignaling pathway. Science 2001;293:1495-1499.

[86] Steelman LS, Pohnert SC, Shelton JG, Franklin RA, Bertrand FE, McCubrey JA. JAK/STAT, Raf/MEK/ERK, PI3K/Akt and BCR-ABL in cell cycle progression and leukemogenesis. Leukemia. 2004; 18(2):189-218.

[87] Steelman LS, Abrams SL, Whelan J, Bertrand FE, Ludwig DE, Basecke J, Libra M, StivalaF, Milella M, Tafuri A, Lunghi P, Bonati A, et al. Contributions of the Raf/MEK/ERK, PI3K/PTEN/Akt/mTOR and Jak/STAT pathways to leukemia. Leukemia 2008;22:686–707.

[88] Silvennoinen O, Witthuhn BA, Quelle FW, Cleveland JL, Yi T,Ihle JN. Structure of the murine Jak2 protein-tyrosine kinase and its role in interleukin 3 signal transduction. ProcNatlAcadSci USA 1993; 90: 8429–8433.

[89] Sozeri O, Vollmer K, Liyanage M, Frith D, Kour G, Mark III GE et al. Activation of the c-Raf protein kinase by protein kinase C phosphorylation. Oncogene 1992; 7: 2259–2262.

[90] Staal SP. Molecular cloning of the akt oncogene and its human homologues AKT1 and AKT2: amplification of AKT1 in a primary human gastric adenocarcinoma. ProcNatlAcadSci USA 1987;84: 5034–5037.

[91] Staal SP, Huebner K, Croce CM, Parsa NZ, Testa JR. The AKT1proto-oncogene maps to human chromosome 14, band q32. Genomics 1988; 2: 96–98.

[92] Stirewalt DL, Kopecky KJ, Meshinchi S, Appelbaum FR, Slovak ML, Willman CL et al. FLT3, RAS, and TP53 mutations in elderly patients with acute myeloid leukemia. Blood 2001; 97:3589-3595.

[93] Stirewalt DL, Radich JP. The role of FLT3 in hemopoietic malignancies. Nat Rev Cancer 2003;3:650-665.

[94] Tabe Y, Jin L, Tsutsumi-Ishii Y, Xu Y, McQueen T, Priebe W, Mills GB, Ohsaka A, Nagaoka I, Andreeff M, Konopleva M. Activation of integrin-linked kinase is a critical prosurvival pathway induced in leukemic cells by bone marrow-derived stromal cells. Cancer Res 2007;67:684–694.

[95] Takebayashi T, Higashi H, Sudo H, Ozawa H, Suzuki E, Shirado O, et al.NF-kB-dependent induction of cyclin D1 by retinoblastoma protein (pRB) family proteins and tumor derived pRB mutants. J BiolChem 2003;278:14897-14905.

[96] Tamburini J, Elie C, Bardet V, Chapuis N, Park S, Broet P, Cornillet-Lefebvre P, Lioure B, Ugo V, Blanchet O, Ifrah N, Witz F, et al. Constitutive phosphoinositide 3-kinase/Akt activation represents a favorable prognostic factor in de novo acute myelogenousleukemia patients. Blood 2007;110:1025–1028.

[97] Tang ED, Nunez G, Barr FG, Guan KL. Negative regulation of the forkhead transcription factor FKHR by Akt. J BiolChem 1999; 274: 16741–16746.

[98] Tanoue T, Maeda R, Adachi M, Nishida E. Identification of a docking groove on ERK and p38 MAP kinases that regulates the specificity of docking interactions. EMBO J 2001; 20:466–479.

[99] Tazzari PL, Cappellini A, Ricci F, Evangelisti C, Papa V, Grafone T, Martinelli G, Conte R, Cocco L, McCubrey JA, Martelli AM. Multidrug resistance-associated protein 1 expression is under the control of the phosphoinositide 3 kinase/Akt signal transduction network in human acute myelogenousleukemia blasts. Leukemia 2007;21:427–438.

[100] Tefferi A. Novel mutations and their functional and clinical relevance in myeloproliferative neoplasms: JAK2, MLP, TET2, ASXL1,CBL, IDH and IKZF1. Leukemia. 2010;24:1128-1138.

[101] Testa U, Grignani F, Samoggia P, Zanetti C, Riccioni R, Lo Coco F, et al. The PML/RARa fusion protein inhibits tumor necrosis factor-a-induced apoptosis in U937 cells and acute promyelocyticleukemia blasts. J Clin Invest 1998;101:2278-2289.

[102] Testa U and Riccioni R. Deregulation of apoptosis in acute myeloid leukemia. Haematologica. 2007;92(1):81-94.

[103] Turkson J, Bowman T, Garcia R, Caldenhoven E, de Groot RP, Jove R. Stat3 activation by Src induces specific gene regulation and is required for cell transformation. Mol Cell Biol. 1998;18:2545–2552

[104] Wang HG, Rapp UR, Reed JC. Bcl-2 targets the protein kinase Raf-1 to mitochondria. Cell 1996; 87: 629–638.

[105] Whitman SP, Archer KJ, Feng L. Absence of the wild-type allele predicts poor prognosis in adult de novo acute myeloid leukemia with normal cytogenetics and the internal tandem duplication of FLT3: a cancer and leukemia group B study. Cancer Res 2001;61: 7233-7239.

[106] Whitman SP, Maharry K, Radmacher MD, Becker H, Mrózek K, Margeson D, Holland KB, Wu YZ, Schwind S, Metzeler KH, Wen J, Baer MR, Powell BL, Carter TH, Kolitz JE, Wetzler M, Moore JO, Stone RM, Carroll AJ, Larson RA, Caligiuri MA, Marcucci G, Bloomfield CD. FLT3 internal tandem duplication associates with adverseoutcome and gene- and microRNA-expression signatures in patients 60 years of age or older with primary cytogenetically normal acute myeloid leukemia: a Cancer and Leukemia Group B study. Blood. 2010;116(18):3622-3266.

[107] Wojnowski L, Zimmer AM, Beck TW, Hahn H, Bernal R, Rapp UR, Zimmer A. Endothelial apoptosis in Braf-deficient mice. Nat Genet 1997; 16: 293–297.

[108] Wu J, Dent P, Jelinek T, Wolfman A, Weber MJ, Sturgill TW. Inhibition of the EGF-activated MAP kinase signaling pathway by adenosine 30,50-monophosphate. Science 1993; 262: 1065–1069.

[109] Wullschleger S, Loewith R, Hall MN. TOR signaling in growth and metabolism. Cell. 2006 Feb 10;124(3):471-484.

[110] Xu Q, Simpson SE, Scialla TJ, Bagg A, Carroll M. Survival of acute myeloid leukemia cells requires PI3 kinase activation. Blood 2003;102:972–980.

[111] Yu H, Jove R. The STATs of cancer—new molecular targets come of age. Nat Rev Cancer. 2004; 4:97–105.

[112] Zhou BP, Liao Y, Xia W, Zou Y, Spohn B, Hung MC. HER-2/neu induces p53 ubiquitination via Akt-mediated MDM2 phosphorylation. Nat Cell Biol 2001; 3: 973–982.

[113] Zeng Z, Shi YX, Samudio IJ, Wang RY, Ling X, Frolova O, Levis M, Rubin JB, Negrin RR, Estey EH, Konoplev S, Andreeff M, et al. Targeting the leukemia microenvironment by CXCR4 inhibition overcomes resistance to kinase inhibitors and chemotherapy in AML. Blood 2009;113:6215–6224.

[114] Zheng X, Beissert T, Kukoc-Zivojnov N, Puccetti E, Altschmied J, Strolz C, et al. -catenin contributes to leukemogenesis induced by AML-associated translocation products by increasing the self renewal of very primitive progenitor cells. Blood 2004;103:3535-3543.

9

Myeloid Leukemia: A Molecular Focus on Etiology and Risk Within Africa

Muntaser E. Ibrahim and Emad-Aldin I. Osman
Department of Molecular Biology, Institute of Endemic Diseases,
University of Khartoum, Khartoum,
Sudan

1. Introduction

The developing world, Africa included, is witnessing an alarming upsurge of cancer incidence. The annual number of new cancer cases is expected to double by 2020 and up to 70% of the 20 million new cases of cancer predicted to occur yearly will be in the developing world (Jones et al., 1999; Ferlay et al., 2003; Yach et al., 2004).

One startling disparity, however, between cancer in the developing and developed worlds is that although the overall incidence of cancer in the developing world is half of that observed in the developed world, survival rates in the developing world are often less than one third of site-specific cancers in the developed world (Sener et al., 2005). This emphasizes the duality of the cancer problem in Africa, for being largely a disease of modern life style, occurring against a background of socio-economic disparities and greater burden of communicable diseases.

The study of genetic epidemiology of cancers in Africa hence entails the study of peculiar features of gene-environment interaction that may be largely private to Africa. In addition to the state of socio-economic underdevelopment that applies almost to the majority of African states, there is the plethora of extreme environments, wide range of climatic conditions and cultures, but most of all the transition state of the African communities from rural subsistent into urban market oriented life style. Furthermore one has to consider the notorious prevalence of infectious and non infectious diseases that may have a bearing both on the initiation of myeloid leukemia, its prognosis and management, e.g. tuberculosis (Omoti et al., 2009), malaria, other chronic infections, sickle cell disease (Ahmed et al., 2008) and common adaptive traits that could modulate the course of the disease, as well as the role of oncogenic viruses discussed below.

One interesting example of a potential trade-off between malignancies and parasitic diseases is CD36 a multiligand receptor associated with a broad array of physiological processes, believed to be under selective pressure from *Plasmodium falciparum*, and deficient or polymorphic in several African populations. The role of CD36 in sickle cell crises and cerebral malaria is debatable. As a receptor for thrombospondin 1, CD36 plays a role in the regulation of angiogenesis, which may be a therapeutic strategy for controlling the dissemination of malignant neoplasm. Moreover, it is commonly expressed on blasts in acute monocytic leukemia, megakaryoblastic leukemia, and erythroleukemia (Ge and

Elghetany, 2005). However, CD36 negative AML cells could be found especially in those populations that usually do not express CD36 (like in several African populations). CD36 negative cells appeared less susceptible to trombospondin-1 induced apoptosis, which make leukemic cells less vulnerable to death through this promising therapeutic strategy (Li et al., 2003).

On the other hand, due to the transition state, a number of risk factors believed to represent etiologic determinants of leukemia like use of pesticides, radiation etc. are not yet commonplace in Africa or at least its rural environment and may explain the differential distribution and the focal nature of hematological malignancies in the continent or/and individual countries. The potential impact of transition to a modern life style with the accompanying risks on the emergence and distribution of these diseases is worth our utmost attention.

Cancers in their complex etiology makes an ideal arena for the classical gene versus environment controversy. Those who favor an upper hand for the environment had their views strengthened by results of studies showing that people who migrate from one country to another generally acquire the cancer rates of the new host country, suggesting that environmental or lifestyle factors rather than genetic factors are the key determinants of the international variation in cancer rates. As far as Africa is concerned, African Americans' disease data, represent a working model to test the role of changing environment and the effect of life style in complex diseases. Interestingly both sides of the argument seem to find support. Chronic myeloid leukemia (CML) patients show worse survival for African American and Hispanics compared to Americans of European origin (Lee et al., 2009). Although the difference in ethnicity data might be argued to reflect socio-economic differences, the current advances in genomics enable the implication of particular genomic regions and genes that explain the ethnic differences in susceptibility to infectious and chronic diseases.

Environmental determinants also falls short of explaining neither the "focality" of cancer types nor the aggressive course of some cancers in Sudan like the breast cancer, a feature that has been claimed to exist across Africa and even among African American women (reviewed by Morris and Mitchell, 2008).

Nutritional factors have also been implicated, adding an extra layer of complexity to the desperately compound picture of cancer etiology. Data on nutrition is greatly deficient in Africa similar to other aspects of genetic epidemiology, although differences in nutritional practices and culture may be key in providing vital clues to the contribution of life style. A study in China (Zhang et al., 2008), for example, suggested that a higher intake of green tea is associated with a reduced risk of adult leukemia. Furthermore, a study by Ross et al. which involved 35.221 older women provided evidence that increased vegetable consumption may decrease the risk of adult leukemia (Ross et al., 2002). Moreover, AML risk was negatively associated with milk intake among women and tea, and positively associated among women with beer, wine and beef (Li et al., 2006). A prospective cohort study by Ma et al. (2009) showed that smoking and total meat intake were risk factors for AML and those who did not drink coffee appeared to have a higher risk of AML.

Africa is still contains one of the last and few enclaves on the planet to harbor communities with distinctive patterns of traditional life styles that once used to characterize human existence. Farmers, pastoralists and hunter-gatherers- like societies do preserve their life style and culture and often coexist in shared terrains. These communities adopt fundamentally contrasting life styles and their food cultures are different. The significance of such disparity to all aspects of health and disease is of interest and the study of potential preponderance of these community members to chronic diseases including hematological malignancies should be investigated.

2. Incidence and epidemiology

The lowest rates of leukemia reported in sub-Saharan Africa probably represent failure of diagnosis or reporting to some extent (Davies, 1973; Fleming, 1993 and Parkin et al., 2005). We should therefore use caution, when drawing conclusions based on the varying prevalence and incidence, as an indication of clustering of cases or an environmental or genetic effect, as this may simply be due to the deficiency of statistics in Africa. The disparity could also be a reflection of the research milieu and capacity of individual countries or research groups, which indeed seem to be the case as most of the current reports on leukemia emerges from countries with well established science capacities.

Even with the scattered and available data, however, the difference from European and global trends could be observed as well as the evolution of the problem of leukemia. An early report from Uganda found that African children in Uganda showed a great and genuine deficiency of leukemia and an excess of solid lympho-reticular tumors (Davies et al., 1965).

In subsequence, the situation seems to change, a study of pediatric leukemia in Cameroon, showed that Acute Lymphoblastic Leukemia (ALL) comprised 78.6%, while AML 21.4% of all pediatric acute leukemia (Obama et al., 1995). In Egypt, the lymphatic and haemopoietic cancer incidence in 2001 have increased approximately 11-fold compared with the incidence in 1972. Moreover, the incidence of leukemia among infant less than 5 years increased exponentially with a higher incidence among boys (Hosny et al., 2002). In Kenya, leukemia in children below the age of 15 years comprised 37% of leukemia in all ages. Childhood acute leukemia formed 52.3% of all the acute leukemia. AML and ALL occurred, in almost equal proportions 42 % and 46 % respectively (Kasili, 1990). In Ethiopia, a report by Shamebo (1990) showed that the commonest type of leukemia was CML 57.8%, acute leukemia and chronic lymphatic leukemia (CLL) accounted for 21.1% each. Of the acute leukemia, 53.3% were ALL while 46.7% were AML (Shamebo, 1990). A recent study in south Nigeria showed that AML comprises 12.3% and CML 23.9% of all leukemia, with a mean age at diagnosis of 25.6 years and 35.2 years respectively (Nwannadi et al., 2011). In the last 25 years in Sudan CML became the predominant cancer in men, while lymphomas remained the second most common cancer. In women, breast, cervical and ovarian cancer remained the three most common cancers over both time periods, but there was also an increase in the incidence of CML among women (Hamad, 2006), the causes of this high incidence of CML are not known.

In Europe AML presents as mainly an adult's disease with a median age at presentation of 64 years, accounting for around 30% of all leukemia in adults, and ~18 000 new patients are diagnosed in Europe each year, representing ~0.6% of all cancers. The annual incidence rate in Europe ranges from two per 100 000/year to four per 100 000/year. In the past decade, the trend in overall incidence of AML has generally been stable or slowly increasing in most European countries, while most cases of CML occur in adults with a median age at presentation around age 60. CML comprises only around 2%–3% of all the leukemia diagnosed in patients <20 years of age but the incidence increases with age slowly until the mid-40s, then more rapidly from about one per 1000 000/year in children <10 years to two per 100 000 in people in the fifth decade to one per 10 000 at age 80. The disease is more common in males. There is no clear evidence of to geographic or ethnic background that predisposes to CML; however, in the United States the incidence is slightly higher in Caucasians than in Blacks or Hispanics (Lee et al., 2009), and it exhibits a male preponderance, in South African Coloured and Black people, and African Americans in comparison to whites but the reason for this is unexplained. (Jacobs et al., 1983). Furthermore, several reports showed an increased incidence of CML during the first 2 decades of life in African subjects (Haddock , 1967; Lowe et al., 1971; Lowenthal et al., 1975), but other reports by Leibowitz et al., (1976) and Jacobs et al., (1983) disagree with this. Jacobs et al. reported that in comparison with Whites and Coloureds, however, the peak incidence for Blacks was lower, lying between the 3rd and 4th decades. The peak incidence for Coloureds was in the 4th and 5th decades, and that for Whites in the 5th and 6th (Jacobs et al., 1983.)

An interesting study in United Arab Emirate (UAE) found that the rate of AML among UAE female nationals was higher than in nationals male and expatriates. The study proposed that chemicals in henna dye, which is used to decorate the body, as well as a lack of sunlight could be behind the increased incidence (Hassan et al., 2009). Henna is applied in many African countries especially Sudan where it is used by vast majority of Sudanese married women.

3. Molecular etiology

Leukemia in common with other cancers arises from mutations in a single cell, which enable the cell to reproduce excessively, emerging as a dominant clone. A large number of different mutant genes contribute to leukaemogenesis singly or, more often, in combination and many are leukemia sub-type specific (Greaves, 1986). The number of genetic abnormalities is believed to reflect the number of genes that control distinct developmental stages of blood formation and the multiple routes to clonal dominance. These include changes not only in proliferative activity, but in ability to differentiate, in resistance to cell death, in DNA repair activity and in general stability of the genes. Whether any particular mutant genes, or hot spots' for mutations within a gene, are linked to particular DNA damaging agents is a topic of considerable relevance to the molecular epidemiology of cancer in general. For these changes to happen some culprit agents has to come into action namely ionizing radiation, chemicals such as polycylic hydrocarbons and certain drugs, and viruses.

The way how these extrinsic factors affect the cell genetically and epigenetically is the core of the functional research in cancer. Although multiple risk factors have been linked to the development of leukemia, however these known risk factors account for only a small number of observed cases. Few epidemiological studies have explored the relation between lifestyle, dietary factors and the incidence of adult Leukemia, and almost none has addressed the molecular and genetic aspects of these interactions.

3.1 Role of viruses
For several reasons pertaining to ecology and the human history in Africa, several pathogens have gained access into human genomes through the African gate. This includes major parasites, viral and bacterial diseases. It is not coincidence that the first well proven

case of viral oncogenesis that of Epstein Barr Virus (EBV) was established in Africa. EBV is a highly prevalent infection in the adult population in Africa and has been associated with a heterogeneous group of lymphomas, including Burkitt's lymphoma (especially the endemic form in Africa), Hodgkin's disease, NK, and T malignancies with cytotoxic phenotypes, and lymphomas in the immune-compromised patient (congenital immunodeficiency, organ transplantation, AIDS). (Rodriguez-Abreu et al., 2007) but not unequivocally with leukemia. Of the oncogenic retroviruses, the Human T-cell leukemia virus (HTLV) type-1 and type-2 have been identified as being related to the development of rare types of leukemia and lymphoma. HTLV-1 is endemic in certain areas including central Africa, and is associated with the development of adult T-cell leukemia or lymphoma (ATLL), which accounts for about half of the lymphoid malignancies in the endemic areas. The virus is transmitted mainly from mother to child, especially by breastfeeding. Sexual transmission and blood transfusion are minor routes of infection and cell-free blood products are not infectious (Rodriguez-Abreu et al., 2007).

The importance of oncogenic viruses stems not only from their transforming oncogenic properties but also from the potential methylating properties of selfish DNA.

Environmental determinant including infection with high-risk viruses are necessary but not sufficient alone in the development of cancer, as most infections regress without intervention. Thus, genetic host factors and cellular immune responses could be potential modifiers for the risk of developing cancer. In particular, p53 and Rb are considered as the most critical tumor suppressor genes involved in regulating cell division. The polymorphism on p53, which encodes either a Proline or an Arginin amino acid residue at codon 72, has been reported as a possible risk factor for several cancers including breast and cervical cancer in Sudan (Eltahir et al, submitted.).

3.2 Population and ethnic diversity

In the last decade the importance of ethnicity, socio-economic and gender differences in relation to disease incidence, diagnosis, and prognosis has been realised. Gender and ethnic differences in these areas should have a focus in health policy in Africa. A study by Lee et al. examined the demographic and clinical features of CML in an ethnically diverse population and found that Hispanic patients present with lower risk profile CML and achieve better treatment responses compared to non-Hispanic patients. The vast majority of their non-Hispanic patients were African American or Asian. This study proposed that biological/genetic factor can contributes to this observed ethnic differences in disease presentation and behavior. Hispanic ethnic group is thought to be the least diverse ethnic group, at the opposite site the African descent is the most diverse ethnic group. African populations are characterized by greater levels of genetic diversity, extensive population substructure, and less linkage disequilibrium (LD) among loci compared to non-African populations (Reich et al., 2001; Campbell and Tishkoff, 2008). Due to the long evolutionary history in Africa there is more genetic diversity within and between populations in the African continent, than between Africans and other peoples in the world (Cavalli-Sforza, 1997). African populations thus vary considerably in their genes. Moreover Africa shows a wide range of environments, climatic, vegetative and zoological. Thus human cancer patters are expected to show a similar degree of diversity, the study of which would contribute to our understanding of their causes.

The majority of cancers as genetic disease of complex nature involve a multiplicity of genetic loci that cooperates to make the disease happen (the multiple -hit theory). It is expected that such genetic component will be influenced by the genetic background of the population at risk. In one of the few studies on a cancer susceptibility genes background mutational profile in different populations, Africans were found to harbor more mutations in their BRCA2 than populations from the rest of the world (Wagner et al., 1999.) which is expected given their larger effective population size.

Africans also possess a number of genetic adaptations that have evolved in response to diverse climates and diets, as well as exposure to infectious disease (Campbell & Tishkoff, 2008), that diversity may carry great challenge in leukemia presentation and behavior/ prognosis and treatment. Moreover, experimental studies using synthetic peptides identical to the BCR-ABL fusion region in CML patients region have revealed the capability of specific peptides to bind to human leukocyte antigen (HLA) class I molecules (HLA-A2, A3, A11, B8) and class II molecules (HLA-DR1, DR2, DR3, DR4 and DR11). Individuals expressing HLA-A3, B8 or DR4 have a diminished risk for the development of CML in Caucasian populations. A statistically significant increase in the frequency of Cw3 and Cw4 antigens in Caucasians and European CML patients has been reported. Another report in Indian population showed that expression of HLA-Cw6 may result in a protective effect on CML acquisition (Chhaya, 2006). A study in Chinese population indicated that the expression of HLA-A*30, DRB1*07 might imply a protective effect on CML acquisition, while B*81 might be associated with CML susceptibility factors in that population (Miao et al., 2007). These results suggest that the development of CML is apparently associated with HLA phenotypes specific to each population. These data is missed in Africa and we intend to investigate this in Sudanese population.

Common polymorphism like the codon 72 in p53 has been argued to unlikely have major genetic effect since polymorphism in loci with major deleterious nature will not be selected for to reach such frequencies unless it is a balanced polymorphism. (i.e. selected for under the influence of the other allele possessing an favorable adaptive trait). Interestingly It has been proposed that the p53 polymorphism at times when the risk of tumors was not a Human concern, gave a reproductive leverage by increasing reproductive success (Kang et al., 2008). The cost of such trade off will not be visible as long as the conditions that predispose for tumors are absent. In fact the derived allele (arginine), almost reached fixation in some populations.

The p53 codon 72 was studied both in normal Sudanese (Bereir et al., 2002) and in the distribution of the polymorphism in different cancers in Sudan, (not including leukemia). The results show that the different alleles pose different risk ratios in different cancer. The Arg allele which is known to be more resistant to cell death was overrepresented breast carcinoma patients from different linguistic groups as compared to controls with an Odd ratio of 19.44 CI 6.6 – 78.3 $P<0.0001$. In cervical cancer the homozygous Arg genotype was detected in 42.3% (33/78) in cervical cancer patients while the heterozygous arg/pro in 38.5% (30/78) and only 19.2% (15/78) had the pro/pro genotype, with an allele effect of 2.4 (CI 1.12 – 5.33, P 0.015). In Burkitt's lymphoma the opposite seems to be true with a major effect from the Pro allele, where the homozygous Arg accounted for only 6.9%, (OR 0.18 CI 0.02 – 0.89, P= 0.018) while the Arg/Pro was 51.7% and pro/pro 41.4% (OR: 0.57, CI 0.23-1.42, P= 0.1). Possibly indicating the different biological pathways of tumorigenesis (Eltahir et al., submitted).

3.3 Gene and chromosomal rearrangements

Cancers as a group of diseases display the entire range of inheritance modes from the single gene like disorder to the complex inheritance pattern seen in chronic diseases. The paucity of genetic investigation in Africa of cancer susceptibility genes and chromosomal aberrations linked to cancer, makes the picture even more opaque. The few examples discussed above and below demonstrate the great relevance of studying the genetic population structure of African populations and establishing the frequencies of the individual SNPs, Ins/dels and chromosomal abnormalities associated with diseases that may be necessary to define the molecular etiological basis of each cancer. In fact both molecular and genetic abnormalities became an important factor for characterising, treating and risk stratifying of myeloid leukemia. In 2002 the WHO classification of Myeloid Neoplasms showed that AML classification includes specific genetic subcategories; thus, determination of genetic features of the neoplastic cells must be performed if possible. Many recurring genetic abnormalities in the myeloid neoplasms can be identified by advanced molecular and cytogenetic techniques. In the WHO classification, the blast threshold for the diagnosis of AML is reduced from 30% to 20% blasts in the blood or marrow. In addition, patients with the clonal, recurring cytogenetic abnormalities t(8;21)(q22;q22), inv(16)(p13q22) or t(16;16)(p13;q22), and t(15;17)(q22;q12) should be considered to have AML regardless of the blast percentage. On the other hand, according to the WHO classification, CML is defined specifically as a myeloproliferative disease that is characterized by the invariable presence of the Philadelphia (Ph) chromosome or the BCR-ABL fusion gene. Although in most cases the diagnosis is easily made from morphologic evaluation of the blood smear, confirmation by genetic studies is essential, particularly in view of the advent of therapy that targets the BCR-ABL fusion protein (Vardiman et al., 2002)

Despite their diagnostic and prognostic values, studies on gene and chromosomal rearrangements associated malignancies is greatly lacking on the African continent, and in spite of the mandatory genotyping of the BCR-ABL as a prerequisite of administering the drug imatinib, in several African countries, there are very few reports on its frequencies. Among the few reports on its association with other leukemias, a multi-country study comprising 181 children with newly diagnosed ALL were tested in laboratories in India, Pakistan, Myanmar, and Sudan, following a common protocol. Across the four countries, the ETV6-RUNX1 (TEL-AML1) fusion gene was present in only 5% of cases. All the positive samples were from children aged 1 to 10 years, in whom the prevalence of this fusion gene, which is associated with good prognosis, was 7.4% (9 out of 121 samples), a much lower rate than reported from Western populations. In the 18 ALL cases tested in Sudan, a notable excess of MLL-AF4 (17%) and BCR-ABL1 (22%) fusion genes was found (Siddiqui et al., 2010).

The significance of studying the frequency of these rearrangements and their relation to pathology, is to establish the level of culpability of the molecular events. A study on Nigerian breast cancer patients suggest that while BRCA1 genomic rearrangement exists, it does not contribute significantly to BRCA1-associated risk in the Nigerian population (Zhang et al., 2011).

Chromosomal translocations in myeloid leukemia yield hybrid RNAs capable of encoding fusion chimeric proteins. The unique amino acid sequences found in these oncogenic fusion proteins represent true tumor-specific antigens that are potentially immunogenic. Although these leukemia-specific fusion proteins have an intracellular location, they might be recognized immunologically by T lymphocytes if peptides derived from the unique sequences are capable of presentation by the major histocompatibility complex (MHC) molecules on Leukemic cells (Bocchia *et al.*, 1995). The ability of a series of synthetic peptides corresponding to the junctional sequences of CML-derived BCR-ABL fusion proteins spanning the b3a2 and b2a2 breakpoints to bind to purified class I molecules was studied by Bocchia *et al.* Four peptides derived from b3a2 CML breakpoint bound with high or intermediate affinity to HLA A3, A11, and B8. None of the CML b2a2 junctional peptides showed affinity of this magnitude for the HLA class I molecules tested. Which draw another important conclusion on the significance of the types of BCR-ABL fusion transcripts among populations in relation to vaccine development? The frequencies of the types of the fusion transcript in Ecuadorian population for example consist of 95% b2a2 (Paz-y-Mino et al., 2002) indicating that they may not benefit much from such vaccine.

Several studies estimated the types of BCR-ABL fusion transcript in CML in different populations. The distribution of transcript type has been studied in European and some other populations (Eisenberg et al., 1988; Lee et al., 1989) with frequencies for b2a2 and b3a2 transcripts being roughly of the order of 40% and 55%, and that for co-expression of b3a2 and b2a2 representing 5% of the cases. A study on an Ecuadorian population, however, registered very different frequencies: 5% for b3a2 and 95% for b2a2 (Paz-y-Mino et al., 2002). In our report in Sudanese patients (Osman et al., 2010), a frequency of 53.5% and 41.9% for b2a2 and b3a2, respectively, was reported, values that are relatively closer to those from a Mexican population (Arana- Trejo et al., 2002). This difference in frequencies may be due to the genetic differences of the populations. Many Controversial reports about the clinical significant of the transcript type in CML were published; however it has a considerable importance in the diagnosis and follow up.

Recently, a polymorphic base in exon 13 of the BCR gene (exon b2 of the major breakpoint cluster region) has been identified in the eighth position before the junctional region of BCR-ABL cDNA. Cytosine replaces thymidine; the corresponding triplets are AAT (T allele) and AAC (C allele), respectively, both coding for asparagine. Therefore, this polymorphism has no implication in the primary structure of BCR and BCR-ABL proteins.

Co-expression of b2a2 and b3a2 transcripts has been linked to two polymorphisms, T to C at exon 13 and A to G at intron 13 (Meissner et al., 1998; Branford et al., 2002). However, in our study by Osman et al. (2010) six PCR products from four patients were sequenced to confirm the products of four b2a2 and two b3a2 and one was found to harbor T to C at exon 13 and expressed only b2a2 transcript which might indicate that this exonic polymorphism is not obligatory for co-expression, as reported by Mondal et al. (2006). Moreover, this polymorphism has no implication on the primary structure of BCR and BCR-ABL proteins. However, since the alteration is located close to the fusion region, it may have a significant influence on the annealing of PCR primers, probes for real time PCR, and antisense oligonucleotides. This polymorphism could be also a useful marker for the differentiation of normal and rearranged BCR alleles in heterozygotes patients and during follow up of minimal residual disease. The allele frequency for this SNP varied markedly between different world populations, with European attaining intermediate values between African and Asians (Table 1)

The molecular basis of CML is well defined and highly consistent, yet prognosis varies considerably. This could reflect the biological diversity occurring in normal populations.

Population	T allele	C allele
African American	0.55	0.45
Sub-Saharan African	0.425	0.575
Asians	0.922	0.078
Chinese	0.91	0.09
Japanese	0.98	0.02
European	0.70	0.30

Data from NCBI/dbSNP/Short Genetic Variations

Table 1. The frequencies of T and C alleles of BCR exon 13 SNP in different populations andethnic groups

The study by Gordon et al 2003 suggest that variation among normal individuals may contribute to inter patient heterogeneity in CML. Differences in behaviour of haemopoietic progenitor cells from different normal individuals may be attributable to genetic diversity or other variables. de Haan et al. (2002) concluded that the expression levels of a large number of genes might be responsible for controlling stem cell behaviour. These collections of genes may be analogous to those responsible for the inter-individual diversity in progenitor cell behaviour

In CML, the occurrence of additional specific cytogenetic and molecular changes subsequent to the initiation of t(9;22) translocation herald disease progression prior to haematologic and clinical manifestation. These events occur in 50 to 80 percent of patients during the transition from the chronic phase of the disease to the accelerated and blast phases. Minor cytogenetic changes include monosomies of chromosomes 7, 17, and Y; trisomies of chromosomes 17 and 21; and translocation t(3;21)(q26;q22) (Mitelman, 1993). Major changes include trisomy 8, isochromosome i(17q), trisomy 19, and an extra Ph chromosome (double Ph). Trisomy 8 is most common, and isochromosome i(17q) occurs almost exclusively in the myeloid type blast phase (Kantarjian et al., 1987; Derderian et al., 1993; Mitelman, 1993).

Molecular abnormalities may correspond to cytogenetic changes. These include abnormalities in p53 (on chromosome 17p13); RB1 (13q14); c-MYC (8q24); p16INK4A (9p21); RAS; and AML–EVI-1, a fusion protein resulting from translocation t(3;21) (q26;q22). Alterations of p53 (deletions, rearrangements, and mutations) occur in 20 to 30 percent of patients with CML in the blast phase (Ahuja et al.,1989) and are associated exclusively with myeloid transformation (Stuppia et al., 1997), whereas abnormalities of RB1 are associated more with lymphoid transformation, although the association is weaker than it was between p53 and myeloid transformation. Mutations of p53 in the progression of CML are associated with an aberrant methylation status of CML cells (Guinn et al., 1997). The introduction of a methyl group causing transcriptional silencing of the calcitonin gene has been found in the transition of chronic-phase CML to blast-phase CML (Malinen et al., 1991). Altered methylation was also described within the M-bcr of cells from patients with chronic-phase CML (Litz et al., 1996). Up to 50 percent of patients with lymphoid transformation have homozygous deletion of p16INK4A (Sill et al., 1995). Alterations of RB1, amplifications of c-MYC, and mutations of RAS are less frequent (Faderl et al., 1999).

The genetic variation in Africa is poised to constitute major challenge for diagnosis and management. In a world where the diagnosis and prognosis of diseases and particularly cancer is increasingly dependent on molecular approaches such diversity might constitute a hurdle for future intervention against cancer in general. The anticancer drug imatinib has shown remarkable success in treatment of CML. Though a variety of resistance mechanisms can arise, in the majority of patients resistance coincides with reactivation of the tyrosine kinase activity of the BCR-ABL fusion oncoprotein. This can result from gene amplification and, more importantly, point mutations that disrupt the bind of imatinib to BCR-ABL itself (Nardi et al., 2004). Although there are no indication of resistance so far in Sudan (Alkhatib, 2011), perhaps due to the limited use of the drug, the risk of resistance is proportional to the number of mutations that exist within the kinase domain and even outside the domain which are expected to be higher in Africa given the increased genetic diversity of African populations. The risk of resistance increases with the identification of Novel potential signaling pathways associated with drug resistance (Duy et al., 2011).

The significance of population genetic background extends to diagnostic and prognostic markers that may be applied to populations and to individuals. This is expected to form a trend in the management of diseases of complex inheritance as we learn more of the biological networks in function during diseases and the role of each individual molecule. In a study by Elamin et al., (submitted), aimed at developing biomarkers for breast cancer, Peroxyredoxin V turned to be a potentially useful marker both as a prognostic and treatment marker in Sudanese breast cancer but not among Chinese.

3.4 Drug metabolizing enzymes

The drug metabolizing enzymes system has been shown to influence the susceptibility, sequel and outcome of cancer treatment. These systems include the Glutathione transferases a family member of genes encoding enzymes involved in the metabolism of many chemicals and shown to be polymorphic with *GSTM1* and *GSTT1* being deleted in proportion of individuals where in the homozygous state results in a phenotypic absence of the corresponding enzyme. These enzymes are considerably important in the detoxification of many environmental compounds and reactive oxygen species, and hence may constitute important cancer predisposition genes.

It includes also the cytochrome P450 enzymes one of the best studied for risk association with cancer (Aqundez, 2004). The P450 shows conflicting and variable degree of association with cancer, possibly reflecting, variation in the role played by these enzymes in carcinogenesis and the genetic background of the population.

In some populations like those of the Indian subcontinent, the frequencies of homozygous 3/3 genotype and CYP3A5*3 allele were elevated significantly in the CML group compared to controls (χ^2=93.15, df=2, p=0.0001) (Sailaja et al., 2010).

In India also, a statistically significant difference between an AML group and normal control was observed in the case of glutathione-S-transferase M1 null (odds ratio 3.25, 95% confidence interval 1.9-5.58, P<0.001) and N-acetyl transferase 2*6B (odds ratio 3.04, 95% confidence interval 1.79-5.16, P<0.001) genotypes. Combined deficiency of N-acetyl transferase 2 and glutathione-S-transferase M1 genes produced an odds ratio of 11.91 (95% confidence interval 4.06-34.96, P<0.001). Those with glutathione-S-transferase M1 null genotype and N-acetyl transferase 2*6B allele are at increased risk of developing AML, and the risk is considerably enhanced in persons with both glutathione-S-transferase M1 and N-acetyl transferase 2 deficiency (Majumdar et al., 2008).

Increased risk of AML has also been reported for combined polymorphisms in detoxification and DNA repair enzymes (Voso et al., 2007), and patients that achieved complete molecular response following administration of imatinib showed significantly (p=0.013) higher in vivo CYP3A activity than patients achieving partial molecular response (Green et al., 2010).

In Sudan impact of the distribution of the GSTM1 and GSTT1 genotype leukemic patients was studied in 77 leukemic patients and 107 controls by Tagelsir et al., (Submitted). The results suggest that these genotypes could play a role in the development of leukemia particularly AML. Statistical analysis showed a significant preponderance of null genotype of both genes among pooled cases [GSTM1 OR 3.45 (95% CI, 1.65 - 7.19); P = 0.001] for; GSTT1 OR 8.57 (95% CI, 3.68 -19.93); P < 0.0001]. Double null was also higher in patients compared to controls (P = 0.01). When the cases were stratified according to the disease type, AML showed the highest positive predictive value for both loci (GSTM1 P < 0.0001, GSTT1 P < 0.0001), ALL and CLL showed similar patterns for GSTT1 (P = 0.001) while the P-values for GSTM1 were (0.01) and (0.007) respectively. CML displayed the least positive predictive value for GSTM1 (0.02), while for GSTT1 the result was as same as AML (P < 0.0001). Double null, however, showed only association with AML (P < 0.0001).

When the distribution of the GSTM1 and GSTT1 null genotypes were compared between linguistic groups of the control subjects, different percentages were obtained and GSTT1 null genotypes was statistically different between the Afro-Asiatic and the Nilo-Saharan groups (P = 0.01). Difference in frequencies between Africans population is reported; Egyptians 15-29% (Abdel-Rahman, 1996; Hamdy et al., 2003), Tunisians 29% (Hanene et al., 2007) and Zimbabweans 26% (Masimirembwa, et al., 1998). generally speaking the GSTM1 frequency (10.3%) is close to sub-Saharan Africa range; Nigerians 22% (Zhao et al., 1994) and Zimbabweans 24% (Masimirembwa, et al., 1998). while the previously reported frequency from Sudan is 39% (Tiemersma et al., 2001) . Other African populations frequencies are; Egyptians 44-55% [Abdel-Rahman, 1996 Hamdy et al., 2003), Tunisians 50% (Hanene et al., 2007).

The Tagelsir study suggests an increased risk for leukemia associated with GSTM1 and GSTT1 null genotypes and highlights a potential role of genetic make up in leukaemogensis. The most statistically significant association for GSTT1 observed for both AML and CML may highlight a possible role of GSTT1 enzyme in protection of the myeloid series. Allelic variation in the gene encoding the GST isoform theta (GSTT1) enzymes was found to modulate the rate of benzene metabolism and excretion (Rossi et al., 1999) as well as benzene-induced myelotoxicity (Wan et al., 2002; Chen et al., 2007). AML – which showed the strongest association with both genes– comprises a distinct type of leukemia with different subtypes and is shown to be to somewhat associated with environmental exposure. Epidemiological studies have shown association between AML (M2, M4, and M5) and maternal exposure to marijuana and alcohol, and maternal and paternal exposures to pesticides, (Buckley et al., 1989; Robison et al., 1989; Severson et al., 1993; Shu et al., 1996). In addition to that AML is shown to be associated with exposure to benzene and may arise as therapy related complication after treatment of other cancers (Hoffbrand & Pettit, 2001).

Paradoxically, the presence of these genes could not be excluded as a possible risk factor for leukemia as some times these enzymes are involved in bioactivation of some chemicals producing more reactive metabolites that could confer threat to the cell. An example of such risk in other cancer was found in a study on Chinese population which showed that the genotype combination of GSTM1 and GSTT1 double positive confers a 4.2-fold higher risk for developing esophageal cancer and a 2.6-fold for esophageal hyperplasia (Lin et al., 1998).

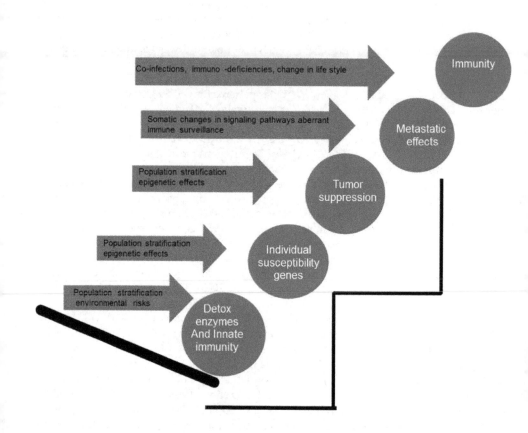

Fig. 1. The ladder and lever mechanism towards carcinogenesis. As the cancer cell struggles through multiple accumulative genetic events leading to cancer (the ladder), the cell will gain the upper hand in its surrounding tissue environment and eventually metastasize, it encounters various modifications and modulating effects that vary between individuals and communities. The variety of effects and the modifier action is expected to be greater in Africa. The up scaling of the ladder requires a lifting effect from the Environment (lever).

3.5 Epigenetics

DNA promoter methylation and histone modification are increasingly recognized as of primary importance in carcinogenesis. The two forms of aberrant methylation, hypomethylation and hypermethylation, are both well documented features of tumor cells (Hanahan and Weinberg, 2000; Jones and Baylin, 2002). The transcriptional silencing of tumor suppressor genes via promoter CpG island hypermethylation constitutes a key tumorigenic process contributing to all the typical hallmarks of a cancer cell that can result from tumor suppressor inactivation. Profiles of tumor suppressor methylation vary according to tumor type (Esteller et al., 2001) and each tumor apparently displays a distinct 'DNA hypermethylation pattern.

Recent studies revealed that specific patterns of DNA methylation characterize AML and help to distinguish AML subtypes. The contribution of this epigenetic dysregulation to leukemogenesis in AML is currently unclear. However, interactions between mutated transcription factors and epigenetic networks have already been shown to be partially responsible for leukemic transformation, for e.g. in acute promyelocytic leukemia (APL). Also, direct mutations in the epigenetic master regulators EZH2 and DNMT3A were recently identified in AML and in diseases leading to secondary leukemia (Schoofs and Muller-Tidow, 2011).

New studies reveal that 20% of individuals with AML harbor somatic mutations in DNMT3A (encoding DNA methyltransferase 3A). Although these leukemia have some gene expression and DNA methylation changes, a direct link between mutant DNMT3A, epigenetic changes and pathogenesis remains to be established.

The disruption of key protective genes through methylation is not confined to tumor suppression, it extends to other vital genes in protection /susceptibility to cancer like drug metabolizing enzymes, as been reported for the glutathione-S-transferase P1 gene silencing (Karius et al., 2011)

4. Future directions

The burden of myeloid leukemia is expected to rise as part of a global trend of increase in cancer incidence. In Africa the cost of this rise given the compound problems of health systems will be devastating. One pressing need is to challenge the preconception of cancer being a disease of the developed societies and show how this image is changing under the rapid sweep of "globalization. Even now the limited data available on leukemia indicate that the incidence of CML in some African countries may exceed those of the industrialized world. The understanding of cancer complex etiology is a prerequisite for successful management and control efforts.

Myeloid leukemia including the chronic subset that behave like a single gene disorder with the predominance of the Ph chromosome, posses complex etiology that includes multiple steps from environmental switches to inactivation of tumor suppression and other guardians of genome integrity and stability and ending with the impact of immune competence. Such complexity renders the handling of each of these potential culprits a daunting task especially in Africa. Without research into the etiology and genetic epidemiology of myeloid leukemia with all possible risk factors considered, including the genetic structure of population at risk, individual genetic effects, role of chronic and concomitant infections, and the possible trade off between infections and malignancies. For diagnosis and management an integrated genomic approach is the way forward. The vision for this approach entails an integrated and automated approach to these analyses, bringing the possibility of formulating an individualized treatment plan within days of a patient's initial presentation. With these expectations comes the hope that such an approach will lead to decreased toxicities and prolonged survival for patients (Godley et al., 2011). Such integrated approaches are expected to meet challenges pertinent to the peculiarity of African genetics.

5. Acknowledgment

The authors acknowledges financial support from the International Centre of Genetic Engineering and Biotechnology (ICGEB)

6. References

Abdel-Rahman SZ, El-zein RA, Anwar WA, Au WW. (1996). A multiplex PCR procedure for polymorphic analysis of GSTM1 and GSTT1 genes in population studies. *Cancer Lett*; 107: 229-33.

Abuidris, D.O., M.E. Ahmed, E.M. Elgaili, & R.S. Arora. (2008). Childhood cancer in Sudan: 1999-2007. *Trop Doct* 38: 208-210.

Ahmed, S.G. & U.A. Ibrahim. (2007). Significance of haemoglobin-S in the pathogenesis of hyperleucocytic syndromes in Nigerian patients with chronic myeloid leukaemia. *Eur J Haematol* 79: 174-176.

Ahuja, H., Bar-Eli, M., Advani, S.H., Benchimol, S. & Cline, M.J. (1989). Alterations in the p53 gene and the clonal evolution of the blast crisis of chronic myelocytic leukemia. Proc Natl Acad Sci U S A, 86:6783-7.

Alkhatib, M.A. (2010). Pattern of pediatric chronic myeloid leukemia in Sudan and hematological response to imatinib. *Pediatr Hematol Oncol* 28: 100-105.

Aplenc, R., T.A. Alonzo, R.B. Gerbing, F.O. Smith, S. Meshinchi, J.A. Ross, J. Perentesis, W.G. Woods, B.J. Lange & S.M. Davies. (2006). Ethnicity and survival in childhood acute myeloid leukemia: a report from the Children's Oncology Group. *Blood* 108: 74-80.

Aqundez J A (2004) Cytochrome P450 gene polymorphisms and cancer. *Curr Drug Metab* 5 (3) 211-24

Arana Trejo, R.M., Ruiz Sanchez, E., Ignacio-Ibarra, G., Baez de la Fuente, E., Garces, O., Gomez Morales, E., Castro Granados, M., Ovilla Martinez, R., Rubio-Borja, M.E., Solis Anaya, L., Herrera, P., Delgado Llamas, J. & Kofman, S. (2002). BCR/ABL p210, p190 and p230 fusion genes in 250 Mexican patients with chronic myeloid leukaemia (CML). *Clin Lab Haematol*, 24, 145-150-.

Bereir R.E.H., Mohamed1 H.S., Seielstad M, El Hassan A.M., Khalil1 E.A.G., Peacock C.S.,. Blackwell J.M & Ibrahim M.E.(2003). Allele frequency and genotype distribution of polymorphisms within disease-related genes is influenced by ethnic population sub-structuring in Sudan. *Genetica* 119: 57–63.

Bocchia, M., Wentworth, P.A., Southwood, S., Sidney, J., McGraw, K., Scheinberg, D.A., & Sette, A. (1995). Specific binding of leukemia oncogene fusion protein peptides to HLA class I molecules. *Blood*, 85, 10, 2680-2684.

Branford, S., T.P. Hughes, & Z. Rudzki. (2002). Dual transcription of b2a2 and b3a2 BCR-ABL transcripts in chronic myeloid leukaemia is confined to patients with a linked polymorphism within the BCR gene. *Br J Haematol* 117: 875-877.

Buckley JD, Robison LL, Swotinsky R, Garabrant DH, LeBeau M, Manchester P, Nesbit ME, Odom L, Peters JM, Woods WG, & Hammond GD.(1989) Occupational exposures of parents of children with acute nonlymphocytic leukemia: a report from the Children's Cancer Study Group. *Cancer Res* 49: 4030-4037.

Campbell, M.C. & S.A. Tishkoff. (2008). African genetic diversity: implications for human demographic history, modern human origins, and complex disease mapping. *Annu Rev Genomics Hum Genet* 9: 403-433.

Cavalli-Sforza, L.L. (1998). The DNA revolution in population genetics. *Trends Genet* 14: 60-65.

Chen Y, Li G, Yin S, Xu J, Ji Z, Xiu X, Liu L, & Ma D. (2007). Genetic polymorphisms involved in toxicant-metabolizing enzymes and the risk of chronic benzene poisoning in Chinese occupationally exposed populations. *Xenobiotica*; 37:103-112.

Chhaya, S.U .(2006). Human leukocyte antigens in Indian patients with chronic myeloid leukemia. *Leuk Lymphoma* 47: 291-295.Davies, J.N. & R. Owor. (1965). Chloromatous Tumours in African Children in Uganda. *Br Med J* 2: 405-407.

Davies, J.N.P. (1973) Childhood tumors. In: Templeton, A.C., ed., Tumors in a Tropical Country *(Recent Results in Cancer Research No. 41)*, Berlin, Springer Verlag

Derderian, P.M., Kantarjian, H.M., Talpaz, M., O'Brien, S., Cork, A., Estey, E., Pierce, S. & Keating, M. (1993). Chronic myelogenous leukemia in the lymphoid blastic phase: characteristics, treatment response, and prognosis. *Am J Med*, 94, 69-74.

Duy C, Hurtz C, Shojaee S, Cerchietti L, Geng H, Swaminathan S, Klemm L, Kweon SM, Nahar R, Braig M, Park E, Kim YM, Hofmann WK, Herzog S, Jumaa H, Koeffler HP, Yu JJ, Heisterkamp N, Graeber TG, Wu H, Ye BH, Melnick A & Müschen M (2011). BCL6 enables Ph+ acute lymphoblastic leukaemia cells to survive BCR-ABL1 kinase inhibition. *Nature*. 19;473(7347):384-8.

Eisenberg, A., R. Silver, L. Soper., Z. Arlin, M. Coleman, B. Bernhardt, & P. Benn.. (1988). The location of breakpoints within the breakpoint cluster region (bcr) of chromosome 22 in chronic myeloid leukemia. *Leukemia*, 2, 642-647.

Elghannam, D.M., N.K. Abousamra, D.A. Shahin, E.F. Goda, H. Azzam, E. Azmy, M.S. El-Din, and M.F. El-Refaei. (2009). Prognostic implication of N-RAS gene mutations in Egyptian adult acute myeloid leukemia. *Egypt J Immunol* 16: 9-15.

Faderl, S., Talpaz, M., Estrov, Z., O'Brien, S., Kurzrock, R. & Kantarjian, H.M. (1999) The biology of chronic myeloid leukemia. *New Engl J Med*, 341(3):164-72.]

Fleming AF (1993). Leukaemias in Africa. *Leukemia*. 7 Suppl 2:S138-41.

Ge, Y. & M.T. Elghetany. (2005). CD36: a multiligand molecule. *Lab Hematol* 11: 31-37.

Gmidene, A., H. Sennana, P. Fenaux, A. Laatiri, M. Zarrouk, H. Bouaziz, I. Harrabi, & A. Saad. (2008). Cytogenetic abnormalities in Tunisian de novo myelodysplastic syndrome: a comparison with other populations. *Leuk Res* 32: 1824-1829.

Godley LA, Cunningham J, Dolan ME, Huang RS, Gurbuxani S, McNerney ME, Larson RA, Leong H, Lussier Y, Onel K, Odenike O, Stock W, White KP & Le Beau MM (2011). An integrated genomic approach to the assessment and treatment of acute myeloid leukemia. *Semin Oncol.* 38(2):215-24.

Gordon, M.Y., S.B. Marley, J.F. Apperley, D. Marin, J. Kaeda, R. Szydlo, and J.M. Goldman. (2003). Clinical heterogeneity in chronic myeloid leukaemia reflecting biological diversity in normal persons. *Br J Haematol* 122: 424-429.

Greaves, M.F. (1993). A natural history for pediatric acute leukemia. *Blood*, 82:1043.

Greaves, M F. (1986). Differentiation-linked leukaemogenesis in lymphocytes. *Science*, 234:697.

Green, H., K. Skoglund, F. Rommel, R.A. Mirghani, & K. Lotfi. (2010) CYP3A activity influences imatinib response in patients with chronic myeloid leukemia: a pilot study on in vivo CYP3A activity. *Eur J Clin Pharmacol* 66: 383-386.

Guinn, B.A. &Mills, K.I. (1997). p53 Mutations, methylation and genomic instability in the progression of chronic myeloid leukaemia. *Leuk Lymphoma*, 26: 221-6.

de Haan, G., Bystrykh, L.V., Weersing, E., Dontje, B., Geiger, H., Ivanova, N., Lemischka, I., Vellenga, E. & Van Zant, G. (2002). A genetic and genomic analysis identifies a cluster of genes associated with hematopoietic cell turnover. Blood, 100, 2056-2062.

Haddock, D.R. (1967). The pattern of leukaemia in Accra, Ghana. *J Trop Med Hyg* 70: 60-62.

Hamad, H.M. (2006). Cancer initiatives in Sudan. *Ann Oncol* 17 Suppl 8: viii32-viii36.

Hamdy SI, Hiratsuka M, Narahara K, Endo N , El-Enany M , Moursi N , Ahmed MS-E & Mizugaki M. (2003). Genotype and allele frequencies of TPMT, NAT2, GST, SULT1A1 and MDR-1 in the Egyptian population. *British J Clin Pharmacol*; 55:560-569.

Hanahan D, & Weinberg RA. (2000) The Hallmarks of Cancer. *Cell* 100, 57-70.

Hanene C, Jihene L, Jamel A, Kamel H & Agnès H (2007) Association of *GST* Genes Polymorphisms with Asthma in Tunisian Children. *Mediators Inflamm* 2007:19564.

Hassan, I.B., S.I. Islam, H. Alizadeh, J. Kristensen, A. Kambal, S. Sonday, & R.M. Bernseen. (2009). Acute leukemia among the adult population of United Arab Emirates: an epidemiological study. *Leuk Lymphoma* 50: 1138-1147.

Hoffbrand AV, Pettit JE & Moss PAH (2001) Essential haematology. 4th edition, Blackwell science Inc.

Hosny, G. and S.M. Elkaffas. (2002). Patterns in the incidence of pediatric cancer in Alexandria, Egypt, from 1972 to 2001. *J Egypt Public Health Assoc* 77: 451-468.

Jacobs, P., H.S. King, and D.M. Dent. (1983). Chronic granulocytic leukaemia. A 10-year experience in the Black, Coloured and White populations of the south-western Cape Province. *S Afr Med J* 63: 879-882.

Jones SB (1999). Cancer in the developing world: a call to action. *BMJ*. 21;319(7208):505-8.

Jones PA & Baylin SB. (2002) The fundamental role of epigenetic events in cancer. *Nat Rev Genet*. 3(6):415-28..

Kang HJ, Feng Z, Sun Y, Atwal G, Murphy ME, Rebbeck TR, Rosenwaks Z, Levine AJ & Hu W (2009). Single-nucleotide polymorphisms in the p53 pathway regulate fertility in humans. *Proc Natl Acad Sci U S A*. 16;106(24):9761-6.

Kantarjian, H.M., Keating, M.J., Talpaz, M., Walters, R.S., Smith, T.L., Cork, A., McCredie, K.B. & Freireich, E.J. (1987). Chronic myelogenous leukemia in blast crisis. Analysis of 242 patients. *Am J Med*, 83, 445-454.

Kasili. E. G. (1990). Childhood Leukaemia: Is it a Problem in Tropical Africa? *Leukemia & Lymphoma*, Vol. 1, No. 3-4 , 187-193

Lee, M.S., LeMaistre, A., Kantarjian, H.M., et al. (1989). Detection of two alternative bcr/abl mRNA junctions and minimal residual disease in Philadelphia chromosome positive chronic myelogenous leukemia by polymerase chain reaction. *Blood*, 73, 2165-2170.

Lee, J.P., E. Birnstein, D. Masiello, D. Yang, & A.S. Yang. (2009). Gender and ethnic differences in chronic myelogenous leukemia prognosis and treatment response: a single-institution retrospective study. *J Hematol Oncol* 2: 30.

Leibowitz, M.R., D.P. Derman, R. Jacobson, K. Stevens, & J. Katz. (1976). Chronic myeloid leukaemia in South African blacks. *S Afr Med J* 50: 2035-2037.

Li, K., M. Yang, P.M. Yuen, K.W. Chik, C.K. Li, M.M. Shing, H.K. Lam, & T.F. Fok. (2003). Thrombospondin-1 induces apoptosis in primary leukemia and cell lines mediated by CD36 and Caspase-3. *Int J Mol Med* 12: 995-1001.

Li, Y., K.B. Moysich, M.R. Baer, J.R. Weiss, J. Brasure, S. Graham, and S.E. McCann. (2006). Intakes of selected food groups and beverages and adult acute myeloid leukemia. *Leuk Res* 30: 1507-1515.Lin D, Tang Y & Lu S. (1998) Glutathione S-transferase M1, T1 genotypes and the risk of esophageal cancer: a case-control study. *Chung Hua Liu Hsing Ping Hsueh Tsa Chih*; 19 :195-199.

Litz, C.E., Vos, J.A., Copenhaver, C.M. (1996). Aberrant methylation of the major breakpoint cluster region in chronic myeloid leukemia. *Blood* 88:2241-9.

Lowe, R.F. (1971). Chronic myelocytic leukaemia in African children. *Trans R Soc Trop Med Hyg* 65: 840-841.

Lowenthal, M.N. (1975). Chronic myeloid leukaemia in Zambians. *Trop Geogr Med* 27: 132-136.

Ma, X., Y. Park, S.T. Mayne, R. Wang, R. Sinha, A.R. Hollenbeck, A. Schatzkin & A.J. Cross (2009). Diet, lifestyle, and acute myeloid leukemia in the NIH-AARP cohort. *Am J Epidemiol* 171: 312-322.

Malinen, T., Palotie, A., Pakkala, S., Peltonen, L., Ruutu, T., Jansson, S.E. (1991). Acceleration of chronic myeloid leukemia correlates with calcitonin gene hypermethylation. *Blood* , 77, 2435-40

Majumdar, S., B.C. Mondal, M. Ghosh, S. Dey, A. Mukhopadhyay, S. Chandra, and U.B. Dasgupta. (2008). Association of cytochrome P450, glutathione S-transferase and N-acetyl transferase 2 gene polymorphisms with incidence of acute myeloid leukemia. *Eur J Cancer Prev* 17: 125-132.

Masimirembwa CM, Dandara C, Sommers DK, Snyman JR & Hasler JA. (1998) Genetic polymorphism of cytochrome P4501A1, microsomal epoxide hydrolase, and glutathione S-transferases M1 and T1 in Zimbabweans and Venda of Southern Africa. *Pharmacogenetics*; 8:83-85.

Meissner, R.V., P.M. Dias, D.T. Covas, F. Job, M. Leite, & N.B. Nardi. (1998). A polymorphism in exon b2 of the major breakpoint cluster region (M-bcr) identified in chronic myeloid leukaemia patients. *Br J Haematol* 103: 224-226.

Miao, K.R., Q.Q. Pan, M. Xue, S. Fan, X.Y. Wang, M. Pan, X.Y. Zhou, X.M. Fei, X. Zhao, and C.Y. Wang. (2007). Human leukocyte antigens in 295 Chinese patients with chronic myeloid leukemia. *Leuk Lymphoma* 48: 2152-2156.

Mitelman, F. (1993). The cytogenetic scenario of chronic myeloid leukemia. *Leuk Lymphoma*, 11, Suppl 1, 11-15.

Mondal, B.C., A. Bandyopadhyay, S. Majumdar, A. Mukhopadhyay, S. Chandra, U. Chaudhuri, P. Chakrabarti, S. Bhattacharyya, and U.B. Dasgupta. (2006). Molecular profiling of chronic myeloid leukemia in eastern India. *Am J Hematol* 81: 845-849.

Morris GJ and Mitchell EP (2008) Higher incidence pof aggressive breast cancers in African – American women; a review. *J Natl Med Assoc.* 100 (6): 698-702.

Nardi V, Azam M, Daley GQ. (2004 Jan). Mechanisms and implications of imatinib resistance mutations in BCR-ABL. *Curr Opin Hematol.*;11(1):35-43.

Nwannadi, O. Alao, G. Bazuaye, M. Nwagu & M. Borke (2011). Clinical and Laboratory Characteristics of Patients with Leukaemia in South-South Nigeria. *The Internet Journal of Oncology*.7 (2)

Obama, M.T., L. Zekeng, P.K. Ketchiozo, M.B. Owono, B.T. Kouam, & J. Mbede. (1995). Childhood leukemia is still a deadly disease in Yaounde, Cameroon: a report of 14 cases. *Pediatr Hematol Oncol* 12: 301-304.

Omoti, C.E., A.N. Olu-Eddo, & A.I. Nwannadi. (2009). Co-existence of TB and adult haematological cancers in Benin City, Nigeria. *Trop Doct* 39: 205-207.

Osman, E.A., K. Hamad, I.M. Elmula, & M.E. Ibrahim. (2010) Frequencies of BCR-ABL1 fusion transcripts among Sudanese chronic myeloid leukaemia patients. *Genet Mol Biol* 33: 229-231.

Parkin, D.M., F. Bray, J. Ferlay, and P. Pisani. (2005). Global cancer statistics, 2002. *CA Cancer J Clin* 55: 74-108.

Paz-y-Mino, C., Burgo, R., Morillo, S.A., Santos, J.C., Fiallo, B.F. & Leone, P.E. (2002). BCR-ABL rearrangement frequencies in chronic myeloid leukemia and acute lymphoblastic leukemia in Ecuador, South America. *Cancer Genet Cytogenet*, 132, 65–67.

Reich DE, Cargill M, Bolk S, Ireland J, Sabeti PC, Richter DJ, Lavery T, Kouyoumjian R, Farhadian SF, Ward R, Lander ES.(2001).Linkage disequilibrium in the human genome. *Nature.* 10;411:199-204.

Robison LL, Buckley JD, Daigle AE, Wells R, Benjamin D, Arthur DC, Hammond GD. (1989) Maternal drug use and risk of childhood nonlymphoblastic leukemia among offspring. An epidemiologic investigation implicating marijuana (a report from the Children's Cancer Study Group). *Cancer*63:1904–1911.

Rodriguez-Abreu, D., A. Bordoni, & E. Zucca. (2007). Epidemiology of hematological malignancies. *Ann Oncol* 18 Suppl 1: i3-i8.

Ross, J.A., C.M. Kasum, S.M. Davies, D.R. Jacobs, A.R. Folsom, & J.D. Potter. (2002). Diet and risk of leukemia in the Iowa Women's Health Study. *Cancer Epidemiol Biomarkers Prev* 11: 777-781.

Rossi AM, Guarnieri C, Rovesti S, Gobba F, Ghittori S, Vivoli G & Barale R. (1999). Genetic polymorphisms influence variability in benzene metabolism in humans. *Pharmacogenetics*. 9: 445–451.

Sailaja, K., D.N. Rao, D.R. Rao, & S. Vishnupriya. (2010) Analysis of CYP3A5*3 and CYP3A5*6 gene polymorphisms in Indian chronic myeloid leukemia patients. *Asian Pac J Cancer Prev* 11: 781-784.

Schoofs T & Müller-Tidow C (2011). DNA methylation as a pathogenic event and as a therapeutic target in AML Cancer Treat Rev.

Sener SF & Grey N (2005).The global burden of cancer.*J Surg Oncol*. 1;92(1):1-3.

Severson RK, Buckley JD, Woods WG, Benjamin D & Robison LL. (1993) Cigarette smoking and alcohol consumption by parents of children with acute myeloid leukemia: an analysis within morphological subgroups—a report from the Children's Cancer Group. *Cancer Epidemiol Biomark Prev*; 2: 433– 439.

Shamebo. M. (1990). Leukaemia in adult Ethiopians. *Ethiop Med J*, 28(1): 31-7

Shu XO, Ross JA, Pendergrass TW, Reaman GH, Lampkin B & Robison LL. (1996). Parental alcohol consumption, cigarette smoking, and risk of childhood leukemia: a Children's Cancer Group study. *J Natl Cancer Inst* 88: 24–31.

Siddiqui R, Nancy N, Naing WP, Ali S, Dar L, Khan BK, Padua RA & Carr R. (2010) Distribution of common genetic subgroups in childhood acute lymphoblastic leukemia in four developing countries. *Cancer Genet Cytogenet*. 200 (2):149-53.

Sill H, Goldman JM &Cross NCP. (1995). Homozygous deletions of the p16 tumor-suppressor gene are associated with lymphoid transformation of chronic myeloid leukemia. *Blood*;85:2013-6.

Stuppia L, Calabrese G, Peila R, et al. (1997). p53 Loss and point mutations are associated with suppression of apoptosis and progression of CML into myeloid blast crisis. *Cancer Genet Cytogenet*;98:28-35.

Tiemersma EW, Omer RE, Bunschoten A, Veer P, Kok FJ, Idris MO, Kadaru AMY, Fedail SS & Kampman E. (2001) Role of Genetic Polymorphism of Glutathione-*S*-Transferase *T1* and Microsomal Epoxide Hydrolase in Aflatoxin-associated Hepatocellular Carcinoma. *Can Epidemiol Biomar Preven* . 10: 785–791.

Vardiman, J.W., N.L. Harris, & R.D. Brunning. (2002). The World Health Organization (WHO) classification of the myeloid neoplasms. *Blood* 100: 2292-2302.

Voso MT, Fabiani E, D'Alo' F, Guidi F, Di Ruscio A, Sica S, Pagano L, Greco M, Hohaus S & Leone G. (2007). Increased risk of acute myeloid leukaemia due to polymorphisms in detoxification and DNA repair enzymes. *Ann Oncol*. 18(9):1523-8

Wagner TM, Hirtenlehner K, Shen P, Moeslinger R, Muhr D, Fleischmann E, Concin H, Doeller W, Haid A, Lang AH, Mayer P, Petru E, Ropp E, Langbauer G, Kubista

E, Scheiner O, Underhill P, Mountain J, Stierer M, Zielinski C & Oefner P. (1999). Global sequence diversity of BRCA2: analysis of 71 breast cancer families and 95 control individuals of worldwide populations. *Hum Mol Genet.* 8(3):413-23.

Wan J, Shi J, Hui L, Wu D, Jin X, Zhao N, Huang W, Xia Z & Hu G. (2002) Association of genetic polymorphisms in CYP2E1, MPO, NQO1, GSTM1, and GSTT1 genes with benzene poisoning. *Envirom Health Perspect* . 110: 1213–1218.

Yach D, Hawkes C, Gould CL & Hofman KJ (2004) The global burden of chronic diseases: overcoming impediments to prevention and control. *JAMA*.2;291(21):2616-22.

Zhang, M., X. Zhao, X. Zhang, & C.D. Holman. (2008). Possible protective effect of green tea intake on risk of adult leukaemia. *Br J Cancer* 98: 168-170.

Zhang J, Fackenthal JD, Huo D, Zheng Y & Olopade OI. (2010). Searching for large genomic rearrangements of the BRCA1 gene in a Nigerian population. *Breast Cancer Research and Treatment* 124, 2: 573-577.

Zhao L, Alldersea J, Fryer A, Tighe A, Oilier B, Thomson W, Jones P & Strange R (1994) Polymorphism at the glutathione S-transferase *GSTMI* locus: a study of the frequencies of the GSTMI A, B, A/B and null phenotypes in Nigerians. *Clin Chim Acta*; 225: 85-88.

10

Epigenetic Changes Associated with Chromosomal Translocation in Leukemia

Soraya Gutierrez[1], Amjad Javed[2], Janet Stein[3],
Gary Stein[3], Sandra Nicovani[4], Valentina Fernandez[1],
Ricardo Alarcon[1], Marcela Stuardo[1], Milka Martinez[1],
Marcela Hinojosa[1] and Boris Rebolledo-Jaramillo[1]
[1]Universidad de Concepcion, Departamento de Bioquimica y Biologia Molecular,
[2]University of Alabama Department of Oral and Maxillofacial Surgery
[3]University of Massachusetts
[4]Universidad Santo Tomás;
[1,4]Chile,
[2,3]USA

1. Introduction

Chromosome translocation reflects an abnormality caused by rearrangement of DNA fragments between non-homologous chromosomes. These rearrangements can be visualized by cytogenetic analysis of affected cells. Non-random chromosomal translocations are frequently associated with a variety of cancers, particularly hematological malignancies and childhood sarcomas although recent evidence demonstrates that such translocations are also common in epithelial tumors (Aplan, 2006; Mitelman et al., 2005). Initially considered as random events that get selected, it has become increasingly apparent that chromosomal translocations are influenced by cell type, cell stage and genomic context. Most commonly, these non-random chromosomal translocations are associated with specific hematopoietic cell types. Such chromosomal translocations are commonly used as diagnostic tool and are increasingly utilized to guide therapeutic decisions. Although, the mechanism that causes chromosomal translocations remains largely unknown, it is commonly accepted that they arise from DNA double strand breaks (DSBs) that are misrepaired (Aplan, 2006; Digweed and Sperling, 2004; Betti et al., 2003; Povirk, 2006). For a translocation to occur there are several mechanistic factors required: First there needs to be at least two DSBs in different chromosomes. Second the DSBs must arise close enough both in three-dimensional space and in time. Finally, DNA repair pathways must be available to join the two broken DNA fragments to form the translocation. It is estimated that everyday a normal cell in our body is exposed to approximately 20,000 DNA damaging events (Ames and Shigenaga, 1992). A major source of DNA damage is oxygen free radicals; however there are other endogenous and exogenous sources of DNA damage such as replication, transcription, and genotoxic stress. All of these processes can induce DSBs, but for two DNA fragments to be joined they must necessarily come in close proximity of each other (less than 1.3μm) (Chen et al., 1996;

Misteli, 2010). These requirements are accommodated in two competing models to explain DSBs proximity in the nucleus: the position first and the breakage first (Figure 1). The position first model suggests that the DNA regions involved in the translocation are in close proximity before DSBs generation. Support for this model comes from the observation that translocation frequencies differ among tissues and is paralleled by tissue-specific organization of the involved chromosomes (Mitelman et al., 2007). For example, the frequency of c-myc translocations to IgH, Igκ, or Igλ locus in Burkitt's lymphomas correlates with reciprocal distance (Roix et al., 2003). In contrast, the breakage first model proposes that DSBs are produced far apart and then move into close proximity to be repaired. In yeast for example, independent DNA lesions move and colocalize in repair factories (Lisby et al., 2003a; Lisby et al., 2003b). In mammalian cells experimental evidence, ranging from no or limited movement to an extensive movement and clustering of these DSBs breaks, provides support for both models (Kruhlak et al., 2006).

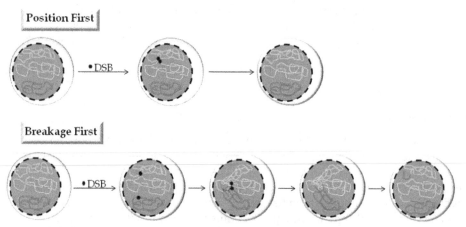

Fig. 1. **Models for Chromosomal Translocation Formation.** In the position first model two DSB that are nearby in the nuclei can be erroneously repair and give rise to a chromosomal translocation. In the breakage first model two DSB that are far apart in the nuclei are brought close together, probably to be repaired, resulting in a translocation.

In eukaryotic cells, DSBs are repaired by two different repair pathways: homologous recombination (HR) and non-homologous end joining (NHEJ) (Figure 2). HR is a relative error-free repair pathway that required information from a template sequence to repair the damage. This pathway is active during S and G2 phases of the cell cycle when the sister chromatid template is easily available and it can also take place during both mitosis and meiosis. NHEJ is a template independent DSBs repair mechanism. It is an error-prone pathway active throughout the cell cycle and the most commonly used DBSs repair pathway in multicellular eukaryotes. NHEJ is subdivided in classical (C-NHEJ) and alternate (A-NHEJ). The C-NHEJ is responsible for individual intrachromosomal DSBs repair in an homology independent manner, while A-NHEJ works in a micro-homology dependent manner, is more error-prone and seems to be the primary pathway responsible for the generation of chromosomal translocations (Simsek and Jasin, 2010; Boboila et al., 2010).

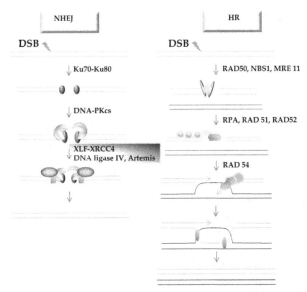

Fig. 2. **DNA Double Strand Break Repair Pathways**. Schematic representation of the two main DNA repair pathways: non homologous end joining (NHEJ) and homologous recombination (HR). The key regulatory proteins involved at multiple stages of each pathway are indicated.

Most of the chromosome translocations that have been analyzed to date show no consistent homologous sequences at the breakpoints regions. However, several structural features like DNase I hypersensitivity, topoisomerase II cleavage sites, DNA fragile sites and matrix or scaffold attachment regions (MARs or SARs) often colocalize with the mapped breakpoints. These observations suggest that chromatin organization may play a role in generation of translocations (Zhang et al., 2002; Strissel et al., 1998; Tanabe et al., 1996; Felix et al., 1995; Stanulla et al., 1997; Zhang and Rowley, 2006). Moreover, chromatin organization also has a prominent role in DNA repair process and therefore may influence both the selection of a DNA repair pathway and the eventual outcome of the DNA repair (Fernandez-Capetillo et al., 2004; Verger and Crossley, 2004; Tsukuda et al., 2005; Murr et al., 2006; Falk et al., 2008; Falk et al., 2010; Misteli and Soutoglou, 2009). Here we will focus on the current knowledge of the role that genomic structural features may have on formation of chromosomal translocations. Particularly we will analyze epigenetic marks associated with chromosome breakpoint regions and unusual DNA conformations among other structural features that may alter genomic structural stability.

2. Higher-order genome organization and translocations

The higher order organization of genomes architecture during interphase of the cell cycle forms chromosomes territories; which are defined as the nuclear space occupied by the DNA of a given chromosome (Cremer and Cremer, 2001; Cremer et al., 2006; Meaburn and Misteli, 2007; Misteli, 2007). Individual chromosomes are organized into open and closed chromatin domains that occupy different spatial compartments. A similar concept of nonrandom nuclear positioning applies to single loci and may be relevant to their translocation potential. For example the BCR and ABL genes, located on chromosomes 9 and 22, whose translocation leads to formation of a fusion protein involved in leukemia, are located in close proximity in normal hematopoietic cells at much higher frequency than would be expected based on a random distribution (Lukasova et al., 1997; Neves et al., 1999; Bartova et al., 2000). The same is true for the human chromosomes 12 and 16, which are frequently translocated in liposarcoma and are found in close proximity in differentiated adipocytes (Kuroda et al., 2004). Similarly, the frequency of c-myc translocations to IgH, Igκ or Igλ locus in Burkitt's lymphomas correlates with reciprocal nuclear distance. However, it is important to note that clonal oncogenic translocations in tumors are highly selected and therefore cannot be used to unequivocally determine the actual translocation frequency. More unbiased examinations may yet reveal translocations between loci that are not frequently in close proximity. The proximity of two particular loci within the interphase nucleus can be cell-type or tissue-specific. In this context, substantial colocalization of IgH and Igλ occurs in activated splenic B cells but not in embryonic stem cells or thymocytes (Wang et al., 2009). Notably, colocalization with IgH is not a characteristic of the entire chromosome 16 on which Igλ locus resides. In fact, about 15Mb sequences on either side of Igλ do not colocalize; therefore, proximity can be determinant in the context of more narrow areas around specific genes and not with broad chromosome territories.

The internal structure of the chromosomal territories is poorly understood but most probably is formed by a network of looping chromatin fibers. This relatively open structure allows access to gene regulatory factors while simultaneously protect the DNA from the continuous attack of damaging agents. Supporting this view, data from several different loci involved in genomic rearrangements exhibit an altered chromatin conformation in their breakpoint regions. For example, the MLL gene exhibits a strong topoisomerase II cleavage site near exon 12 where genomic breakpoint from therapy related AML (t-AML) patients and infant leukemia patient with MLL translocation have been mapped. Moreover, the same region also exhibit hypersensitivity to DNaseI and is cleaved by S1 and Mung Bean nuclease which specifically recognize and cleave single-strand regions in supercoiled DNA (Strissel et al., 1998; Felix et al., 1995; Stanulla et al., 1997). These features however are not exclusive to MLL gene, as topoisomerase II and DNaseI hypersensitive sites has also been found at the breakpoint regions of AF9, BCL, ABL, RUNX1, ETO and CBP among other genes (Greaves, 1996; Zhang et al., 2002; Strissel et al., 1998; Aplan et al., 1996; Relling et al., 1998; Strick et al., 2006; Sperry et al., 1989). However, not all breakpoint regions identified to date for genes involved in translocations colocalize with either topoisomeraseII cleavage sites or DHS, suggesting that other chromatin structural properties maybe involved in determining the location of chromosome breakage.

3. Chromatin organization and DNA repair

Higher order chromatin structure is not only important for global susceptibility of DNA to damage but may also be relevant for DNA repair. It is well documented that the earliest response to a DSB is the phosphorylation of the histone H2A variant histone H2AX on its C-terminus. Within seconds of DSB formation, the phosphorylated H2AX is present over surrounding regions, spanning thousand to millions of base pairs (Rogakou et al., 1998; Rogakou et al., 1999; Leatherbarrow et al., 2006; Kinner et al., 2008). H2AX is not present in lower eukaryote, but the domain that is phosphorylated in response to DSB is present in the C-terminus of other H2A-family members like H2A in S. cerevisiae and H2AZ in D. melanogaster (Downs et al., 2007). Although loss of H2AX does not abrogate DNA-damage checkpoints or repair, it impairs the joining of programmed DNA lesions during immunoglobulin class-switch recombination. These observations suggest that chromatin modifications at a distance are required for bringing together the DNA ends (Petersen et al., 2001; Reina-San-Martin et al., 2003). Moreover, failing to rejoin these programmed DSB in the absence of H2AX result in frequent chromosomal abnormalities (Franco et al., 2006; Ramiro et al., 2006). In addition to phosphorylation, H2A is also modified by acetylation in its N-terminal tail by NuA4, a histone acetyl transferase (HAT). Acetylation seems to be important for the ability of cells to survive after DNA damage (Bird et al., 2002).

The findings that DSB induces a rapid local decrease in the density of the chromatin fiber (Kruhlak et al., 2006) and that nearby nucleosomes are repositioned (Shim et al., 2007) support the idea that ATP-dependent chromatin remodeling factors have an early role in the DNA damage response. Indeed, several reports have demonstrated that the ATP-dependent chromatin remodeling complexes RSC (Remodels the Structure of Chromatin), SWI/SNF (SWItch/Sucrose NonFermenting), INO80 (INOsitol requiring) and SWR (Sick with Rat8 ts) are recruited to DSB, although at different time after the DNA damage. The first complex recruited to the DSB is RSC, which mobilize the nucleosomes near a DSB to new positions. Interestingly, in the absence of RSC the phosphorylation of H2AX is delayed. The other three chromatin remodeling complexes, SWI/SNF, INO80 and SWR, are enriched at sites of DSB at later times suggesting that they are not required for the initial detection or signaling of the DSB, but for the subsequent stages of the repair process.

Additionally, acetylation of conserved residues in the N-terminal tails of H3 and H4 has been found to contribute to both homologous and non-homologous recombination processes. For example, in mammalian cells, the TIP60 and the HAT cofactor TRRAP (transformation/transcription-domain associated protein) are recruited to sites of DSB, where they induce acetylation of H4 and facilitate homologous recombination. Similarly, another HAT, MOF (also known as MYST1) contributes to irradiation-induced acetylation of H4 at lysine 16 (H4K16). Defects on H3 and H4 acetylation have been linked to sensitivity to ionizing radiation and alteration in cell cycle checkpoints (Gupta et al., 2005). Complexes catalyzing the reverse process, i.e. histone deacetylation, have been shown to be enriched at late times at the DSB regions. If the acetylation of histones in the vicinity of DNA damage facilitate the repair process, then it is possible that the role of these histone deacetylase complexes might be to restore the chromatin to its original state once the DNA has been repaired.

4. Histone post-translational modifications in chromosomal rearrangements

The role of histone modifications on genomic rearrangements has been extensively studied in the V(D)J recombination process. This assembly process depends on a series of site-specific recombination reactions that are initiated by DSBs produced by RAG1 and RAG2 complex (Bassing et al., 2002). Each rearranging gene segment is flanked by a recombination signal sequence (RSS). The recombinase complex recognizes pair of compatible RSS, introduce DSBs and then channel the reaction products to a DNA repair pathway. Aberrant targeting of RAG proteins can produce chromosomal translocations that are associated with many forms of leukemia or lymphoma. In general, genes segments within recombinationally active loci are mark by the same histone modifications that characterize transcriptionally active genes, i.e. H3 and H4 acetylation as well as H3 trimethylation at lysine 4 (H3K4me3). More recently, it has become evident that the predominant effect of these histone modifications is to recruit the RAG complex to the RSS. In fact, RAG2 through its PHD domain specifically binds to H3K4me3 and mutations that abolish this binding results in greatly impaired V(D)J recombination activity (Liu et al., 2007; Matthews et al., 2007). Additional support for the epigenetic role on V(D)J recombination comes from the observation that in V genes H3 acetylation, although lower than in J genes, exhibit a gradient of enrichment that mirrored the rearrangement frequency. Interestingly, a reciprocal pattern is observed for the repressive modification H3 dimethylation at lysine 9 (H3K9me2) (Espinoza and Feeney, 2005; Espinoza and Feeney, 2007).

H3 trimethylation at lysine 4 (H3K4me3) is also implicated in meiotic recombination. In fact PRDM9, a zinc finger protein that catalyze the trimethylation of H3 at lysine 4, has recently been identified as a major determinant of sequence-specific meiotic recombination (Cheung et al., 2010).

Another histone modification, H3 methylation at lysine 79 (H3K79me), is associated with recombinationally active loci both in yeast and mammalian cell lines (Ng et al., 2003). Moreover, overexpression of DOT1L (a H3K79me specific methyltransferase) together with genotoxic stress and dihydrotestosterone significantly increases formation of chromosomal rearrangement involving the ETS genes, which are a distinguishing feature of prostate cancer (Kumar-Sinha et al., 2008; Lin et al., 2009).

Lin and colleagues (Lin et al., 2009), using prostate cancer as a model to study translocation mechanisms, have shown that after irradiation far more translocations are formed in androgen treated than in control cells. They also demonstrated that the translocation regions, TMPRSS2, ERG and ETV all contain binding sites for the androgen receptor (AR) near their breakpoints and that, after treatment with androgen, there is a rapid recruitment of AR to these sites. Moreover, AR recruitment induces changes in higher-order chromatin structure and epigenetic modifications establishing an open chromatin conformation characteristic of transcribed genes. Another consequence of AR binding was the recruitment of the activation-induced cytidine deaminase (AID), a key factor in somatic hypermutation (SHM) and class switch recombination (CSR) where it contributes to formation of DSB during the process of generating antibody diversity.

Additional data supporting the role of chromatin structure in genomic rearrangements comes from the analysis of the mechanisms involved in formation of t(2;5), a chromosomal translocation associated with anaplastic large cell lymphoma (ALCL). Mathas et al (Mathas et al., 2009) found up-regulation of several genes located near the ALCL translocation breakpoint, regardless of the presence of t(2;5) in the tumor. Moreover, their increased transcriptional activity promotes cell survival and repression of T-cell specific gene expression programs, both characteristics are a hallmark of ALCL (Mathas et al., 2009). Interestingly, cells isolated from ALCL patients lacking t(2;5) were more susceptible to form the (2;5) translocation than control cells. Together these data suggest that deregulation of breakpoint-proximal genes occurs before the formation of translocations and that similar to V(D)J recombination, transcriptional activity and altered chromatin structure predispose cells to chromosomal translocation.

This pattern of highly accessible chromatin structure characterized by H3 and H4 acetylation is also found at the breakpoint regions of other genes involved in translocations like MLL (Khobta et al., 2004), *RUNX1* (Stuardo et al., 2009) and ETO (our unpublished data). Using chromatin immunoprecipitation assays (ChIPs) we analyzed the chromatin structure at intrón 5 of the *RUNX1* gene, where all the translocation points for the (8;21) translocation has been mapped (Figure 3). Our results demonstrate that chromatin organization at intron 5 is completely different in HL-60 hematopoietic cells than in a non-hematopoietic cell (Stuardo et al., 2009). In fact, two distinct features mark the intron 5 in HL-60: a complete lack or significantly reduced levels of histone H1 and an increased association of hyperacetylated histone H3.

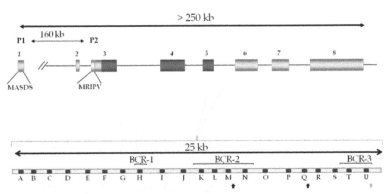

Fig. 3. **Diagrammatic representation of the *RUNX1* gene.** Top panel show the exon-intron organization of the gene as well as the two promoters that regulate its expression. Bottom panel show a magnification of intron 5 of the *RUNX1* gene. The three breakpoint clusters (BCR) are indicated as well as the amplification fragments analyzed by ChIP assays (purple blocks labeled A-U). Dark gray arrows indicate topoisomerase II sites and light gray arrow DNase I hypersensitive site.

The decreased association of histone H1, may indicate an overall enhanced accessibility and hence an increased availability to nucleases or DNA damaging agents. Notably, the region where the DNaseI hypersensitive site has been mapped presents one of the lowest rates of association of histone H1 in myeloid HL-60 cells (Figure 4, region U). Although the complete intron 5 is enriched in acetylated histone H3 (Figure 5), the chromatin organization is not homogeneous throughout the intron, suggesting that particular regions of intron 5 may play a regulatory role in transcription, subnuclear localization or compaction of the *RUNX1* gene. Interestingly, the chromatin organization at intron 5 resembles the chromatin structure adopted by the V(D)J gene segment. During V(D)J recombination, gene segments encoding the variable regions for immunoglobulins and T-cell receptors (TCR) are recombined and assembled in a new configuration. The same recombinase is present in both T and B cells, however recombination of immunoglobulins loci happens only in B cells while TCR loci rearrange only in T cells. Targeting of recombinase activity to specific gene segments is controlled largely by changes in chromatin accessibility in a spatio-temporal manner, and acetylation of histone tails has been shown to be a key event in this process. In fact, acetylation of histone H3 or H4 is elevated in B or T cell type at gene segments that can recombine, and reduced at segments that do not undergo recombination (Maes et al., 2006;

Maes et al., 2001; McMurry and Krangel, 2000). Moreover, hyperacetylation induced by inhibitors of histone deacetylase complexes (HDAC) rescues recombination defects caused by the elimination of extracellular signals that induce recombination (Durum et al., 1998). These studies suggest that histone hyperacetylation precedes recombination by opening chromatin and promoting access to the recombinase. Thus regardless of the molecular mechanism involved, it seems that an open chromatin conformation is a common requirement for a translocation to take place (Figure 6).

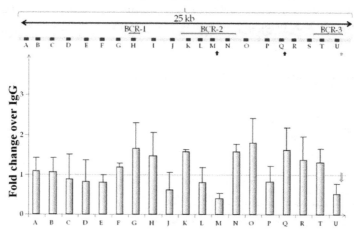

Fig. 4. Intron 5 of *RUNX1* gene exhibit decreased association of histone H1. Chromatin immunoprecipitation assays were performed with formaldehyde cross-linked chromatin isolated form HL-60 cells. Real-time PCR amplification of ChIP-DNA is shown as fold change over IgG in bar graph for immunoprecipitation with anti H1 antibody. Light gray arrow indicates DNaseI hypersensitive site.

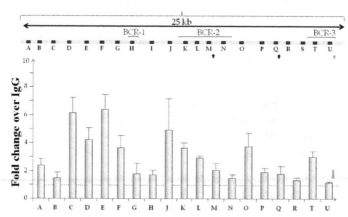

Fig. 5. Intron 5 of *RUNX1* gene is enriched in acetylated histone H3. Chromatin immunoprecipitation assays were performed with formaldehyde cross-linked chromatin isolated form HL-60 cells. Real-time PCR amplification of ChIP-DNA is shown as fold change over IgG for immunoprecipitation with anti acetylated H3 antibody. Light gray arrow indicates DNaseI hypersensitive site.

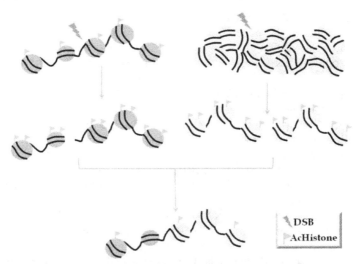

Fig. 6. **Summary of chromatin structure and histone modification in the regions involed in chromosomal translocation.** DSB can occur either in euchromatin or heterochromatin, but they must arise close enough both in time and in space to give rise to a chromosomal translocation. In both cases the regions surrounding the DSB will exhibit an open chromatin conformation either due to its presence in euchromatin or as result of the DNA repair process.

5. DNA conformation

In addition to the classical B-DNA structure described by Watson and Crick (Watson and Crick, 1953), more than 10 different DNA conformations are documented to date. These alternative DNA conformations include Z-DNA, hairpins/cruciforms, H-DNA (triplexes), slipped DNA and sticky DNA among others (Felsenfeld and RICH, 1957; Wang et al., 1979; Lilley, 1980; Panayotatos and Wells, 1981; Lyamichev et al., 1983; Sen and Gilbert, 1988; Mirkin, 2008). Several studies have shown that these non-canonical DNA structures affect DNA replication and transcription, and contribute to genome instability. For example non-B forming sequences located in c-MYC and BCL-2 genes localize with translocation breaking points. Studies have demonstrated that the H-DNA structure from the human c-MYC gene can induce DSBs in mammalian cells and stimulate genomic instability on mouse chromosomes in transgenic mice (Wang et al., 2008). However, the same sequences are not mutagenic in bacteria, suggesting a requirement for host-specific trans-acting factors to generate genomic instability.

Palindromic sequences, including palindromic AT-rich repeats (PATRRs), have the potential to form stem-loop structures by intrastrand base pairing within single-stranded DNA. In fact, PATRRs mapped on chromosome 22q11 and other chromosomes, such as 11q23 and 17q11, were found to cause non random chromosomal translocation in sperm cells in the general population (Kato et al., 2006) as well as in cell culture (Inagaki et al., 2009). Polymorphisms within the PATRRs affect the susceptibility to translocation *in vitro*, with longer and more symmetric PATRRs showing a stronger predisposition to translocation events (Kato et al., 2006; Kogo et al., 2007; Inagaki et al., 2009). Therefore, it has been proposed that the secondary structures adopted by palindromic DNA induce a greater susceptibility to DSBs thus leading to translocations in human (Kurahashi et al., 2000).

There have also been identified chromosomal fragile sites, which are genomic regions especially susceptible to DNA breakage. These fragile sites are non-random specific loci that are stable under normal conditions, but under conditions of partial replication stress can form visible gaps or breaks in metaphase chromosomes (Durkin and Glover, 2007; Richards, 2001). Many different studies have established a connection between DNA fragile sites and the formation of cancer-specific genome rearrangements. However, only recently there has been direct evidence linking breakage at DNA fragile sites to the formation of a cancer specific translocation. Using as model RET/PTC rearrangements; which are commonly found in the papillary thyroid carcinoma (PTC) and in all cases result in the fusion of the tyrosine kinase domain of RET (rearranged in transformation) to the 5' portion of various unrelated genes (Nikiforov, 2008) Gandhi et al (Gandhi et al., 2010) demonstrate that fragile site-inducing chemicals can create DNA breaks within the RET/PTC partner genes and ultimately lead to the formation of RET/PTC rearrangements. Moreover, aphidicolin induced DNA breaks at RET gene were located within intron 11, which is the breakpoint cluster region identified in thyroid cells. Clinical studies have shown that two different rearrangements, RET/PTC1 and RET/PTC3, are more frequent in sporadic and radiation-induced tumors respectively (Fenton et al., 2000; Fugazzola et al., 1995; Nikiforov et al., 1997; Motomura et al., 1998). Interestingly, treatment of cells with aphidicolin (APH), 2-aminopurine (2-AP) and 5-bromodeoxyuridine (BrdU) resulted in the generation of RET/PTC1 but not RET/PTC3 suggesting that sporadic PTC tumors may result from breakage at fragile sites. Although no consensus sequence have been identified in the fragile sites until now, the majority of them can form highly stable non-B DNA structures.

6. Concluding remarks

Traditionally it has been assumed that translocations arise randomly by stochastic DSB and that enrichment of particular translocations was result of the survival advantage acquired by the cells bearing the translocation. However, more recent results suggest that breaks in the genome occur in a nonrandom fashion and that higher-order chromatin organization maybe, at least in part, responsible for the formation of recurrent translocations. Although, significant progresses have been made in understanding formation of chromosomal translocation, particularly in the area of VDJ recombination, many more questions remain unanswered. For instance, it is still not known what proteins or pathways are involved in formation and maintenance of structure at the breakpoint regions, if these regions have a role in some cellular processes and what signaling pathways or environmental conditions promote chromosomal translocations. The response to these basic research questions may greatly improve diagnostic and therapeutic and may help to develop preventive measures for disorders associated with genomic instability such as chromosomal translocations.

7. Acknowledgments

This work has been supported by Fondo Nacional de Desarrollo Cientifico y Tecnologico (FONDECYT, Grant 1100670) (to SEG);National Institute of Health (Grant R03 TW007170-01A2) (JLS and SEG).

8. References

Ames, B.N. and Shigenaga, M.K. (1992). Oxidants are a major contributor to aging. Ann. N. Y. Acad. Sci. *663*, 85-96.

Aplan, P.D., Chervinsky, D.S., Stanulla, M., and Burhans, W.C. (1996). Site-specific DNA cleavage within the MLL breakpoint cluster region induced by topoisomerase II inhibitors. Blood *87*, 2649-2658.

Aplan, P.D. (2006). Causes of oncogenic chromosomal translocation. Trends in Genetics *22*, 46-55.

Bartova, E., Kozubek, S., Kozubek, M., Jirsova, P., Lukasova, E., Skalnikova, M., and Buchnickova, K. (2000). The influence of the cell cycle, differentiation and irradiation on the nuclear location of the abl, bcr and c-myc genes in human leukemic cells. Leuk. Res *24*, 233-241.

Bassing, C.H., Swat, W., and Alt, F.W. (2002). The mechanism and regulation of chromosomal V(D)J recombination. Cell *109 Suppl*, S45-S55.

Betti, C.J., Villalobos, M.J., Diaz, M.O., and Vaughan, A.T. (2003). Apoptotic stimuli initiate MLL-AF9 translocations that are transcribed in cells capable of division. Cancer Res *63*, 1377-1381.

Bird, A.W., Yu, D.Y., Pray-Grant, M.G., Qiu, Q., Harmon, K.E., Megee, P.C., Grant, P.A., Smith, M.M., and Christman, M.F. (2002). Acetylation of histone H4 by Esa1 is required for DNA double-strand break repair. Nature *419*, 411-415.

Boboila, C., Jankovic, M., Yan, C.T., Wang, J.H., Wesemann, D.R., Zhang, T., Fazeli, A., Feldman, L., Nussenzweig, A., Nussenzweig, M., and Alt, F.W. (2010). Alternative end-joining catalyzes robust IgH locus deletions and translocations in the combined absence of ligase 4 and Ku70. Proc. Natl. Acad. Sci. U. S. A *107*, 3034-3039.

Chen, A.M., Lucas, J.N., Hill, F.S., Brenner, D.J., and Sachs, R.K. (1996). Proximity effects for chromosome aberrations measured by FISH. Int. J Radiat. Biol *69*, 411-420.

Cheung, V.G., Sherman, S.L., and Feingold, E. (2010). Genetics. Genetic control of hotspots. Science *327*, 791-792.

Cremer, T. and Cremer, C. (2001). Chromosome territories, nuclear architecture and gene regulation in mammalian cells. Nat. Rev. Genet. *2*, 292-301.

Cremer, T., Cremer, M., Dietzel, S., Muller, S., Solovei, I., and Fakan, S. (2006). Chromosome territories--a functional nuclear landscape. Curr. Opin. Cell Biol *18*, 307-316.

Digweed, M. and Sperling, K. (2004). Nijmegen breakage syndrome: clinical manifestation of defective response to DNA double-strand breaks. DNA Repair (Amst) *3*, 1207-1217.

Downs, J.A., Nussenzweig, M.C., and Nussenzweig, A. (2007). Chromatin dynamics and the preservation of genetic information. Nature *447*, 951-958.

Durkin, S.G. and Glover, T.W. (2007). Chromosome fragile sites. Annu. Rev Genet *41*, 169-192.

Durum, S.K., Candeias, S., Nakajima, H., Leonard, W.J., Baird, A.M., Berg, L.J., and Muegge, K. (1998). Interleukin 7 receptor control of T cell receptor gamma gene rearrangement: role of receptor-associated chains and locus accessibility. J Exp. Med *188*, 2233-2241.

Espinoza, C.R. and Feeney, A.J. (2005). The extent of histone acetylation correlates with the differential rearrangement frequency of individual VH genes in pro-B cells. J Immunol. *175*, 6668-6675.

Espinoza, C.R. and Feeney, A.J. (2007). Chromatin accessibility and epigenetic modifications differ between frequently and infrequently rearranging VH genes. Mol Immunol. 44, 2675-2685.

Falk, M., Lukasova, E., and Kozubek, S. (2008). Chromatin structure influences the sensitivity of DNA to gamma-radiation. Biochim. Biophys. Acta 1783, 2398-2414.

Falk, M., Lukasova, E., and Kozubek, S. (2010). Higher-order chromatin structure in DSB induction, repair and misrepair. Mutat. Res 704, 88-100.

Felix, C.A., Lange, B.J., Hosler, M.R., Fertala, J., and Bjornsti, M.A. (1995). Chromosome band 11q23 translocation breakpoints are DNA topoisomerase II cleavage sites. Cancer Res 55, 4287-4292.

Felsenfeld, G. and RICH, A. (1957). Studies on the formation of two- and three-stranded polyribonucleotides. Biochim. Biophys. Acta 26, 457-468.

Fenton, C.L., Lukes, Y., Nicholson, D., Dinauer, C.A., Francis, G.L., and Tuttle, R.M. (2000). The ret/PTC mutations are common in sporadic papillary thyroid carcinoma of children and young adults. J Clin. Endocrinol. Metab 85, 1170-1175.

Fernandez-Capetillo, O., Lee, A., Nussenzweig, M., and Nussenzweig, A. (2004). H2AX: the histone guardian of the genome. DNA Repair (Amst) 3, 959-967.

Franco, S., Gostissa, M., Zha, S., Lombard, D.B., Murphy, M.M., Zarrin, A.A., Yan, C., Tepsuporn, S., Morales, J.C., Adams, M.M., Lou, Z., Bassing, C.H., Manis, J.P., Chen, J., Carpenter, P.B., and Alt, F.W. (2006). H2AX prevents DNA breaks from progressing to chromosome breaks and translocations. Mol Cell 21, 201-214.

Fugazzola, L., Pilotti, S., Pinchera, A., Vorontsova, T.V., Mondellini, P., Bongarzone, I., Greco, A., Astakhova, L., Butti, M.G., Demidchik, E.P., and . (1995). Oncogenic rearrangements of the RET proto-oncogene in papillary thyroid carcinomas from children exposed to the Chernobyl nuclear accident. Cancer Res 55, 5617-5620.

Gandhi, M., Dillon, L.W., Pramanik, S., Nikiforov, Y.E., and Wang, Y.H. (2010). DNA breaks at fragile sites generate oncogenic RET/PTC rearrangements in human thyroid cells. Oncogene 29, 2272-2280.

Greaves, M.F. (1996). Infant leukaemia biology, aetiology and treatment. Leukemia 10, 372-377.

Gupta, A., Sharma, G.G., Young, C.S., Agarwal, M., Smith, E.R., Paull, T.T., Lucchesi, J.C., Khanna, K.K., Ludwig, T., and Pandita, T.K. (2005). Involvement of human MOF in ATM function. Mol Cell Biol 25, 5292-5305.

Inagaki, H., Ohye, T., Kogo, H., Kato, T., Bolor, H., Taniguchi, M., Shaikh, T.H., Emanuel, B.S., and Kurahashi, H. (2009). Chromosomal instability mediated by non-B DNA: cruciform conformation and not DNA sequence is responsible for recurrent translocation in humans. Genome Res 19, 191-198.

Kato, T., Inagaki, H., Yamada, K., Kogo, H., Ohye, T., Kowa, H., Nagaoka, K., Taniguchi, M., Emanuel, B.S., and Kurahashi, H. (2006). Genetic variation affects de novo translocation frequency. Science 311, 971.

Khobta, A., Carlo-Stella, C., and Capranico, G. (2004). Specific histone patterns and acetylase/deacetylase activity at the breakpoint-cluster region of the human MLL gene. Cancer Res 64, 2656-2662.

Kinner, A., Wu, W., Staudt, C., and Iliakis, G. (2008). Gamma-H2AX in recognition and signaling of DNA double-strand breaks in the context of chromatin. Nucleic Acids Res 36, 5678-5694.

Kogo, H., Inagaki, H., Ohye, T., Kato, T., Emanuel, B.S., and Kurahashi, H. (2007). Cruciform extrusion propensity of human translocation-mediating palindromic AT-rich repeats. Nucleic Acids Res 35, 1198-1208.

Kruhlak, M.J., Celeste, A., Dellaire, G., Fernandez-Capetillo, O., Muller, W.G., McNally, J.G., Bazett-Jones, D.P., and Nussenzweig, A. (2006). Changes in chromatin structure and mobility in living cells at sites of DNA double-strand breaks. J Cell Biol 172, 823-834.

Kumar-Sinha, C., Tomlins, S.A., and Chinnaiyan, A.M. (2008). Recurrent gene fusions in prostate cancer. Nat Rev Cancer 8, 497-511.

Kurahashi, H., Shaikh, T.H., Hu, P., Roe, B.A., Emanuel, B.S., and Budarf, M.L. (2000). Regions of genomic instability on 22q11 and 11q23 as the etiology for the recurrent constitutional t(11;22). Hum. Mol Genet 9, 1665-1670.

Kuroda, M., Tanabe, H., Yoshida, K., Oikawa, K., Saito, A., Kiyuna, T., Mizusawa, H., and Mukai, K. (2004). Alteration of chromosome positioning during adipocyte differentiation. J Cell Sci 117, 5897-5903.

Leatherbarrow, E.L., Harper, J.V., Cucinotta, F.A., and O'Neill, P. (2006). Induction and quantification of gamma-H2AX foci following low and high LET-irradiation. Int. J Radiat. Biol 82, 111-118.

Lilley, D.M. (1980). The inverted repeat as a recognizable structural feature in supercoiled DNA molecules. Proc. Natl. Acad. Sci. U. S. A 77, 6468-6472.

Lin, C., Yang, L., Tanasa, B., Hutt, K., Ju, B.G., Ohgi, K., Zhang, J., Rose, D.W., Fu, X.D., Glass, C.K., and Rosenfeld, M.G. (2009). Nuclear receptor-induced chromosomal proximity and DNA breaks underlie specific translocations in cancer. Cell 139, 1069-1083.

Lisby, M., Antunez, d.M., Mortensen, U.H., and Rothstein, R. (2003a). Cell cycle-regulated centers of DNA double-strand break repair. Cell Cycle 2, 479-483.

Lisby, M., Mortensen, U.H., and Rothstein, R. (2003b). Colocalization of multiple DNA double-strand breaks at a single Rad52 repair centre. Nat Cell Biol 5, 572-577.

Liu, Y., Subrahmanyam, R., Chakraborty, T., Sen, R., and Desiderio, S. (2007). A plant homeodomain in RAG-2 that binds Hypermethylated lysine 4 of histone H3 is necessary for efficient antigen-receptor-gene rearrangement. Immunity. 27, 561-571.

Lukasova, E., Kozubek, S., Kozubek, M., Kjeronska, J., Ryznar, L., Horakova, J., Krahulcova, E., and Horneck, G. (1997). Localisation and distance between ABL and BCR genes in interphase nuclei of bone marrow cells of control donors and patients with chronic myeloid leukaemia. Hum. Genet 100, 525-535.

Lyamichev, V.I., Panyutin, I.G., and Frank-Kamenetskii, M.D. (1983). Evidence of cruciform structures in superhelical DNA provided by two-dimensional gel electrophoresis. FEBS Lett. 153, 298-302.

Maes, J., Chappaz, S., Cavelier, P., O'Neill, L., Turner, B., Rougeon, F., and Goodhardt, M. (2006). Activation of V(D)J recombination at the IgH chain JH locus occurs within a 6-kilobase chromatin domain and is associated with nucleosomal remodeling. J Immunol. 176, 5409-5417.

Maes, J., O'Neill, L.P., Cavelier, P., Turner, B.M., Rougeon, F., and Goodhardt, M. (2001). Chromatin remodeling at the Ig loci prior to V(D)J recombination. J Immunol. 167, 866-874.

Mathas, S., Kreher, S., Meaburn, K.J., Johrens, K., Lamprecht, B., Assaf, C., Sterry, W., Kadin, M.E., Daibata, M., Joos, S., Hummel, M., Stein, H., Janz, M., Anagnostopoulos, I., Schrock, E., Misteli, T., and Dorken, B. (2009). Gene deregulation and spatial genome reorganization near breakpoints prior to formation of translocations in anaplastic large cell lymphoma. Proc. Natl. Acad. Sci. U. S. A 106, 5831-5836.

Matthews, A.G.W., Kuo, A.J., Ramon-Maiques, S., Han, S., Champagne, K.S., Ivanov, D., Gallardo, M., Carney, D., Cheung, P., Ciccone, D.N., Walter, K.L., Utz, P.J., Shi, Y., Kutateladze, T.G., Yang, W., Gozani, O., and Oettinger, M.A. (2007). RAG2 PHD finger couples histone H3 lysine 4 trimethylation with V(D)J recombination. Nature 450, 1106-1110.

McMurry, M.T. and Krangel, M.S. (2000). A role for histone acetylation in the developmental regulation of VDJ recombination. Science 287, 495-498.

Meaburn, K.J. and Misteli, T. (2007). Cell biology: chromosome territories. Nature 445, 379-781.

Mirkin, S.M. (2008). Discovery of alternative DNA structures: a heroic decade (1979-1989). Front Biosci. 13, 1064-1071.

Misteli, T. (2007). Beyond the sequence: cellular organization of genome function. Cell 128, 787-800.

Misteli, T. (2010). Higher-order genome organization in human disease. Cold Spring Harb. Perspect. Biol 2, a000794.

Misteli, T. and Soutoglou, E. (2009). The emerging role of nuclear architecture in DNA repair and genome maintenance. Nat Rev Mol Cell Biol 10, 243-254.

Mitelman, F., Mertens, F., and Johansson, B. (2005). Prevalence estimates of recurrent balanced cytogenetic aberrations and gene fusions in unselected patients with neoplastic disorders. Genes Chromosomes. Cancer 43, 350-366.

Mitelman, F., Johansson, B., and Mertens, F. (2007). The impact of translocations and gene fusions on cancer causation. Nat Rev Cancer 7, 233-245.

Motomura, T., Nikiforov, Y.E., Namba, H., Ashizawa, K., Nagataki, S., Yamashita, S., and Fagin, J.A. (1998). ret rearrangements in Japanese pediatric and adult papillary thyroid cancers. Thyroid 8, 485-489.

Murr, R., Loizou, J.I., Yang, Y.G., Cuenin, C., Li, H., Wang, Z.Q., and Herceg, Z. (2006). Histone acetylation by Trrap-Tip60 modulates loading of repair proteins and repair of DNA double-strand breaks. Nat Cell Biol 8, 91-99.

Neves, H., Ramos, C., da Silva, M.G., Parreira, A., and Parreira, L. (1999). The nuclear topography of ABL, BCR, PML, and RARalpha genes: evidence for gene proximity in specific phases of the cell cycle and stages of hematopoietic differentiation. Blood 93, 1197-1207.

Ng, H.H., Ciccone, D.N., Morshead, K.B., Oettinger, M.A., and Struhl, K. (2003). Lysine-79 of histone H3 is hypomethylated at silenced loci in yeast and mammalian cells: a potential mechanism for position-effect variegation. Proc. Natl. Acad. Sci. U. S. A 100, 1820-1825.

Nikiforov, Y.E. (2008). Thyroid carcinoma: molecular pathways and therapeutic targets. Mod. Pathol. 21 Suppl 2, S37-S43.

Nikiforov, Y.E., Rowland, J.M., Bove, K.E., Monforte-Munoz, H., and Fagin, J.A. (1997). Distinct pattern of ret oncogene rearrangements in morphological variants of radiation-induced and sporadic thyroid papillary carcinomas in children. Cancer Res *57*, 1690-1694.

Panayotatos, N. and Wells, R.D. (1981). Cruciform structures in supercoiled DNA. Nature *289*, 466-470.

Petersen, S., Casellas, R., Reina-San-Martin, B., Chen, H.T., Difilippantonio, M.J., Wilson, P.C., Hanitsch, L., Celeste, A., Muramatsu, M., Pilch, D.R., Redon, C., Ried, T., Bonner, W.M., Honjo, T., Nussenzweig, M.C., and Nussenzweig, A. (2001). AID is required to initiate Nbs1/gamma-H2AX focus formation and mutations at sites of class switching. Nature *414*, 660-665.

Povirk, L.F. (2006). Biochemical mechanisms of chromosomal translocations resulting from DNA double-strand breaks. DNA Repair (Amst) *5*, 1199-1212.

Ramiro, A.R., Jankovic, M., Callen, E., Difilippantonio, S., Chen, H.T., McBride, K.M., Eisenreich, T.R., Chen, J., Dickins, R.A., Lowe, S.W., Nussenzweig, A., and Nussenzweig, M.C. (2006). Role of genomic instability and p53 in AID-induced c-myc-Igh translocations. Nature *440*, 105-109.

Reina-San-Martin, B., Difilippantonio, S., Hanitsch, L., Masilamani, R.F., Nussenzweig, A., and Nussenzweig, M.C. (2003). H2AX is required for recombination between immunoglobulin switch regions but not for intra-switch region recombination or somatic hypermutation. J Exp. Med. *197*, 1767-1778.

Relling, M.V., Yanishevski, Y., Nemec, J., Evans, W.E., Boyett, J.M., Behm, F.G., and Pui, C.H. (1998). Etoposide and antimetabolite pharmacology in patients who develop secondary acute myeloid leukemia. Leukemia *12*, 346-352.

Richards, R.I. (2001). Fragile and unstable chromosomes in cancer: causes and consequences. Trends Genet *17*, 339-345.

Rogakou, E.P., Boon, C., Redon, C., and Bonner, W.M. (1999). Megabase chromatin domains involved in DNA double-strand breaks in vivo. J Cell Biol *146*, 905-916.

Rogakou, E.P., Pilch, D.R., Orr, A.H., Ivanova, V.S., and Bonner, W.M. (1998). DNA double-stranded breaks induce histone H2AX phosphorylation on serine 139. J Biol Chem. *273*, 5858-5868.

Roix, J.J., McQueen, P.G., Munson, P.J., Parada, L.A., and Misteli, T. (2003). Spatial proximity of translocation-prone gene loci in human lymphomas. Nat Genet *34*, 287-291.

Sen, D. and Gilbert, W. (1988). Formation of parallel four-stranded complexes by guanine-rich motifs in DNA and its implications for meiosis. Nature *334*, 364-366.

Shim, E.Y., Hong, S.J., Oum, J.H., Yanez, Y., Zhang, Y., and Lee, S.E. (2007). RSC mobilizes nucleosomes to improve accessibility of repair machinery to the damaged chromatin. Mol Cell Biol *27*, 1602-1613.

Simsek, D. and Jasin, M. (2010). Alternative end-joining is suppressed by the canonical NHEJ component Xrcc4-ligase IV during chromosomal translocation formation. Nat Struct Mol Biol *17*, 410-416.

Sperry, A.O., Blasquez, V.C., and Garrard, W.T. (1989). Dysfunction of chromosomal loop attachment sites: illegitimate recombination linked to matrix association regions and topoisomerase II. Proc. Natl. Acad. Sci. U. S. A *86*, 5497-5501.

Stanulla, M., Wang, J., Chervinsky, D.S., Thandla, S., and Aplan, P.D. (1997). DNA cleavage within the MLL breakpoint cluster region is a specific event which occurs as part of higher-order chromatin fragmentation during the initial stages of apoptosis. Mol Cell Biol *17*, 4070-4079.

Strick, R., Zhang, Y., Emmanuel, N., and Strissel, P.L. (2006). Common chromatin structures at breakpoint cluster regions may lead to chromosomal translocations found in chronic and acute leukemias. Hum. Genet *119*, 479-495.

Strissel, P.L., Strick, R., Rowley, J.D., and Zeleznik, L. (1998). An in vivo topoisomerase II cleavage site and a DNase I hypersensitive site colocalize near exon 9 in the MLL breakpoint cluster region. Blood *92*, 3793-3803.

Stuardo, M., Martinez, M., Hidalgo, K., Montecino, M., Javed, A., Lian, J.B., Stein, G.S., Stein, J.L., and Gutierrez, S.E. (2009). Altered chromatin modifications in AML1/RUNX1 breakpoint regions involved in (8;21) translocation. J Cell Physiol *218*, 343-349.

Tanabe, S., Bohlander, S.K., Vignon, C.V., Espinosa, R., III, Zhao, N., Strissel, P.L., Zeleznik, L., and Rowley, J.D. (1996). AF10 is split by MLL and HEAB, a human homolog to a putative Caenorhabditis elegans ATP/GTP-binding protein in an invins(10;11)(p12;q23q12). Blood *88*, 3535-3545.

Tsukuda, T., Fleming, A.B., Nickoloff, J.A., and Osley, M.A. (2005). Chromatin remodelling at a DNA double-strand break site in Saccharomyces cerevisiae. Nature *438*, 379-383.

Verger, A. and Crossley, M. (2004). Chromatin modifiers in transcription and DNA repair. Cell Mol Life Sci. *61*, 2154-2162.

Wang, A.H., Quigley, G.J., Kolpak, F.J., Crawford, J.L., van Boom, J.H., van der, M.G., and Rich, A. (1979). Molecular structure of a left-handed double helical DNA fragment at atomic resolution. Nature *282*, 680-686.

Wang, G., Carbajal, S., Vijg, J., DiGiovanni, J., and Vasquez, K.M. (2008). DNA structure-induced genomic instability in vivo. J Natl. Cancer Inst. *100*, 1815-1817.

Wang, J.H., Gostissa, M., Yan, C.T., Goff, P., Hickernell, T., Hansen, E., Difilippantonio, S., Wesemann, D.R., Zarrin, A.A., Rajewsky, K., Nussenzweig, A., and Alt, F.W. (2009). Mechanisms promoting translocations in editing and switching peripheral B cells. Nature *460*, 231-236.

Watson, J.D. and Crick, F.H. (1953). Molecular structure of nucleic acids; a structure for deoxyribose nucleic acid. Nature *171*, 737-738.

Zhang, Y. and Rowley, J.D. (2006). Chromatin structural elements and chromosomal translocations in leukemia. DNA Repair (Amst) *5*, 1282-1297.

Zhang, Y., Strissel, P., Strick, R., Chen, J., Nucifora, G., Le Beau, M.M., Larson, R.A., and Rowley, J.D. (2002). Genomic DNA breakpoints in AML1/RUNX1 and ETO cluster with topoisomerase II DNA cleavage and DNase I hypersensitive sites in t(8;21) leukemia. Proc. Natl. Acad. Sci. U. S. A *99*, 3070-3075.

Permissions

The contributors of this book come from diverse backgrounds, making this book a truly international effort. This book will bring forth new frontiers with its revolutionizing research information and detailed analysis of the nascent developments around the world.

We would like to thank Prof. Dr. Steffen Koschmieder and Dr. Utz Krug, for lending their expertise to make the book truly unique. They have played a crucial role in the development of this book. Without their invaluable contribution this book wouldn't have been possible. They have made vital efforts to compile up to date information on the varied aspects of this subject to make this book a valuable addition to the collection of many professionals and students.

This book was conceptualized with the vision of imparting up-to-date information and advanced data in this field. To ensure the same, a matchless editorial board was set up. Every individual on the board went through rigorous rounds of assessment to prove their worth. After which they invested a large part of their time researching and compiling the most relevant data for our readers. Conferences and sessions were held from time to time between the editorial board and the contributing authors to present the data in the most comprehensible form. The editorial team has worked tirelessly to provide valuable and valid information to help people across the globe.

Every chapter published in this book has been scrutinized by our experts. Their significance has been extensively debated. The topics covered herein carry significant findings which will fuel the growth of the discipline. They may even be implemented as practical applications or may be referred to as a beginning point for another development. Chapters in this book were first published by InTech; hereby published with permission under the Creative Commons Attribution License or equivalent.

The editorial board has been involved in producing this book since its inception. They have spent rigorous hours researching and exploring the diverse topics which have resulted in the successful publishing of this book. They have passed on their knowledge of decades through this book. To expedite this challenging task, the publisher supported the team at every step. A small team of assistant editors was also appointed to further simplify the editing procedure and attain best results for the readers.

Our editorial team has been hand-picked from every corner of the world. Their multi-ethnicity adds dynamic inputs to the discussions which result in innovative outcomes. These outcomes are then further discussed with the researchers and contributors who give their valuable feedback and opinion regarding the same. The feedback is then collaborated with the researches and they are edited in a comprehensive manner to aid the understanding of the subject.

Apart from the editorial board, the designing team has also invested a significant amount of their time in understanding the subject and creating the most relevant covers. They scrutinized every image to scout for the most suitable representation of the subject and create an appropriate cover for the book.

The publishing team has been involved in this book since its early stages. They were actively engaged in every process, be it collecting the data, connecting with the contributors or procuring relevant information. The team has been an ardent support to the editorial, designing and production team. Their endless efforts to recruit the best for this project, has resulted in the accomplishment of this book. They are a veteran in the field of academics and their pool of knowledge is as vast as their experience in printing. Their expertise and guidance has proved useful at every step. Their uncompromising quality standards have made this book an exceptional effort. Their encouragement from time to time has been an inspiration for everyone.

The publisher and the editorial board hope that this book will prove to be a valuable piece of knowledge for researchers, students, practitioners and scholars across the globe.

List of Contributors

Valeria Bertagnolo, Federica Brugnoli and Silvano Capitani
University of Ferrara, Section of Human Anatomy, Department of Morphology and Embryology, Italy

Joanna Fares
Laboratory of Cellular Oncology, National Cancer Institute, NIH, Bethesda, Maryland, USA
Georgetown University, Department of Biochemistry and Molecular Biology, Washington DC, USA

Linda Wolff and Juraj Bies
Laboratory of Cellular Oncology, National Cancer Institute, NIH, Bethesda, Maryland, USA

Julia Schanda, Manuel Grez and Christian Wichmann
Georg-Speyer-Haus, Institute for Biomedical Research, Frankfurt am Main, Germany

Reinhard Henschler
Institute of Transfusion Medicine, German Red Cross Blood Center, Frankfurt am Main, Germany

Silvia de la Iglesia Iñigo, María Teresa Gómez Casares and Jezabel López Brito
Servicio de Hematología, Hospital de Gran Canaria Doctor Negrín, Las Palmas de Gran-Canaria, Spain

Carmen Elsa López Jorge
Servicio de Hematología, Hospital de Gran Canaria Doctor Negrín, Las Palmas de Gran-Canaria, Spain
Unit Research, Hospital de Gran Canaria Doctor Negrín, Las Palmas de GranCanaria, Spain

Pedro Martin Cabrera
Secció de Citologia Hematològica, Servei d'Anatomia Patològica Hospital Universitari de Bellvitge, Barcelona, Spain

Claudia Bănescu, Carmen Duicu and Minodora Dobreanu
Univ Med & Pharm Tg-Mures, România

Emma Lång and Stig Ove Bøe
Oslo University Hospital, Oslo, Norway

Maha Abdullah and Zainina Seman
University Putra Malaysia, Malaysia

Muntaser E. Ibrahim and Emad-Aldin I. Osman
Department of Molecular Biology, Institute of Endemic Diseases, University of Khartoum, Khartoum, Sudan

Printed in the USA
CPSIA information can be obtained
at www.ICGtesting.com
JSHW011420221024
72173JS00004B/607

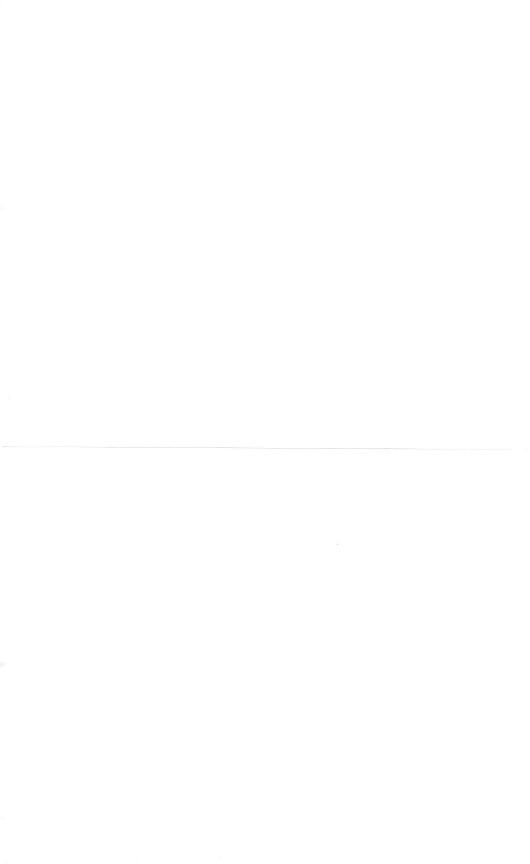